REDEFINING RECOVERY FROM APHASIA

Redefining Recovery from Aphasia

Dalia Cahana-Amitay, PhD
ASSOCIATE DIRECTOR, HAROLD GOODGLASS APHASIA RESEARCH CENTER &
LANGUAGE IN THE AGING BRAIN LABORATORY
DEPARTMENT OF NEUROLOGY
BOSTON UNIVERSITY SCHOOL OF MEDICINE
VA BOSTON HEALTHCARE SYSTEM
BOSTON, MA

Martin L. Albert, MD, PhD
DIRECTOR, HAROLD GOODGLASS APHASIA RESEARCH CENTER &
CO-DIRECTOR, LANGUAGE IN THE AGING BRAIN LABORATORY
DEPARTMENT OF NEUROLOGY
BOSTON UNIVERSITY SCHOOL OF MEDICINE
VA BOSTON HEALTHCARE SYSTEM
BOSTON, MA

OXFORD
UNIVERSITY PRESS

OXFORD
UNIVERSITY PRESS

Oxford University Press is a department of the University of Oxford.
It furthers the University's objective of excellence in research, scholarship,
and education by publishing worldwide.

Oxford   New York
Auckland   Cape Town   Dar es Salaam   Hong Kong   Karachi
Kuala Lumpur   Madrid   Melbourne   Mexico City   Nairobi
New Delhi   Shanghai   Taipei   Toronto

With offices in
Argentina   Austria   Brazil   Chile   Czech Republic   France   Greece
Guatemala   Hungary   Italy   Japan   Poland   Portugal   Singapore
South Korea   Switzerland   Thailand   Turkey   Ukraine   Vietnam

Oxford is a registered trademark of Oxford University Press
in the UK and certain other countries.

Published in the United States of America by
Oxford University Press
198 Madison Avenue, New York, NY 10016

© Oxford University Press 2015

All rights reserved. No part of this publication may be reproduced, stored in
a retrieval system, or transmitted, in any form or by any means, without the prior
permission in writing of Oxford University Press, or as expressly permitted by law,
by license, or under terms agreed with the appropriate reproduction rights organization.
Inquiries concerning reproduction outside the scope of the above should be sent to the
Rights Department, Oxford University Press, at the address above.

You must not circulate this work in any other form
and you must impose this same condition on any acquirer.

Library of Congress Cataloging-in-Publication Data
Cahana-Amitay, Dalia, author.
Redefining recovery from aphasia / Dalia Cahana-Amitay and Martin L. Albert.
    p. ; cm.
Includes bibliographical references.
ISBN 978–0–19–981193–9 (alk. paper)
I. Albert, Martin L., 1939–, author.   II. Title.
[DNLM: 1. Aphasia—rehabilitation.   2. Brain—physiology.   3. Recovery of Function.
4. Speech—physiology. WL 340.5]
RC425
616.85'52—dc23
2014028697

The science of medicine is a rapidly changing field. As new research and clinical experience broaden our
knowledge, changes in treatment and drug therapy occur. The author and publisher of this work have checked
with sources believed to be reliable in their efforts to provide information that is accurate and complete, and
in accordance with the standards accepted at the time of publication. However, in light of the possibility of
human error or changes in the practice of medicine, neither the author, nor the publisher, nor any other party
who has been involved in the preparation or publication of this work warrants that the information contained
herein is in every respect accurate or complete. Readers are encouraged to confirm the information contained
herein with other reliable sources, and are strongly advised to check the product information sheet provided by
the pharmaceutical company for each drug they plan to administer.

9 8 7 6 5 4 3 2 1
Printed in the United States of America
on acid-free paper

Contents

Preface ix

1. What We Know and Do Not Know about Recovery from Aphasia 1
    Defining Recovery from Aphasia 1
    Stating the Problem 4

2. Language in the Healthy Brain: Evidence for Multifunctionality 12
    Where Do We Start? 12
    Models of Functional Neuroanatomy of Language 13
    Psycholinguistic Models of Brain-Language Interlinks 15
    A Call for Multifunctional Brain-Language Models 18
    Future Directions for Neural Multifunctional Models of Language 20
    A Note About Language in the Aging Brain 25

3. Executive Functions and Recovery from Aphasia 36
    Executive Functions and Aphasia: Old Questions, New Light 36
    Defining Executive Functions 37
    Models of Executive Functions 38
    Neural Correlates of Executive Functions 39
    Neural Correlates of Language-Executive Functions: Links to Semantic and Discourse-Level Processes 40
    Executive Functions and Semantic Processing: Semantic Control 40
    Executive Functions and Discourse Processing 42
    Limitations on Neural Mappings 42
    What Do Executive Tasks Really Tell Us? 43
    Assessing Executive Functions in People with Aphasia 43
    Executive Dysfunction in Aphasia: Dissociable from Language Impairment? 47
    Perseveration in Aphasia 48
    Behavioral Findings Related to Language Performance 49
    Semantic Control in Aphasia 49

    Executive Functions and Functional Communication in Aphasia 51
    Neural Correlates of Discourse and Executive Functions in Aphasia 52
    Prognostic Value of Executive Functions in Aphasia 54
    Effects on Neural Reorganization in the Aphasic Brain 56

4. Attention Systems and Recovery from Aphasia 74
    Introduction 74
    Components of Attention 75
    Basic Attention: Sustained Attention, Vigilance, and Arousal 76
    Complex Attention: Selective, Focused, Alternating, Divided Attention 77
    Mechanisms of "Complex" Attention 78
    The Relationship Between Attention and Language 79
    The Neural Basis of Attention 80
    Neural Underpinnings of Attention—Language Interlinks 83
    Attention and Aphasia: Neurobehavioral Evidence 86
    Neural Underpinnings 86
    Behavioral Patterns 86
    Mechanisms of Attention Allocation in Aphasia 88
    Treatment of Attention in Aphasia 89
    Neural Approaches to the Role of Attention in Aphasia Treatment 92

5. The Role of Memory Functions in Recovery from Aphasia 103
    Introduction 103
    Memory: Multiple Classifications 104
    Explicit/Implicit, Declarative/Procedural Memory Systems and Their Neural Underpinnings 105
    Long-Term, Short-Term, and Working Memory: A Window into Memory-Language Dependencies 107
    Short-Term/Working Memory-Language Interlinks: Evidence for Neural Correlates 114
    Memory Deficits and Aphasia 116
    Short-Term Memory/Working Memory Assessment in Aphasia 117
    Behavioral Observations 118
    Neural Correlates of Short-Term Memory/Working Memory in Aphasia 121
    Memory Systems, Aphasia Recovery, and Treatment 123
    Learning in Aphasia Treatment 125
    Neural Structures in Studies of Memory-Related Aphasia Treatment 127

6. The Role of Emotion in Recovery from Aphasia 146
    Introduction 146
    Emotion: Definition and Its Effects on Cognition 147
    Emotion-Language/Cognition-Brain Interlinks 150
    Depression and Anxiety After Stroke 153
    Altered Emotions in Aphasia 155
    Depression and Aphasia 156

Neural and Psychosocial Factors 157
Depression and Aphasia: Recovery and Intervention Effects 159
Anxiety and Stress Reactivity in Aphasia 161
Mechanisms of Stress Responses in Aphasia 161
Targeting Psychophysiological Stress Reactivity in Aphasia Treatment 164

7. *Praxis in Recovery from Aphasia* 186
   Introduction 186
   Praxis, Language, and the Brain 188
   Cognitive Mechanisms Underlying Gesture-Language Interlinks 189
   Neural Mechanisms Underlying Language-Praxis Interconnections 191
   Apraxia and Aphasia: Behavioral and Neural Correlates 196
   Theoretical Accounts of Apraxia 198
   The Role of Frontoparietal Networks in Apraxia and Aphasia 201
   The Relevance of Mirror Neurons to Aphasia 203
   The Role of Gesture (or Lack Thereof) in Aphasia Treatment 204

8. *Visual Processing in Recovery from Aphasia* 224
   Introduction 224
   The Use of Visual Information During Language Performance 226
   Effects of Pictures and Visual Scenes on Language Processing 227
   Looking the Other Person in the Mouth: Audiovisual Language Processing 229
   Visual Processing of Pictures/Visual Scenes in Aphasia: Behavioral and Neural Correlates 235
   Interactions with Other Cognitive Domains 238
   Audiovisual Processing in Aphasia: Behavioral and Neural Correlates 238
   Aphasia Assessment/Treatment Studies Incorporating Visual Components 240
   Use of Pictorial Stimuli 240
   Audiovisual Cueing 241

9. *Redefining Recovery from Aphasia* 255
   What Have We Learned? 255
   An Argument for the Neural Multifunctionality of Language: Converging Evidence 257
   Rethinking the Neural Organization of Language: What Is New? 261
   Redefining Recovery from Aphasia 263

INDEX 271

Preface

Learn from yesterday, live for today, hope for tomorrow.
The important thing is not to stop questioning.
                                                    EINSTEIN

THE STUDY OF recovery from aphasia has taught us two important lessons: (1) people with aphasia do not stop improving their language skills over time; (2) each person with aphasia follows a different, unique path to recovery. Neurobiological mechanisms underlying these changes have eluded researchers and clinicians for, now, almost 200 years, as experts in the field have attempted to describe, deconstruct, and reconstruct profiles of language change during recovery from aphasia. We believe the predominant focus on language over these years has not done justice to the full story. In this book we argue that recovery from aphasia is necessarily more than recovery of language functions alone. This claim, of course, begs the question of what pieces are missing from the puzzle of aphasia recovery and how one might go about finding them.

It is with this question in mind that we approached the writing of this book. Our goal was to compile the now impressive body of evidence that could serve to shift the focus of clinical and research perspectives on recovery from aphasia from a language-centric understanding of brain-language relations to one in which the interaction among an array of cognitive phenomena and neural events paves the way to recovery from aphasia. In this sense, our book diverges from most other books on aphasia, which focus almost exclusively on language, language disorders, and treatment of language disorders. Our aim here is not to propose new therapies for aphasia but rather to highlight nonlinguistic factors that participate in reshaping the neural networks supporting recovery of language functions in aphasia. We are proposing that the neural representation of language in the healthy brain engages neural structures that mediate nonlinguistic functions, such as cognition, emotion, and sensorimotor processing that, together, give rise to language as we know it. We call this view of language *neural multifunctionality*, which we propose guides the reshaping of the neural circuitry contributing to recovery from aphasia. This new perspective on brain-language relations, we hope, will provide a solid scientific basis for development of a comprehensive, theory-driven characterization of aphasia, which can then serve as a guide to future clinical practice for management and treatment of aphasia.

During the process of writing this book we worked closely with many people who were extremely helpful in different ways at different times. We would like to take this opportunity to thank them. First is Prof. Sung-Bom Pyun, a neurorehabilitation specialist from the Department of Physical Medicine and Rehabilitation Korea University, who during his stay as a visiting scholar at our research center helped gather the materials for the chapters on executive function, attention, and memory. Second is Sarah Wolford who, during her work with us as a research assistant and long after she moved on to graduate school, processed these materials, sifting through articles, summaries, and chapter outlines. We thank Ted Jenkins, who helped compile the materials for the chapter on emotion while working with us as a research assistant and, while pursuing his doctoral studies, continued to volunteer his time to help shape the chapter on praxis. In addition, we thank Dr. Kevin Black, Assistant Professor of Physics at Boston University, for helping us crystalize some of the ideas we included in the final chapter.

We also thank those people without whom this project would not have been possible. First are the many individuals living with aphasia who came to the Harold Goodglass Aphasia Research Center over the years and with whom we had the privilege of working. Then there is our "hard-core support" team, led by Abigail Oveis, our dedicated research assistant, who did anything and everything we asked of her in relation to this book and did it exceptionally well. As the book was nearing completion, our summer interns, Madeline Piela and Daniel Albert-Rozenberg, worked relentlessly on compiling the bibliography, formatting, and last-minute configuring of the different documents comprising the manuscript. In addition, there are our dear colleagues Professors Loraine K. Obler and Avron Spiro III, who provided us not only with moral support but also with insightful comments about the new ideas expressed in the book. Finally, we thank our beloved families, Oved, Shahar, and Inbar Amitay and Phyllis Albert, who were simply there for us at all times!

DCA
MLA
Boston, Massachusetts

1

What We Know and Do Not Know about Recovery from Aphasia

Defining Recovery from Aphasia

The idea that people with aphasia can continue to improve their language skills over many years (e.g., Allen et al., 2012; Holland, Fromm, De Ruyter, & Stein, 1996; Kiran & Sandberg, 2011), possibly even throughout their lives, is the premise for much of the research and clinical work carried out in today's world of aphasiology. Efforts to account for these long-term gains have appealed to neurobiological explanations that, together, point to a dynamic process by which language networks in the aphasic brain reorganize adaptively to compensate functionally for the effects of brain damage on language performance (e.g., Hillis, 2007). The history of recovery from aphasia has focused—obviously, naturally, and defensibly—on language. In a similar vein, studies of the cognitive neuroscience underlying recovery from aphasia have focused—obviously, naturally, and defensibly—on language. We believe this predominant focus on language over the years has not done justice to the full story.

The goal of this book is to refocus clinical and research approaches to recovery from aphasia: to move from a language-centric understanding of brain-language relations to one in which the entire panoply of cognitive phenomena and neural events interact, thereby influencing recovery. Our aim here is not to propose new therapies for aphasia, language- or cognition-based, but rather to consider the weight of nonlinguistic factors in reshaping the neural networks supporting the recovery of language functions in aphasia, which are steadily emerging as critical players in this process. We will attempt to achieve this goal in three ways: first by considering psycholinguistic models of language in the healthy brain, which will serve as a baseline against which the neural reorganization of language networks in the compromised brain can be assessed; second by exploring the neural substrates of nonlinguistic functions—such as memory, attention, perception, action, and the ways in which nonlinguistic cognitive, emotional, and action phenomena—influence the adaptive reorganization of language networks in the brain during recovery from aphasia; and finally by providing a synthetic theory of the cognitive neuroscience of recovery from aphasia that focuses on the concept of multifunctionality.

The word "multifunctionality" and the concept of multifunctionality in cognitive neuroscience deserve particular consideration here as they represent a principal theme of this book, and have been variously used throughout the decades. There is, for example, neural multifunctionality, suggesting that presumably specialized regions or networks of the brain can be recruited for new functions (e.g., Noë, 2004). There is also linguistic multifunctionality, which occurs in language any time that a single linguistic element is used in more than one distinct context (e.g., Bateman, Matthiessen, & Zeng, 1999; Halliday, 1994). Vygotsky famously used the term multifunctionality to talk about language, philosophy, and the philosophy of language (Vygotsky, 1986), as did Jakobson in his writings on the structure of language (Jakobson, 1980). Use of the word multifunctionality could also tease our readers into believing that we are reopening the old debate in early modern neuropsychology between those who believed in the equipotentiality of brain function (e.g., Lashley, 1929) and those who believed in highly localized cerebral specificity (e.g., Nielsen, 1946; see also Holmes, Teuber, & Weinstein, 1958).

Specifically for the purposes of this book, as we reevaluate current concepts of recovery from aphasia, we will be using the term multifunctionality to refer to aspects of neural multifunctionality, focusing on the dynamic development of new neural support systems in the aphasic brain in service of new functions (Cahana-Amitay & Albert, 2014). We propose that this multifunctionality operates in a multidirectional and reciprocal fashion, such that neural networks engaged in language recovery continuously influence—but at the same time are also reshaped by—neural supports of nonlinguistic functions so as to give rise to new functional neuroanatomies (i.e., newly established or newly reinforced neural networks) in the neurologically compromised brain (Cahana-Amitay & Albert, 2014).

With the help of increasingly skilled testing of cognition in clinical populations and the use of increasingly sophisticated technology—such as functional imaging, diffusion tensor imaging, perfusion imaging, magnetoencephalography, and transcranial magnetic stimulation—researchers have shown that the neural processes involved in recovery from aphasia implicate cognitive systems beyond those devoted strictly to language and engage neural networks not only in regions immediately surrounding cerebral lesions but also in widely dispersed regions bilaterally (e.g., Marsh & Hillis, 2006; Turkeltaub,

Messing, Norise, & Hamilton, 2011). Our use of the term multifunctionality refers to these cognitive and neural interactions that influence recovery from aphasia.

As we discuss throughout the book, the neural and cognitive mechanisms involved in the recovery of language functions in aphasia have remained largely an open question despite the surge of studies exploring this topic (e.g., Anglade, Thiel, & Ansaldo, 2014; Ansaldo, Arguin, & Lecours, 2002; Baker, Rorden, & Frisriksson, 2010; Basso et al., 1998; Belin et al., 1996; Crinion & Leff, 2007; Fridriksson et al., 2009; Meizner et al., 2004, 2008; Mimura et al., 1998; Naeser et al., 2005; Price & Crinion, 2005; Rosen et al., 2006; Saur et al., 2006; Saur & Hartwigsen, 2012; Thompson & den Ouden, 2008). In attempting to address this question, we will also examine one of the thorniest of issues plaguing research on aphasia recovery: the extreme variability in recovery patterns even in the face of comparable etiologies and similar clinical presentations (Lazar & Antoniello, 2008). Indeed, the extent to which an aphasic patient is able to recover his or her language abilities varies considerably (Lazar & Antoniello, 2008), with studies reporting complete recovery in 11% to 50% of patients (e.g., Enderby et al., 1987; Marquarsden, 1969; Pedersen et al., 1995) and in mild cases up to 70% (Laska et al., 2001). Among those in whom aphasia persists for more than a year, milder forms of the disorder are observed over time (Pedersen et al., 1995), with 40% of patients showing excellent improvement, 13% good, 19% fair, and 28% poor (Kertesz & McCabe, 1977).

Successful recovery from aphasia is affected by multiple prognostic factors, including but not limited to aphasia type, severity, lesion characteristics (location/size), sex, age, and premorbid intelligence (e.g., Lazar & Antoniello, 2008). Results from these studies are mixed but several generalizations have been made. For example, people diagnosed with anomia, transcortical aphasia, and conduction aphasia reportedly make a better recovery than those with Broca's or Wernicke's aphasia, who demonstrate a greater range of recovery patterns (Kertesz & McCabe, 1977). Or people initially diagnosed with severe aphasia show poorer language outcomes over time than patients with less severe aphasia, although results in this regard are quite varied, with some severe cases showing excellent recovery (Pedersen et al., 1995; Pedersen, Vinter, & Olsen, 2004). Also, being young and male has been found to positively affect chances of aphasia recovery (McClung, Gonzalez-Rothi, & Nadeau, 2010).

In a recent study, McClung, Gonzalez-Rothi, & Nadeau (2010) proposed relevant prognostic factors grouped into endogenous, referring primarily to neurobiological processes, and exogenous, relating to experiential processes of the aphasic patient. These experiential factors are further divided into those that are therapy-related and those that are ambient (i.e., external to it), as shown in Table 1.1. Although the factors listed in this extremely useful and detailed diagram can help to explain some of the variability observed in recovery, the authors point out that the effects of some have yet to be verified empirically (e.g., languages spoken, educational level, handedness, genetic influences, expectations, time postonset, living environment, occupational status). In addition, as

TABLE 1.1
PROGNOSTIC FACTORS IN APHASIA RECOVERY

Brain-Related Processes (Endogenous)	Experiential Processes (Exogenous)			
	Therapeutic Experience	*Ambient Experience (External to Therapy)*		
		Within the Individual		**Between Individuals**
		Prestroke Factors	*Poststroke Factors*	*Personal Context* / *Social Context*
		Gender	Lesion size	/ Communication partners—spouses
		Age		/ Communication partners—family
		Prestroke depression	Depression	Leisure / Communication partners—friends
		Ethnic/cultural background		/ Communication partners—society
		Language(s) spoken	Exercise	/ Communication partners—psychosocial attributes
		Socioeconomic status		

Source: Adapted from McClung, J. S., Gonzalez-Rothi, L. J., & Nadeau, S. E. (2010). Ambient experience in restitutive treatment of aphasia. *Frontiers in Human Neuroscience, 4*(183), 1–19. doi: 10.3389/fnhum.2010.00183.

we shall emphasize in this book, other poststroke factors not included in this list, such as cognitive and emotional status and their underlying neural representations, play a crucial role in determining the course of recovery.

Stating the Problem

What pieces are missing from the neural puzzle of aphasia recovery and how might one go about finding them and putting the puzzle together? Our limited ability to converge on a clear picture of aphasia recovery stems in part from the fact that most recovery studies continue to focus primarily on the evaluation of impaired language functions and their neural correlates with little regard for the neural bases of spared functions or to general cognitive functioning (Rapp et al., 2012).

The idea that nonlinguistic functioning is part and parcel of the behavioral manifestations observed in aphasia is not new (for a recent historical review, see Gainotti, 2014). Head (1915, 1926), for example, proposed that while language deficits are the primary characteristic of aphasia, the disorder also involves, to a certain degree, an "intellectual" problem. He suggested that it is the impaired interaction among memory, intelligence, and symbolic thinking that accounts for the deficits observed in aphasia, where those with the poorest performance on intellectual tasks were the patients with more severe aphasia. Behavioral studies have demonstrated that people with aphasia indeed rely on skills such as attention (e.g., Erickson, Goldinger, LaPointe, 1996; Hula & McNeil, 2008; Lesniak et al., 2008; Murray, 2002, 2012; Murray, Keeton, & Karcher, 2006; Peach, Rubin, & Newhoff, 1994), executive functions (Fridriksson et al., 2006; Keil & Kaszniak, 2002; Lesniak et al., 2008; Purdy, 2002; Ramsberger, 2005; Zinn et al., 2007), and memory (e.g., Albert, 1976; Barba et al., 1996; Caspari et al., 1998; Downey et al., 2004; Freedman & Martin, 2001; Friedmann & Gvion, 2003; Grober, 1984; Helm-Estabrooks, 2002; Lang & Quitz, 2012; Mayrt & Murray, 2012; Murray, Keeton, & Karcher, 2006; Wright et al., 2007; Wright, Newhoff, Downey, & Austermann, 2003; Wright & Shisler, 2005; Sung et al., 2008) for the construction and/or retrieval of linguistic information. For example, the degree of cognitive ability in persons with aphasia can affect their engagement in verbal learning (Freedman & Martin, 2001) or online language performance (Hula & McNeil, 2008) as well as conversational success (Fridriksson et al., 2006; Ramsberger, 2005).

Moreover, the importance of cognitive factors as predictors of treatment outcomes has been widely demonstrated (e.g., Fillingham et al., 2005a,b; Fridriksson et al., 2006; Helm-Estabrooks, 2002; Keil Kaszniak, 2002; Ramsberger, 2005; Vallila-Rohter & Kiran, 2013). Although it is not always the case that a person with aphasia also suffers cognitive decline (Basso et al., 1973; Chertkow et al., 1997; Helm-Estabrooks, 2002), deficits in short-term memory, for example, have been shown to negatively influence aphasic patients' abilities to perform tasks involving new phonological encoding or semantic learning (Freedman & Martin, 2001). Similarly, impaired executive functioning has been shown to adversely affect measures of functional communication in people with aphasia, and spared executive/attentional skills have been reported to have a remedial effect on conversational skills (Ramsberger, 2005).

Our goal in this book is to offer an integrated view of aphasia recovery that relies on current psycholinguistic models elucidating the neural representation of language in the healthy brain and also considers the role of nonlinguistic factors—such as cognition, emotion, and praxis—in reshaping the neural circuitry associated with recovery from aphasia. Specifically, we introduce emerging multifunctional approaches to the neurobiology of language that call for the incorporation of nonlinguistic, cognitive functions into language models of the intact brain as our theoretical foundation (Chapter 2). We then focus on the functionality of executive function systems (Chapter 3), attention (Chapter 4), memory (Chapter 5), emotion (Chapter 6), praxis (Chapter 7), and visual processing (Chapter 8) and their effects on language performance in aphasia, tying them together with aspects of brain plasticity and neural mechanisms of recovery from aphasia (Chapter 9). In this sense, we depart from most other books on aphasia, which focus almost exclusively on language, language disorders, and the treatment of language disorders.

In Chapter 3, for example, we explore the extent to which executive system deficits can interact with aspects of lexical retrieval in aphasia, tying them to current models of semantic control and their proposed neural underpinnings (e.g., Badre & Wagner, 2007). We show that people with aphasia with damage to their prefrontal cortex have deficits on lexical selection tasks when presented with strong semantic competition and/or open-ended task demands, thus impairing their ability to cognitively control task-appropriate responses that activate semantic information within the semantic store (e.g., Badre et al., 2005; Gardner et al., 2012; Thompson-Schill et al., 1997; Whitney et al., 2011). We further demonstrate that such difficulties are also apparent in people with aphasia with lesions in white matter tracts connecting frontal, temporal, and parietal regions (Harvey et al., 2013) as well as those with damaged subcortical circuits (Radanovic et al., 2003). We then conclude Chapter 3 by reviewing aphasia treatment studies showing that targeting specific executive support systems can improve naming in persons with aphasia due to stroke-induced cortical lesions by stimulating activation of the right hemisphere (Crosson et al., 2005, 2007, 2009).

Our description of each behavior considered in this book (cognitive, emotional, and praxic) will follow the same structural plan, designed to inform the reader about underlying mechanisms, biological foundations, particular interactions with language abilities, and manifestations in aphasia. Specifically, we will provide (1) definition(s) of the behavior in question; (2) a description of mechanisms underlying that behavior in the healthy brain and its neural underpinnings; (3) a description of specific models explaining interdependencies between that behavior and language and their neural correlates; (4) the means to assess the behavior in question (tests used to measure it), focusing on specific challenges for evaluating it in people with aphasia; and (5) findings regarding this behavior in aphasia and its neural correlates. To the extent that the literature allows, we will also discuss the prognostic value of each behavior for aphasia treatment as well as neuroimaging studies exploring the contribution of that behavior to the neural reorganization of language function in the aphasic brain.

The organizational principle underlying our book is, to a large extent, an artificial construct imposed for ease of exposition. At the risk of slightly misrepresenting the integrative approach we put forth here, we describe the empirical findings in discrete chapters, fully recognizing that the domains discussed are interconnected and often overlap. We discuss neural plasticity and neural reorganization in recovery from aphasia, demonstrating how concepts of the neuroscience of recovery from aphasia emerge organically from data and analyses provided throughout the book.

We hope this novel view of the neural multifunctionality of language will provide a solid scientific basis for development of a comprehensive and theory-driven characterization of aphasia, which can then serve as a guide to future clinical practice for the management and treatment of aphasia.

References

Albert, M. L. (1976). Short-term memory and aphasia. *Brain and Language, 3,* 28–33.

Allen, L., Mehta, S., McClure, J. A., & Teasall, R. (2012). Therapeutic interventions for aphasia initiated more than six months post stroke: a review of the evidence. *Topics in Stroke Rehabilitation, 19*(6), 523–535.

Anglade, C., Thiel, A., & Ansaldo A. I. (2014). The complementary role of the cerebral hemispheres in recovery from aphasia after stroke: a critical review of the literature. *Brain Injury, 28*(2), 138–145.

Ansaldo, A. I., Arguin, M., & Lecours, A. (2002). Initial right hemisphere take-over and subsequent bilateral participation during recovery from aphasia. *Aphasiology, 16,* 287–304.

Badre, D., Poldrack, R. A., Paré-Blagoev, E. J., Insler, R., & Wagner, A. D. (2005). Dissociable controlled retrieval and generalized selection mechanisms in ventrolateral prefrontal cortex. *Neuron, 47,* 907–918.

Badre, D., & Wagner, A. D. (2007). Left ventrolateral prefrontal cortex and the cognitive control of memory. *Neuropsychologia, 45,* 2883–2901.

Baker, J., Rorden, C., & Fridriksson, J. (2010). Using transcranial direct current stimulation (tDCS) to treat stroke patients with aphasia. *Stroke, 41*(6), 1229–1236.

Barba, G. D., Frasson, E., Mantovan, M. C., Gallo A., & Denes, G. (1996). Semantic and episodic memory in aphasia. *Neuropsychologia, 34*(5), 361–367.

Basso, A., De Renzi, E., Faglioni, P., Scotti, G., & Spinnler, H. (1973). Neuropsychological evidence for the existence of cerebral areas critical to the performance of intelligence tests. *Brain, 96,* 715–728.

Basso, G., Romero S., Pietrini, P., Beeson, P. M., Rapczack, S., & Grafman, J. (1998). Neurofrontal correlates of language reorganization after massive hemisphere stroke. Poster presented at the 4th International Conference on Functional Mapping of the Human Brain, Montreal, Quebec, Canada, June 7–12, 1998. *Neuroimage, 7*(4), S472.

Bateman, J. A., Matthiessen, C.M.I.M., & Zeng, L. (1999). Multilingual natural language generation for multilingual software: a functional linguistic approach. *Applied Artificial Intelligence, 13,* 607–639.

Belin, P., Van Eeckhout, P., Zilbovicius, M., Remy, P., François, C., Guillaume, S., ... & Samson, Y. (1996). Recovery from nonfluent aphasia after melodic intonation therapy: a PET study. *Neurology, 47,* 1504–1511.

Cahana-Amitay, D. & Albert, M. L. (2014). Brain and language: evidence for neural multifunctionality. *Behavioural Neurology,* http://dx.doi.org/10.1155/2014/260381

Caspari, I., Parkinson, S. R., LaPointe, L. L., & Katz, R. C. (1998). Working memory and aphasia. *Brain and Cognition, 37,* 205–223.

Chertkow, H., Bub, D., Deaudon, C., & Whitehead, V. (1997). On the status of object concepts in aphasia. *Brain and Language, 58,* 203–232.

Crinion, J. T., & Leff, A. P. (2007). Recovery and treatment of aphasia after stroke: functional imaging studies. *Current Opinion in Neurology 20*(6), 667–673. doi:10.1097/WCO.ob013e3282f1c6fa.

Crosson, B., Fabrizio, K. S., Singletary, F., Cato, M. A., Wierenga, C. E., Parkinson, R. B., ... Rothi, L. J. (2007). Treatment of naming in nonfluent aphasia through manipulation of intention and attention: a phase 1 comparison of two novel treatments. *Journal of the International Neuropsychological Society, 13*(4), 582–594.

Crosson, B., Moore, A. B., Gopinath, K., White, K. D., Wierenga, C. E., & Gaiefsky, M. E., … Gonzalez Rothi, L. J. (2005). Role of the right and left hemispheres in recovery of function during treatment of intention in aphasia. *Journal of Cognitive Neuroscience, 17*(3), 392–406.

Crosson, B., Moore, A. B., McGregor, K. M., Chang, Y. L., Benjamin, M., Gopinath, K., … & White, K. D. (2009). Regional changes in word-production laterality after a naming treatment designed to produce a rightward shift in frontal activity. *Brain and Language, 111*(2), 73–85.

Downey, R. A., Wright, H. H., Schwartz, R. G., Newhoff, M., Love, T., & Shapiro, L. P. (2004). Toward a measure of working memory in aphasia. Poster presented at Clinical Aphasiology Conference; Park City, UT.

Enderby, P., Wood, V. A., Wade, D. T., & Hewer, R. L. (1987). Aphasia after stroke: a detailed study of recovery in the first 3 months. *International Rehabilitation Medicine, 8*(4), 162–165.

Erickson, R. J., Goldinger, S. D., & LaPointe, L. L. (1996). Auditory vigilance in aphasic individuals: Detecting nonlinguistic stimuli with full or divided attention. *Brain and Cognition, 3*, 244–253.

Fillingham, J. K., Sage, K., & Lambon Ralph, M. A. (2005a). Further explorations and an overview or errorless and errorful therapy for aphasic word-finding difficulties: the number of naming attempts during therapy affects outcome. *Aphasiology, 19*(7), 597–614.

Fillingham, J. K., Sage, K., & Lambon Ralph, M. A. (2005b). Treatment of anomia using errorless versus errorful learning: Are frontal executive skills and feedback important? *International Journal of Language and Communication Disorders, 40*(4), 505–523.

Freedman, M. L., & Martin, R. C. (2001). Dissociable components of short-term memory and their relation to long-term learning. *Cognitive Neuropsychology, 18*(3), 193–226.

Fridriksson, J., Baker, J. M., Whiteside, J., Eoute, D., Moser, D., Vesselinov, R., & Rorden, C. (2009). Treating visual speech perception to improve speech production in nonfluent aphasia. *Stroke, 40*, 853–858.

Fridriksson, J., Nettles, C., Davis, M., Morrow, L., & Montgomery, A. (2006). Functional communication and executive function in aphasia. *Clinical Linguistics and Phonetics, 20*, 401–410.

Friedmann, N., & Gvion, A. (2003). Sentence comprehension and working memory limitation in aphasia: a dissociation between semantic-syntactic and phonological reactivation. *Brain and Language, 86*(1), 23–39.

Gainotti, G. (2014). Old and recent approaches to the problem of non-verbal conceptual disorders in aphasic patients. *Cortex. 53*, 78–89, doi:10.1016/j.cortex.2014.01.009

Gardner, H. E., Lambon Ralph, M. A., Dodds, N., Jones, T., Ehsan, S., & Jefferies, E. (2012). The differential contributions of pFC and temporo-parietal cortex to multimodal semantic control: exploring refractory effects in semantic aphasia. *Journal of Cognitive Neuroscience, 24*(4), 778–793. doi: 10.1162/jocn_a_00184

Grober, E. (1984). Nonlinguistic memory in aphasia. *Cortex, 20*(1), 67–73.

Halliday, M. A. K. (1994). *An introduction to functional grammar.* London: Edward Arnold.

Harvey, D. Y., Wei, T., Ellmore, T. M., Hamilton, A. C., & Schnur, T. T. (2013). Neuropsychological evidence for the functional role of the uncinate fasciculus in semantic control. *Neuropsychology, 51*(5), 789–801. doi: 10.1016/j.neuropsychologia.2013.01.028

Head, H. (1915). Jackson on aphasia and kindred affections of speech. *Brain, 38*, 1–189.
Head, H. (1926). *Aphasia and kindred disorders of speech.* London: Hafner.
Helm-Estabrooks, N. (2002). Cognition and aphasia: a discussion and a study. *Journal of Communication Disorders, 35*(2), 171–186.
Hillis, A. E. (2007). Aphasia: progress in the last quarter of a century. *Neurology, 69*, 200–213.
Holland, A. L., Fromm, D. S., De Ruyter, F., & Stein, M. (1996). Treatment efficacy: aphasia. *Journal of Speech and Hearing Research, 39*(5), S27–S36.
Holmes, J. A., Teuber, H., & Weinstein, S. (1958). Equipotentiality versus cortical localization. *Science, 127*(3292), 241–242.
Hula W. D., & McNeil M. R. (2008). Models of attention and dual-task performance as explanatory constructs in aphasia. *Seminars in Speech and Language, 29*(3), 169–187.
Jakobson, R. (1980). *The framework of language.* Ann Arbor: University of Michigan Press.
Keil, K., & Kaszniak, A. W. (2002). Examining executive function in individuals with brain injury: a review. *Aphasiology, 16*, 305–335.
Kertesz, A., & McCabe, P. (1977). Recovery patterns and prognosis in aphasia. *Brain, 100*(Pt1), 1–18.
Kiran, S., & Sandberg, C. (2011). Treating communication problems in individuals with disordered language. In R. Peach & L. Shapiro (Eds.). *cognition and acquired language disorders: a process-oriented approach* (pp. 298–326). London: Elsevier.
Lang, C. J., & Quitz, A. (2012). Verbal and nonverbal memory impairment in aphasia. *Journal of Neurology, 259*, 1655–1661.
Lashley, K. S. (1929). *Brain mechanisms and intelligence.* Chicago: University of Chicago Press.
Laska, A. C., Hellblom, A., Murray, V., Kahan, T., & Von Arbin, M. (2001). Aphasia in acute stroke and relation to outcome. *Journal of Internal Medicine, 249*(5), 413–422.
Lazar, R. M., & Antoniello, D. (2008). Variability in recovery from aphasia. *Current Neurology and Neuroscience Reports, 8*(6), 497–502.
Lesniak, M., Bak, T., Czepiel, W., Seniow, J., & Czlonkowska, A. (2008). Frequency and prognostic value of cognitive disorders in stroke patients. *Dementia and Geriatric Cognitive Disorders, 26*(4), 356–363.
Marquarsden, J. (1969). *The natural history of acute cerebrovascular disease: a retrospective study of 769 patients.* Copenhagen: Munksgaard.
Marsh E. B., & Hillis, A. E. (2006). Recovery from aphasia following brain injury: the role of reorganization. *Progress in Brain Research, 157*, 143–156.
McClung, J. S., Gonzalez-Rothi, L. J., & Nadeau, S. E. (2010). Ambient experience in restitutive treatment of aphasia. *Frontiers in Human Neuroscience, 4*(183), 1–19. doi: 10.3389/fnhum.2010.00183
Meizner, M., Elbert, T., Wienbruch, C., Djundja, D., Barthel, G., & Rockstroh, B. (2004). Intensive language training enhances brain plasticity in chronic aphasia. *BMC Biology, 2*, 20. doi: 10.1186/1741-7007-2-20
Meinzer, M., Flaisch, T., Breitenstein, C., Wienbruch, C., Elbert, T., & Rockstroh, B. (2008). Functional re-recruitment of dysfunctional brain areas predicts language recovery in aphasia. *NeuroImage, 15*, 2038–2046.
Mimura, M., Kato, M., Kato, M., Sano, Y., Kojima, T., Naeser, M., & Kashima, H. (1998). Prospective and retrospective studies of recovery in aphasia: changes in cerebral blood flow and language functions. *Brain, 121*, 2083–2094.

Murray, L. L. (2002). Cognitive distinctions between depression and early Alzheimer's disease in the elderly. *Aphasiology, 16*, 573–586.

Murray L. L. (2012). Attention and other cognitive deficits in aphasia: presence and relation to language and communication measures. *American Journal of Speech-Language Pathology, 21*, S51–S64.

Murray, L. L., Keeton, R. J., & Karcher, L. (2006). Treating attention in mild aphasia: evaluation of attention process training-II. *Journal of Communication Disorders, 39*, 37–61.

Naeser, M. A., Martin, P. I., Nicholas, M., Baker, E. H., Seekins, H., Kobayashi, M., … & Pascual-Leone, A. (2005). Improved picture naming in chronic aphasia after TMS to part of right Broca's area: an open-protocol study. *Brain and language, 93*(1), 95–105.

Nielsen, J. M. (1946). *Agnosia, apraxia, aphasia: their value in cerebral localization.* New York: Hoeber.

Noë, A. (2004). *Action in perception*. Cambridge, MA: MIT Press.

Peach, R. K., Rubin, S. R., & Newhoff, M. (1994). A topographic event-related potential analysis of the attention deficit for auditory processing in aphasia. *Clinical Aphasiology 22*, 81–96.

Pedersen P. M., Jørgensen H. S., Nakayama H., Raaschou H. O., & Olsen T. S. (1995). Aphasia in acute stroke: incidence, determinants, and recovery. *Annals of Neurology, 38*(4), 659–666.

Pedersen P. M., Vinter K., & Olsen T. S. (2004). Aphasia after stroke: type, severity and prognosis. The Copenhagen aphasia study. *Cerebrovascular Diseases, 17*(1), 35–43.

Price, C. J., & Crinion, J. (2005). The latest on functional imaging studies of aphasic stroke. *Current Opinion in Neurology, 18*(4), 429–434.

Purdy, M. (2002). Executive function ability in persons with aphasia. *Aphasiology, 16*(4–6), 549–557.

Radanovic, M., Azambuja, M., Mansur, L. L., Porto, C. S., & Scaff, M. (2003). Thalamus and language: interface with attention, memory and executive functions. *Arquivos de Neuro-Psiquiatria, 61*(1), 34–42.

Ramsberger, G. (2005). Achieving conversational success in aphasia by focusing on non-linguistic cognitive skills: A potentially promising new approach. *Aphasiology, 19*, 1066–1073.

Rapp, B., Caplan, D., Edwards, S., Visch-Brink, E., & Thompson, C. (2012). Neuroimaging in aphasia treatment research: Issues of experimental design for relating cognitive to neural changes. *NeuroImage, 73*, 200–207.

Rosen, H. J., Petersen, S. E., Linenweber, M. R., Snyder, A. Z., White, D. A., Chapman, L., … Weiller, C. (2006). Dynamics of language reorganization after stroke. *Brain, 129*(6), 1371–1384.

Saur, D., & Hartwigsen, G. (2012). Neurobiology of language recovery after stroke: lessons from neuroimaging studies. *Archives of Physical Medicine and Rehabilitation, 93*(1 Suppl):S15–S25. doi: 10.1016/j.apmr.2011.03.036

Sung, J. E., McNeil, M. R., Pratt, S. R., Dickey, M. W., Hula, W. D., Szuminsky, N. J., & … Den Ouden, D. B. (2008). Neuroimaging and recovery of language in aphasia. *Current Neurology and Neuroscience Reports, 8*(5), 475–483.

Thompson-Schill, S. L., D'Esposito, M., Aguirre, G. K., & Farah, M. J. (1997). Role of left inferior prefrontal cortex in retrieval of semantic knowledge: a reevaluation. *Proceedings of the National Academy of Sciences of the United States of America, 94*(26), 14792–14797.

Turkeltaub, P. E., Messing, S., Norise, C., & Hamilton, R. H. (2011). Are networks for residual language function and recovery consistent across aphasic patients? *Neurology*, *76*, 1726–1734.

Vallila-Rohter, S. M., & Kiran, S. (2013). Non-linguistic learning and aphasia: evidence from a paired associate and feedback-based task. *Neuropsychologia*, *51*(1), 79–90. doi: 10.1016/j.neuropsychologia.2012.10.024

Vygotsky, L. (1986). *Thought and Language*. Cambridge, MA: MIT Press.

Whitney, C., Kirk, M., O'Sullivan, J., Lambon, Ralph M. A., & Jefferies, E. (2011). The neural organization of semantic control: TMS evidence for a distributed network in left inferior frontal and posterior middle temporal gyrus. *Cerebral Cortex*, *21*, 1066–1075.

Wright, H. H., Downey, R. A., Gravier, M., Love, T., & Shapiro, L. P. (2007). Processing distinct linguistic information types in working memory in aphasia. *Aphasiology*, *21*, 802–813.

Wright, H. H., Newhoff, M., Downey, R., & Austermann, S. (2003). Additional data on working memory in aphasia. *Journal of International Neuropsychological Society*, *9*, 302.

Wright, H. H., & Shisler, R. (2005). Working memory in aphasia. *American Journal of Speech-Language Pathology*, *14*, 107–118.

Zinn, S., Bosworth, H. B., Hoenig, H. M., & Swartzwelder, H. S. (2007). Executive function deficits in acute stroke. *Archives of Physical Medicine and Rehabilitation*, *88*(2), 173–180.

2

Language in the Healthy Brain

EVIDENCE FOR MULTIFUNCTIONALITY

Where Do We Start?

In this chapter we provide a brief review of current models of functional neuroanatomy of language in the healthy brain. The purpose of this review is not to summarize all of the available findings describing brain-language relationships—a formidable task in and of itself—but rather to situate the study of aphasia recovery in the context of a "neural" approach to language that would serve as a basis for creating an integrative framework with increased empirical validity and greater clinical utility beyond that which existing models of language impairment currently provide. It is designed to provide the theoretical background against which we propose to develop the concept of neural multifunctionality (Cahana-Amitay & Albert, 2014).

To date, a clear and comprehensive model explaining the functional neuroanatomy of language in the healthy brain is still a work in progress. The newest theoretical accounts reflect a shift toward models with increased empirical and conceptual resolution that consider the dynamic nature of the biological foundations of language (e.g., Blumstein & Amso, 2013; Grimaldi, 2012; Grimaldi & Craighero, 2012; Poeppel et al., 2012). Empirical resolution refers to the high degree of precision with which we can characterize the temporal and spatial features of language-related brain activation patterns. Greater conceptual resolution refers to the increased specificity with which we can describe language-based representations/operations.

Models of Functional Neuroanatomy of Language

Current brain-language models have developed in reaction to the classical groundbreaking Broca-Wernicke-Lichtheim-Geschwind lesion-deficit model of aphasia (Geschwind, 1965). In this model, language was localized in the left hemisphere, where damage to specific regions was thought to result in specific patterns of language deficits. For example, the left posteroinferior frontal region, Broca's area, was argued to mediate speech production (a lesion to this area would result in articulatory impairments); the left posterotemporal region, Wernicke's area, auditory speech recognition (a lesion to this area would yield deficient comprehension); and the arcuate fasciculus connecting these regions, repetition (a lesion in these fibers would result in impaired repetition but preserved comprehension).

This view of brain-language relations has resulted in the creation of a clinical classification of aphasic syndromes, which, to some extent, still guides aphasia research and clinical practice. This classification comprises seven major aphasic syndromes with distinct behavioral and brain damage patterns (e.g., Helm-Estabrooks, Albert, & Nicholas, 2013; Saffran, 2000). These are summarized in Table 2.1. The behavioral patterns are characterized in terms of speech fluency, word and sentence production, word and sentence comprehension, and repetition, as used in many clinical assessment tools (e.g., Goodglass & Kaplan, 1983; Kertesz, 1982; but see Crary, Wertz, & Deal, 1992).

Over the years, however, these mappings have been shown to suffer from serious clinical, biological, and psycholinguistic shortcomings (e.g., Alexander, 1997; Caramazza, 1984; Dronkers et al., 2004; Hickok & Poeppel, 2004a; Poeppel & Hickok, 2007). For example, they cannot explain the entire range of lesion-deficit patterns that persons with aphasia exhibit (e.g., when a lesion to a specific brain region does not lead to the predicted behavioral profile or when lesions to multiple brain areas give rise to behavioral patterns that would be expected from damage to an altogether different area). Or, they cannot account for shifts in behavioral patterns that persons with aphasia demonstrate over time (e.g., Wernicke-like deficits evolving into conduction-like or anomia-like behavioral patterns). Such changes reportedly affect 30% to 60% of aphasic persons (Pashek & Holland, 1988), with anomia being the most common outcome (Kertesz & McCabe, 1977; Pashek & Holland, 1988).

The classical model has been further criticized with the surge of new findings from studies using sophisticated techniques for measuring online brain activity (e.g., hemodynamic changes in the brain through functional magnetic resonance imaging [fMRI], intrinsic brain connectivity through resting-state fMRI, or the time course of brain activation during task performance via electroencephalography [EEG] or magneto-encephalography [MEG]). Through these methods, many new inter- and intrahemispheric language networks have been identified (e.g., Catani et al., 2007, 2012; Catani & ffytche, 2005; Catani, Jones, & ffytche, 2005), extending well beyond the core

TABLE 2.1
MAJOR TYPES OF CLINICAL APHASIC SYNDROMES

Type	Fluency	Production Word	Production Sentence	Comprehension Word	Comprehension Sentence	Repetition	Lesion Site
Global	Nonfluent	Poor	None	Poor	Poor	Poor	Large perisylvian regions, deep into subjacent white matter
Broca's	Nonfluent	Range (poor to good); better with nouns than verbs	Impaired, could be agrammatic	Range (poor to good)	Impaired on syntactically complex sentences	Poor	Lateral frontal, suprasylvian, pre-Rolandic regions, extending into subcortical perventricular white matter
Conduction	Fluent, semantic, phonemic substitutions; repeated attempts (off-target) to produce word	Variable, with substitutions	Good, but filled with substitutions	Good	Variable, especially on syntactically complex sentences	Poor	Supramarginal gyrus and underlying white matter, Wernicke's area, left insula, and auditory cortex
Wernicke's	Fluent, excessive, semantic and/or phonemic substitutions	Poor	Good, but empty of content	Poor	Poor	Poor	Posterior third of superior temporal gyrus
Transcortical sensory	Fluent, excessive, semantic and/or phonemic substitutions	Poor	Good, but empty of content	Poor	Poor	Preserved	Posterior parietotemporal areas
Transcortical motor	Preserved but limited	Variable	Variable	Good	Variable	Preserved	Anterior frontal paramedian area, anterior and superior to Broca's region
Anomia	Fluent but interrupted by word retrieval problems	Poor	Good but filled with word-finding difficulties	Variable	Good	Preserved	Angular gyrus, second temporal gyrus

language areas (e.g., Friederici, 2012; Grodzinsky & Friederici, 2006; Price, 2012; Tomasi & Volkow, 2012; Turken & Dronkers, 2011), including cortical networks bilaterally (e.g., Price, 2012), as well as subcortical circuits (Crosson, 2013; Friederici, 2006; Kotz & Schwatze, 2010; Olivier, Mess, Eckstein, & Friederici, 2011).

Price (2010), for example, reviewed standard coordinates of peak activations in over 100 fMRI studies published in 2009, and delineated a complex set of neural networks of language comprehension and production. For language comprehension, these included the superior temporal gyri bilaterally for prelexical acoustic analysis and phonemic categorization of auditory stimulus; middle and inferior temporal cortex for meaningful speech; left angular gyrus and pars orbitalis for semantic retrieval; superior temporal sulci bilaterally for sentence comprehension; and inferior frontal areas, posterior planum temporale, and ventral supramarginal gyrus for implausible sentences. For language production additional networks were identified, including the left middle frontal cortex for word retrieval independently of articulation; left anterior insula for articulatory planning, left putamen, presupplementary motor area, supplementary motor area, and motor cortex for overt speech initiation and execution; and anterior cingulate and bilateral head of caudate nuclei for response suppression during monitoring of speech output. Such data pointed to a need to propose new models of the neuroanatomy of language with increased neural and psycholinguistic specificity. These models would elucidate specific links between formal language operations and lay out the dynamic spatial and temporal neuronal pathways mediating them (Poeppel, 2011).

PSYCHOLINGUISTIC MODELS OF BRAIN-LANGUAGE INTERLINKS

For nearly a quarter century models have been developed to reconcile neurological findings with psycholinguistic accounts in order to provide a systematic explanation for the biological foundation of language (e.g., Amunts et al., 2010; Ben Shalom & Poeppel, 2008; Friederici, 2006; 2011; 2012; Friederici & Gierhan, 2013; Grodzinsky & Friederici, 2006; Hickok & Poeppel, 2000, 2004, 2007; Poeppel et al., 2012; Price, 2010, 2012). These models have pointed to different functional anatomies underlying different word- and/or sentence-level linguistic processes.

One of the most influential models, already considered in some aphasia recovery studies (e.g., Kümmerer et al., 2013; Saur & Hartwigsen, 2012), is the *dorsal/ventral account* by Hickok and Poeppel (2004b, 2007). This model comprises a dual-route neuroanatomical circuitry for auditory processing—dorsal and ventral streams—inspired by comparable proposals the field of visual processing (Milner & Goodale, 1995; Ungerleider & Mishkin, 1982) and auditory processing in animal studies (Rauschecker, 1998). The ventral stream, known as the "what" pathway, is argued to support auditory recognition processes, including lexical semantic processing through neural networks projecting to regions within the temporal lobe. The dorsal stream, known as the "where" pathway, serves as an interface for sensorimotor integration, where phonological mappings of sound-to-articulatory representations are formed via projections from auditory cortical circuits to temporoparietal and frontal networks. This neural organization is shown in Figure 2.1 below.

This formulation of the dorsal/ventral model does not address the computational nature of frontal networks, which have been argued to interact with the dorsal system (Ben Shalom & Poeppel, 2008). From the perspective of aphasia recovery, this gap is problematic, given findings indicating that neural reorganization in chronic aphasia relies on bilateral activation of temporofrontal networks (e.g., Crinion & Leff, 2007; Thompson & den Ouden, 2008). Later iterations of this model, which we discuss in Chapters 7 and 8, flesh out some of these details, and we discuss their potential relevance to mechanisms of recovery from aphasia.

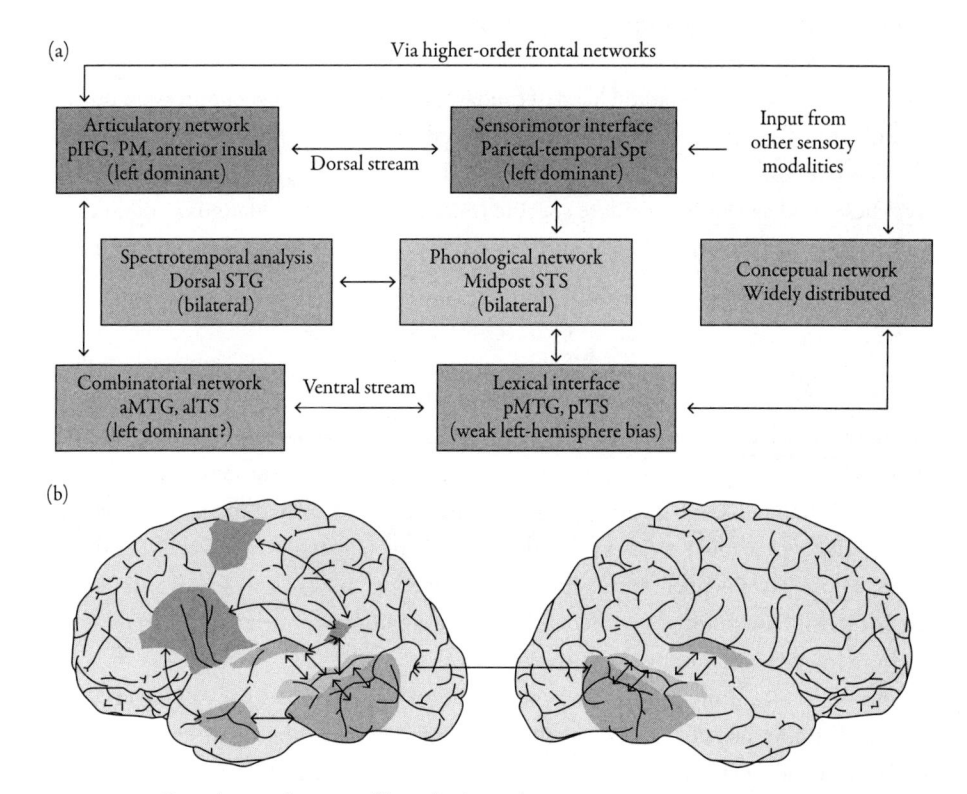

FIGURE 2.1 Dorsal-ventral streams (See color insert.)

Reprinted under the Creative Commons Attribution License from Cahana-Amitay, D., and Albert, M. L. (2014). Brain and language: evidence for neural multifunctionality. Behavioural Neurology, http://dx.doi.org/10.1155/2014/260381. Hindawi, copyright 2014.

STS, superior temporal sulcus; STG, superior temporal gyrus; aITS, anterior inferior temporal sulcus; aMTG, anterior middle temporal gyrus; pIFG, posterior inferior frontal gyrus; PM, premotor cortex.

Source: Adapted from Cahana-Amitay, D., & Albert, M. L. (2014). Brain and language: evidence for neural multifunctionality. *Behavioural Neurology*, Figure 1.

Many psycholinguistic studies have attempted to elucidate the functional neuroanatomy of frontal language networks (e.g., Grodzinsky & Amunts, 2006). These represent different and often opposing characterizations of the processes involved and their underlying neural bases (e.g., Grodzinsky & Friederici, 2006; Hagoort, 2005). The accounts differ primarily in the degree to which they view language as a computationally independent component of the brain (i.e., modular [Fodor, 1983]). Namely, they diverge in terms of "whether there are domain-specific modules associated with different components of the grammar, whether such modules recruit distinct neural structures that are solely dedicated to the processing of that module, and whether the neural systems associated with language are different from those recruited across other cognitive domains" (Blumstein & Amso, 2013, p. 45).

Some proposals have related particular frontal networks to specific semantic and syntactic processes (e.g., Ben-Shachar et al., 2003; Friederici, 2006; Newman et al., 2003), reflecting a fixed module-specific neural organization (Blumstein & Amso, 2013). Friederici (2006), for example, demonstrated that during language comprehension the pars opercularis and pars triangularis (areas BA 44/45) within Broca's area mediate reconstruction of sequential input into hierarchical syntactic structures, whereas BA6 and the frontal operculum subserve the processing of local structures. Her proposal was based on brain activation patterns induced by sentence comprehension tasks involving canonical and noncanonical word orders of varying lengths and processing demands as well as syntactic violations at the phrase level.

A different approach has been proposed by Hagoort (2005), who argued for a model involving distributed neural networks, where language processing in Broca's area, the left inferior frontal gyrus, engages parallel processing of semantic, syntactic, and phonological information through three functional components: memory, unification, and control. Memory serves to retrieve language information from long-term memory, unification functions to integrate the retrieved information into larger phrasal units, and control selects a language "action." Based on findings from EEG and MEG studies, he specified the temporal features of unification and memory retrieval, and suggested that language functions are supported by neuronal synchronization that reflects functional interrelatedness rather than domain-specificity (Bastiaansen & Hagoort, 2006).

Our discussion of Hagoort's framework is not meant to endorse his view and its implications for neural reorganization in aphasia recovery but rather intends to highlight the importance of at least one implication of his model: *that the processing of linguistic information necessarily interacts with the processing of other types of information at different points in time*. This implication suggests reevaluating strict modular views of language representation in the brain (Fodor, 1983), which attributes language processing to discrete neurofunctional components rather than to multiple functionally overlapping neural networks (Blumstein & Amso, 2013).

Cumulative evidence speaks to the existence of functionally diverse neural networks in the left inferior frontal gyrus (e.g., Amunts et al., 2010), which subserve several language functions, including speech processing (e.g., Myers, Blumstein, Walsh, & Eliassen, 2009), processing of syntactic complexity (Grodzinsky & Friederici, 2006), plausibility (e.g., Caplan et al., 2000; Rogalsky et al., 2008), and semantic processing (Binder et al., 2009). These frontal networks have also been associated with nonlinguistic functions, such as processing of math operations, mental rotations, and music (Baldo & Dronkers, 2007; Jordan et al., 2001; Maess, Koelsch, Gunter, & Friederici, 2001; Podzebenko et al., 2002). Similarly, posterior portions of left temporal networks have been found to mediate both syntactic (e.g., Cooke et al., 2002; Constable et al., 2004; Hasson, Nusbaum, & Small, 2006) and nonsyntactic processing (e.g., Graves, Grabowske, Mehta, & Gupta, 2008; Hicock, Okada, & Serences, 2009; Noppeney, Phillips, & Price, 2004).

Researchers have been able to tease apart some these overlapping functions, supporting a weaker version of modularity, termed by some multifunctional modularity (Grodzinsky, 2010), where independent functional components of language and their neural correlates can be identified and then incorporated into a model that would integrate them. Such a model would account for findings such as those reported by Makuuchi and colleagues (Makuuchi, Bahlmann, & Friederici, 2012), who found an anterior-to-posterior functional network within the prefrontal cortex that supports domain-general hierarchical structuring in language, arithmetic, and working memory tasks as well as a domain-specific neural substrate implicating the dorsal pars opercularis that mediates processing of hierarchically complex sentences. This syntactic-specificity was evidenced in patterns of reduced brain activation in the pars opercularis in response to language tasks only.

A CALL FOR MULTIFUNCTIONAL BRAIN-LANGUAGE MODELS

The findings reviewed here indicate a need to develop an integrative brain-language model that explains multifunctionality across shared neural networks (Blumstein & Amso, 2013). A multifunctional neural model of language would require brain-language mappings that reflect the functional diversity of the neural networks subserving language, including the roles of nonlinguistic skills. To use the words of Fedorenko, Nieto-Castañón, and Kanwisher (2012):

> In order to claim that a particular brain region R supports a particular cognitive function, it is necessary not only to formulate predictions about the kinds of cognitive operations that should result in activity in region R, but also to be able to explain why other kinds of cognitive operations result in activity in region R. (p. 188)

This task, of course, is easier said than done. The greatest challenge is to characterize the nature of these nonlinguistic contributions and identify their respective neural correlates. Carpenter, Just, and Reichle (2000) have long noted that the neural organization of executive functions and working memory comprises widely and dynamically distributed networks in prefrontal cortices, which do not afford clearly identifiable mechanisms that allocate functions to different neural regions.

In spite of this challenge, recent attempts to formulate accounts that elucidate neural interfaces among language, cognitive, motor, and sensory processes have, in fact, been made (e.g., Friederici, 2011, 2012; Friederici & Gierhan, 2012; Gierhan, 2013; Price, 2012). Fridereici (2012), for example, proposed a model consisting of two dorsal and ventral streams (Friederici & Gierhan, 2012), which presumably mediate spoken language processing from auditory perception to sentence comprehension and interface at certain points with working memory functions. Her arguments are based primarily on neuroimaging and electrophysiological studies, where facets of language functions were assessed through tasks contrasting specific features (e.g., comparison of words and pseudowords or semantically plausible sentences to implausible ones) to help create detailed brain maps for phonological, semantic, and sentential processes.

The two ventral pathways are assumed to subserve semantic processing (e.g., word-level semantic categorization, lexical-semantic access, sentential plausibility), through networks involving BA 45/47 and the frontal operculum, as well as basic syntactic operations (e.g., local phrase structure building), through the uncinate fasciculus (UF), which connects the frontal operculum and temporal areas. The role of the UF in relation to language, however, has not been widely demonstrated (Kho et al., 2008; Papagno, 2011; Papagno et al., 2011).

The two dorsal pathways are argued to mediate sensory-to-motor integrations engaging the temporal cortex, the primary motor region, and the pars opercularis (area BA 44) as well as the processing of structurally complex sentences, during which BA 44 transfer information to the posterior temporal cortex in a top-down manner—for example, when examination of sentential context is required. Because involvement of both BA 44 and the temporal cortex has been observed during syntactic processing and because the dorsal portion of BA 44 and the inferior frontal sulcus have been related to syntactic working memory, Friederici proposed incorporating working memory into her model as a functional component of processing of syntactically complex sentences (as in Caplan & Waters, 1999; Makuuchi et al., 2009), which we also address in Chapter 5. However, the specification of the precise cognitive mechanisms that would link prefrontal and parietal regions, which also partake in sentence comprehension, remained underdetermined. In a later study using dynamic causal model, Makuuchi and Friederici (2013) attempted to clarify this issue by analyzing the processing of complex syntax during reading. They proposed hierarchical connectivity, whereby linguistic information is processed via the activation of visual word form regions (fusiform gyrus), working memory areas (inferior frontal sulcus and intraparietal sulcus), and language cortices (pars opercularis and the middle temporal gyrus), with connectivity increasing as processing load does.

As noted in Cahana-Amitay and Albert (2014), another model of the functional neuroanatomy of language that makes room for nonlinguistic contributions to language processing has been proposed by Price (2012), who reviewed over 1,000 positron emission and neuroimaging studies published over the past 20 years (1992–2011). She found converging evidence for neural networks for heard speech, speech production, and reading, which interact with sensory and motor processes localized to specific structures and with distributed activations shared across several functions.

Price (2012) reviewed the neural data for nine major language functions, including auditory speech processing of sounds (speech and nonspeech), phonological processing, speech comprehension (semantic and syntactic), word retrieval, covert articulatory planning and overt articulation, auditory and motor feedback in speech production, visual word processing, and orthographic-phonological mapping, divided into 36 cytoarchitectonic regions, as shown in Figure 2.2. Each function presumably interacts with specific nonlinguistic processes—such as acoustic processing of all types of auditory stimuli, rate of transitions in rapidly changing auditory stimuli, short-term memory to maintain auditory imagery when no auditory input is available, influence of general multimodal context on sentence comprehension (e.g., to guide guessing), selection of motor commands from several options, ordering complex motor commands, and timing of motor output to ensure execution of motor plan—thus engaging specific neural networks.

These complex interconnections reflect the integrative nature of Price's model, where multiple networks are recruited to support language processing (e.g., phonological or orthographic), involving functional integration of multiple bottom-up and top-down processes.

However, there is more to the neural organization of language in the brain than neuroimaging techniques typically reveal (Cahana-Amitay & Albert, 2014; Price, 2010). Most studies continue to focus on characterizing language functions that engage cortical-cortical connections, although more and more evidence is accumulating to suggest the involvement of additional neural structures in language processing. These include language networks in the cerebellum, which have been associated with articulation (e.g., Brown et al., 2009), acquisition of novel words (e.g., Davis et al., 2009), auditory self-monitoring (e.g., Zheng, Munhall, & Johnsrude, 2010), and working memory (e.g., Koelsch et al., 2009). Or they may include networks associated with subcortical circuitry, which provide bilateral support for language functions (e.g., Price, 2010). Yet there is evidence that the left caudate is involved in the control/selection of motor sequences necessary for articulation and, in language comprehension tasks, during nonautomatized processing (Friederici, 2006). The "control" function of the caudate has been associated with a neural circuit linking the caudate to prefrontal, premotor, and temporal, and parietal cortices reciprocally through the thalamus. We return to their role in Chapter 3, which discusses the neural contributions of executive functions to language processing.

FUTURE DIRECTIONS FOR NEURAL MULTIFUNCTIONAL
MODELS OF LANGUAGE

Neural models of language such as those just discussed do not usually take into account interindividual variability in the neuroanatomical representation of language, thus

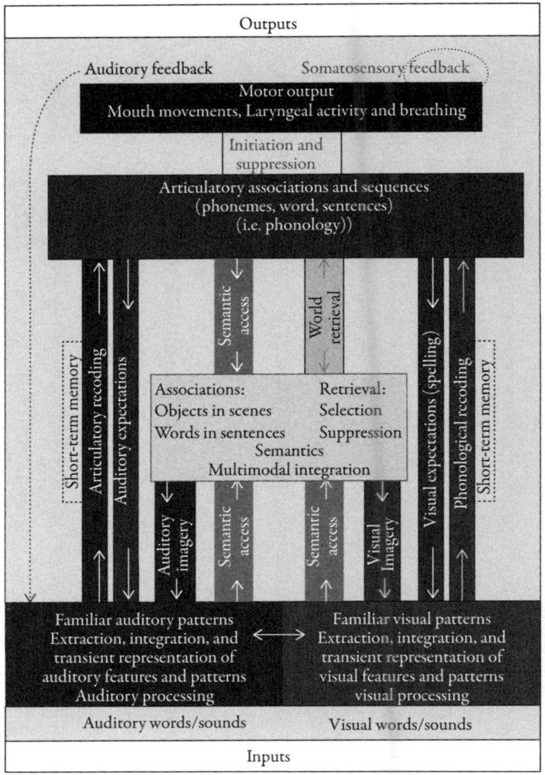

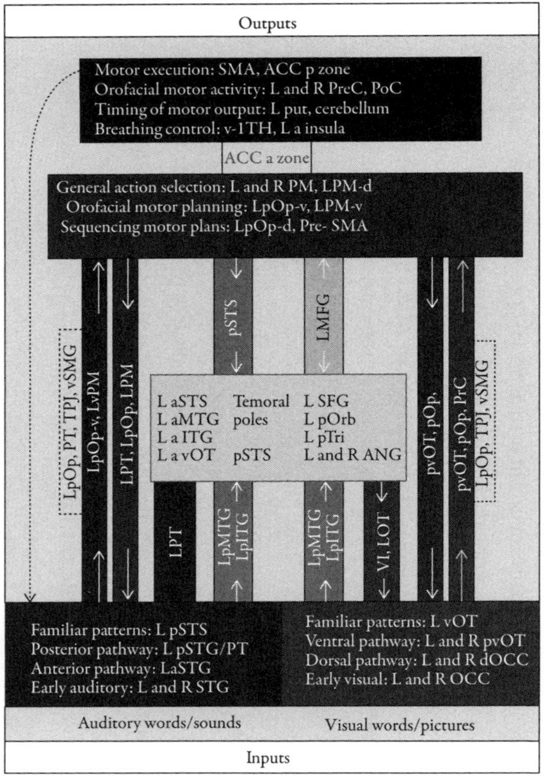

FIGURE 2.2 Brain-function mappings (See color insert.)

Reprinted under the Creative Commons Attribution License from Cahana-Amitay, D. and Albert, M.L. (2014). Brain and language: evidence for neural multifunctionality. *Behavioural Neurology*, http://dx.doi.org/10.1155/2014/260381. Hindawi, copyright 2014.

a, anterior; A, auditory cortex; ACC, anterior cingulate; AG, angular gyrus; c, caudate; CB, cerebellum; d, dorsal; GP, globus pallidus; IFS, inferior frontal sulcus; IOG, inferior occipital gyrus; ITG, inferior temporal gyrus; MFG, middle frontal gyrus; Occ, occipital; OT, occipitotemporal; p, posterior; PO, parietal operculum; pOp, pars opercularis; pOrb, pars orbitalis; pTri, pars triangularis; PT, planum temporale; poC, postcentral; preC, precentral; PM, premotor; PUT, putamen; SFG, superior frontal gyrus; SMA, supplementary motor cortex; STG, superior temporal gyrus; STS, superior temporal sulcus; SMG, supramarginal gyrus; TPJ, temporoparietal junction; Th, thalamus; v, ventral; VI, lobule VI (medial anterior); VII, lobule VII (lateral posterior).

Source: Adapted from Cahana-Amitay, D., & Albert, M. L. (2014). Brain and language: evidence for neural multifunctionality. *Behavioural Neurology*, Figure 2.

undermining their ability to create a clearly discernible functional neuroanatomical map for language (e.g., Fedorenko et al., 2010; Fedorenko, Nieto-Castañón, & Kanwisher, 2012). This limitation is anchored in part in the fact that most neuroimaging studies of language use data obtained from meta-analyses or group analysis maps that do not capture the entire range of brain activity in specific target regions (e.g., when brain activation patterns in a voxel-based analysis are averaged over participants in whom no effects are found) and so necessarily underestimate their functional specificity (Fedorenko & Kanwisher, 2009). To address this problem, Fedorenko et al. (2010) developed a "functional localizer," which has been used in neuroimaging studies in other domains, including vision (Kanwisher, 2010) and social cognition (Saxe & Kanwisher, 2003). This technique enables quick mappings of language-sensitive regions within a person that could then be pooled across persons in order to identify functional rather than anatomical regions of interest.

In response to this proposal, Grodzinsky (2010) noted that the source of interindividual variability to which Fedorenko and colleagues refer rests, to a large extent, on the differences among the linguistic tasks chosen to demonstrate functional distinctions. Furthermore, he pointed out that despite individual differences, group studies have generated robust and clear findings that allow for the creation of reasonably reliable brain-language mappings within the limits of current neuroimaging methods (evidenced, for example in Price's [2012] work).

However, is the available resolution of current neuroimaging techniques sufficient for uncovering the yet-to-be-determined brain-language interlinks? Our limited ability to identify the full scope of cortical-subcortical correlates of language functions might be related to the fact that most studies consider only the cytoarchitectonic organization of brain structures without taking into account the potential role of neurochemical mechanisms of neurotransmission in relation to language functions. This gap is highlighted in the work of Amunts et al. (2010), who characterized the neural organization of the frontal cortex at the neuronal level, using a multireceptor analysis. The emerging picture portrayed a circuitry connecting premotor, prefrontal, and Broca's cortices as well as previously unexplored neural structures containing left-lateralized cholinergic receptors (M_2) in the dorsal and ventral areas 44v and 44d.

Studies exploring brain-language relations at the neuronal level have started proliferating both in the healthy (e.g., Bastiaansen & Hagoort, 2006) and neurologically compromised brain (e.g., Pulvermüller & Berthier, 2008). We will discuss these in more detail in Chapters 7 and 8, where we review ideas about sensorimotor integration during language processing. The central argument in many of these studies is that language models comprising abstract representations are incapable of detailing neuronal circuitry and therefore cannot be applied in neurobiological studies of language (e.g., Pulvermüller & Berthier, 2008).

A most recent example of such a study, however, comes from the work of Duffau et al. (2014), who proposed a delocalized dynamic model of language processing in which semantic, phonological, and syntactic processing are mediated by parallel (not serial), segregated, but interconnected cortical-subcortical widespread networks of synchronized neurons—a model based on brain stimulation mapping performed during surgery in awake participants. This stimulation creates transient virtual lesions of up to 4 seconds in the brain that allow for the recreation of linguistic errors and the exploration of their neuronal foundation. These researchers analyzed errors that participants produced during picture naming and, based on the patterns they found, determined that large-scale subnetworks support language functions, which functionally compensate one another following the induction of the lesions. They then developed a model that explicitly lays out these neuronal patterns, including the neural substrates associated with the processing of visual input, working memory, and executive function, as shown in Figure 2.3.

Studies adhering to this theoretical perspective typically use models that directly simulate brain activation (e.g., models of parallel distributed processing), which argue that the most basic functional unit in the brain is "the neural network," consisting of operational units that correspond to the firing rates of neurons, whose spreading activation yields a given behavior (e.g., Nadeau, 2012). This neural activity reflects experience-based statistical regularities that explain a range of cognitive functions rather than discrete

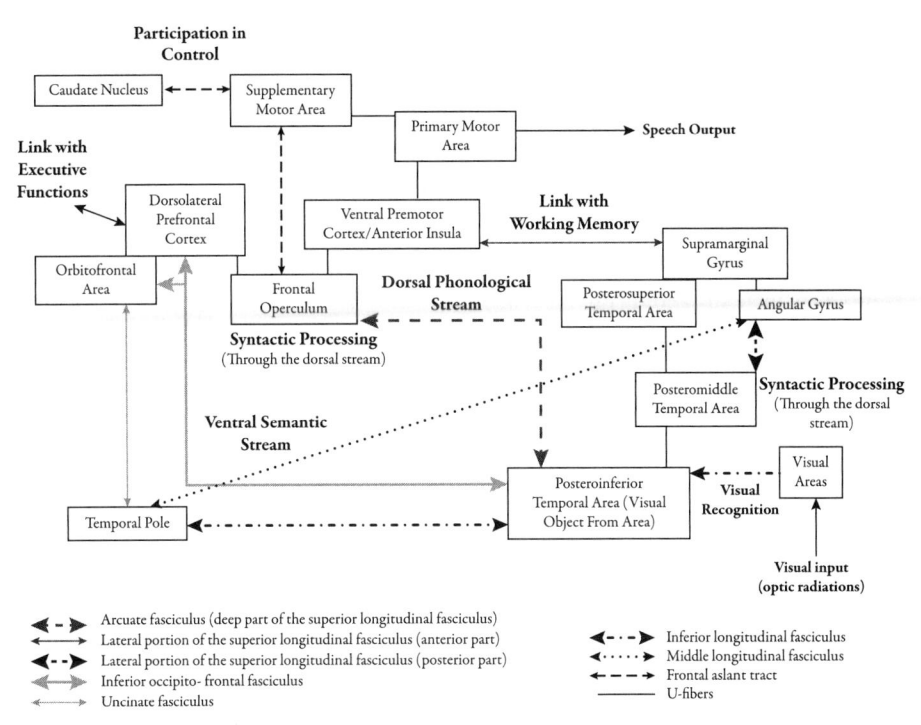

FIGURE 2.3 Neural correlates of visual-working memory-executive functions-language interlinks (See color insert).

Source: Reprinted by permission from Elsevier Limited [Brain and Language] from Figure 2 in Duffau, H., Moritz-Gasser, S., & Mandonnet, E. (2014). A re-examination of neural basis of language processing: proposal of a dynamic hodotopical model from data provided by brain stimulation mapping during picture naming. *Brain and Language, 131*, 1–10, copyright 2014.

linguistic compositional operations. We return to this idea in Chapter 5, where we discuss language-memory interlinks.

However, to explain the neurobiological bases of language, there is no need to resolve the irreconcilable gap between abstract linguistic representations and neural data (Poeppel & Embick, 2005). Efforts should be directed at distinguishing the temporal and spatial features underlying functional relations (Fuster, 2003; Schnelle, 2010), where neuronal bundles combine into groups within and outside of cortical networks to yield specific operations/computations (Grimaldi & Craighero, 2012). Such an approach could involve the study of the biological bases of language at the neurochemical level, which would allow us in the future to capture that dynamic nature—temporal and spatial—of the language system, where broadly distributed networks, with a biological predisposition to language organization, can recruit shared neurobiological mechanisms in service of language functions (Blumstein & Amso, 2013).

Although a neural model of language functions at the neurochemical level has yet to be proposed, an explicit and therefore important contribution to this endeavor is the declarative/procedural model postulated by Ullman (2004). In this model, he has systematically laid out commonalities and possible interdependencies between memory and language circuits, proposing that "brain systems which subserve declarative and procedural memory play analogous roles in language as in their nonlanguage functions" (p. 244). Specifically, temporal networks—which subserve the encoding, consolidation, and retrieval of new memories in declarative memory—are also assumed to support the mental lexicon, which comprises noncompositional, irregular, unpredictable forms. Similarly, neural networks implicating frontal, basal ganglia, parietal, and cerebellar circuits, in contrast, mediate learning, the execution of motor actions, and the performance of cognitive operations, which contribute to the combinatory functions of grammar (i.e., sequencing and hierarchical organization of structures).

In support of his proposal, Ullman elucidates the potential neurochemical underpinnings of his system, citing studies that report positive effects of cholinergic pharmacological manipulations on lexical/declarative memory (Ballard, 2002; Hammond et al., 1987; Nissen, Knopman, & Schacter, 1987; Rammsayer, Rodewald, & Groh, 2000). These findings are consistent with comparable claims made in other pharmacotherapy studies (e.g., Cahana-Amitay, Albert, & Oveis, 2014), in which cholinergic deficiency has been tied to impaired verbal memory (e.g., Klein & Albert, 2004; Mimura et al., 1995). These include, for example, impaired naming and reduced verbal fluency among healthy young women who received a drug blocking cholinergic activity (Aarsland, Larsen, Reinvang, & Aasland, 1994) as well as perseverative and paraphasic errors among aphasic patients with cholinergic deficiencies (Berthier, Hinojosa, & Moreno-Torre, 2004; Corbett, Jefferies, & Lambon Ralph, 2008; Gotts, della Rocchetta, & Cipolotti, 2002; McNamara & Albert, 2004).

Ullman's system is assumed to interact competitively, where access to a representation in the declarative system, such as an irregular noun form (e.g., 'feet'), blocks the compositional computation in the procedural component (e.g., '*feets'). Ullman speculates that in the case of brain damage, such a model would have at least two consequences: (1) damage to one component would lead to enhanced learning in the other and (2) learning in one component would suppress the functionality of the other. How this system would provide neural support for the compositionality of sentences is not stated as clearly; Ullman even mentions that this aspect of grammar might be handled more modularly. The question of whether his specific predictions are borne out empirically has yet to be tested, but his proposal opens new possibilities for aphasia intervention targets, which can change the course of recovery and so affect neural reorganization in the aphasic brain.

A NOTE ABOUT LANGUAGE IN THE AGING BRAIN

Modeling of brain-language interlinks has clearly made considerable progress since the early days of the classical Broca-Wernicke-Lichtheim-Geschwind model, showing much greater neural resolution and empirical power. However, the emerging brain-language maps are typically based on neural data collected from young healthy adults (e.g., usually college-aged students), whose functional neuroanatomy is likely distinct from that of older adults in certain important ways. As we point out below, evidence suggests that certain aspects of language and related nonlinguistic cognitive functions decline over time, pointing to underlying changes in their neural correlates—which is usually overlooked in neural studies of aphasia.

Age-related language changes typically involve the emergence of difficulties with lexical retrieval and sentence processing. Older adults' impaired retrieval of nouns and verbs, for example, has been related to problems in accessing phonological information encoded on words (e.g., Albert et al., 1988; Au et al., 1995; Barresi et al., 2000; Connor et al., 2004; Cross & Burke, 2004; Goral et al., 2007; Mackay et al., 2002; Morrison et al., 2003; Mortensen et al., 2006; Nicholas et al., 1985; Obler et al., 2002). Their reduced sentence processing abilities (lower accuracy and/or slower reaction times) have been attributed to syntactic complexity, low plausibility, decreased predictability, or increased background noise (e.g., Cahana-Amitay et al., 2013; Caplan, Dede, Waters, Michaud, & Tripodis, 2011; DeDe, Caplan, Kemtes, & Waters, 2004; Goral et al., 2011; Kemtes & Kemper, 1997; Obler, Nicholas, Albert, & Woodward, 1985; Obler, Fein, Nicholas, & Albert,1991; Schneider, Daneman, Murphy, & See, 2000; Waters & Caplan, 2005; Wingfield, Peelle, & Grossman, 2003).

Many accounts of age-related language difficulties have proposed considering interactions with other neurocognitive domains in aging to account for the observed behaviors. These include reduction in processing speed (e.g., Boyle, Wilson, Schneider, Bienias, & Bennett, 2008; Eckert et al., 2010; Salthouse, 1996) as well as decreases in cognitive functions, such as working memory, divided attention, inhibitory control, or set shifting (e.g., Goral et al., 2011; Just & Carpenter, 1992; Kane, Bleckley, Conway, & Engle, 2001;

Kane & Engle, 2002; Lustig, May, & Hasher, 2001; Wingfield, Lindfield, & Kahana, 1998). Findings indicate that slower processing speed among older adults adversely affects picture naming (e.g., Cotelli et al., 2010), particularly of actions as compared with objects (Druks et al., 2006; Szekely et al., 2005). Reduced working memory span, which interferes with one's ability to store and process information simultaneously (e.g., Just & Carpenter, 1992), has been linked to decreased success in the syntactic processing of complex sentences (e.g., processing stimuli containing embedded clauses or more than a single negative marker) (e.g., Goral et al., 2011).

Relatedly, successful language performance among older adults has been associated with the preservation of cognitive abilities such that the combined contribution of spared cognitive functions serves as a compensatory mechanism to support a compromised linguistic function (e.g., Goffaux, Phillips, Sinai, & Pushkar, 2008; Wingfield & Grossman, 2006). Thus, better-performing adults are those in whom a larger number of cognitive functions remain intact (e.g., Boyle et al., 2008; Cabeza, Andersen, Locantore, & McIntosh, 2002).

These age-based compensatory mechanisms have been associated with neural changes in hemispheric asymmetry in the aging brain (e.g., Cabeza et al., 2002), typically measured in terms of changes in gray matter volume and/or white matter integrity (e.g., Antonenko et al., 2013; Obler et al., 2010; Shafto et al., 2007, 2009; Stamatakis et al., 2011; Wierenga et al., 2008; Wingfiled & Grossman, 2006). The claim is that language functions among older adults increasingly rely on ancillary networks outside the core language networks, including right homologous counterparts (e.g., Wingfield & Grossman, 2006). Neuroimaging studies of lexical retrieval among older adults have demonstrated, for example, frontal bilateral involvement (Ellis, Burani, Izura, Bromiley, & Venneri, 2006; Obler et al., 2010; Wierenga et al., 2008), with some variability in the brain regions identified, likely related to differences among the tasks used in each study (e.g., Kan & Thompson-Schill, 2004). Similar arguments have been made in studies exploring the neural underpinnings of sentence processing in aging (e.g., Bahlemann et al., 2011; Caplan et al., 2000; Cooke et al., 2002; 2006; Friederici, 2002, 2012; Luke et al., 2002; Pelle et al., 2004; Wingfield & Grossman, 2006).

From the perspective of the study of aphasia recovery, understanding the functional neuroanatomy of language in the aging brain is clearly relevant, as the average person with aphasia is not a college student. Recent findings indicate that over 50% of aphasic persons who are referred to aphasia therapy are aged 70 years or older (Basso & Macis, 2011). Age is an important prognostic factor that influences the course and outcome of recovery (McClung, Gonzalez Rothi, & Nadeau, 2010). Although evidence is inconclusive (Code, 2001), the consensus is that young age is a predictor of positive recovery, depending on aphasia severity (Ross & Wertz, 2001; Smith, 1971) and possibly also on aphasia type, fluent aphasia showing, on average, later age of onset, 56.5 years, compared with nonfluent aphasia, 45.3 years (Brown & Grober, 1983; Eslinger & Damasio, 1981; Obler, Albert, Goodglass et al., 1978). Functional gains have been measured in terms of language outcomes (e.g., Jorgense et al., 1999) and activities of daily living, especially of physical recovery (e.g., Ahlsio et al., 1984).

Neuroimaging data from both young and older adults clearly indicate that neural networks susberving language functions also partially mediate nonlinguistic functions, such as working memory, which contribute to certain aspects of language performance. These data are extremely valuable, even if at present the degree of overlap between brain-language maps derived from young adults and those obtained from older adults remains unclear. They open up new possibilities of exploring the neural underpinning of language that can reshape our thinking about aphasic language deficits and the clinical interventions designed to ameliorate them.

References

Aarsland, D., Larsen, J. P., Reinvang, I., & Aasland, A. M. (1994). Effects of cholinergic blockade on language in healthy young women: implications for the cholinergic hypothesis in dementia of the Alzheimer type. *Brain, 117*(Pt 6), 1377–1384.

Albert, M. S., Heller, H. S., & Milberg, W. (1988). Changes in naming ability with age. *Psychology and Aging, 3*(2), 173–178.

Alexander, M. P. (1997). Aphasia: clinical and anatomic aspects. In T. E. Feinberg & M. J. Farah (Eds.), *Behavioral neurology and neuropsychology* (pp. 133–150). New York: McGraw-Hill.

Amunts, K., Lenzen, M., Friederici, A. D., Schleicher, A., Morosan, P., Palomero-Gallagher, N., & Zilles, K. (2010). Broca's region: novel organizational principles and multiple receptor mapping. *PLoS Biology, 8*(9), pii: e1000489. doi: 10.1371/journal.pbio.1000489

Antonenko, D., Brauer, J., Meizner, M., Fengler, A., Kerti, L., & Friederici, A. (2013). Functional and structural syntax networks in aging. *NeuroImage, 83*, 513–523.

Au, R., Joung, P., Nicholas, M., Obler, L. K., Kass, R., & Albert, M. L. (1995). Naming ability across the adult life span. *Aging, Neuropsychology, and Cognition, 2*(4), 300–311.

Baldo, J. V., & Dronkers, N. F. (2007). Neural correlates of arithmetic and language comprehension: a common substrate? *Neuropsychologia, 45*(2), 229–235.

Ballard, C. G. (2002). Advances in the treatment of Alzheimer's disease: benefits of dual cholinesterase inhibition. *European Neurology, 47*(1), 64–70.

Barresi, B., Nicholas, M., Connor, L. T., Obler, L. K., & Albert, M. L. (2000). Semantic degradation and lexical access in age-related naming failures. *Aging, Neuropsychology, and Cognition, 7*(3), 169–178.

Bastiaansen, M., & Hagoort, P. (2006). Oscillatory neuronal dynamics during language comprehension. In C. Neuper & W. Klimesch (Eds.), *Event-related dynamics of brain oscillations* (pp. 179–196). Amsterdam: Elsevier.

Ben-Shachar, M., Hendler, T., Kahn, I., Ben-Bashat, D., & Grodzinsky, Y. (2003). The neural reality of syntactic transformations: evidence from fMRI. *Psychological Science, 14*(5), 433–440.

Ben Shalom, D., & Poeppel, D. (2008). Functional anatomic models of language: assembling the pieces. *The Neuroscientist, 14*(1), 119–127. doi: 10.1177/1073858407305726

Berthier, M. L., Hinojosa, J., & Moreno-Torre, I. (2004). Beneficial effects of donepezil and modality-specific language therapy on chronic conduction aphasia. *Neurology, 62*(Suppl 5), A462.

Binder, J. R., Desai, R. H., Graves, W. W., & Conant, L. L. (2009). Where is the semantic system? a critical review and meta-analysis of 120 functional neuroimaging studies. *Cerebral Cortex, 19*(12), 2767–2796.

Blumstein, S. E., & Amso, D. (2013). Dynamic functional organization of language: insights from neuroimaging. *Perspectives on Psychological Science, 8*(1), 44–48.

Boyle, P. A., Wilson, R. S., Schneider, J. A., Bienias, J. L., & Bennett, D. A. (2008). Processing resources reduce the effect of Alzheimer pathology on other cognitive systems. *Neurology, 70*(17), 1534–1542.

Brown, S., Laird, A. R., Pfordresher, P. Q., Thelen, S. M., Turkeltaub, P., & Liotti, M. (2009). The somatotopy of speech: phonation and articulation in the human motor cortex. *Brain and Cognition, 70*(1), 31–41.

Brown, J. W., & Grober, E. (1983). Age, sex and aphasia type. Evidence for a regional cerebral growth process underlying lateralization. *The Journal of Nervous and Mental Disease, 171*(7), 431–434.

Cabeza, R., Anderson, N. D., Locantore, J. K., & McIntosh, A. R. (2002). Aging gracefully: compensatory brain activity in high-performing older adults. *NeuroImage, 17*(3), 1394–1402.

Cahana-Amitay, D., & Albert, M. L. (2014). Brain and language: evidence for neural multifunctionality. *Behavioural Neurology*, http://dx.doi.org/10.1155/2014/260381.

Cahana-Amitay, D., Albert, M. L., Ojo, E. A., Sayers, J., Goral, M., Obler, L. K., & Spiro, A. (2013). Effects of hypertension and diabetes on sentence comprehension in aging. *The Journals of Gerontology. Series B, Psychological Sciences and Social Sciences. 68*(4), 513–521.

Cahana-Amitay, D., Albert, M. L., & Oveis, A. (2014). Psycholinguistics of aphasia pharmacotherapy: asking the right questions. *Aphasiology, 28*(2), 133–154.

Caplan, D., Alpert, N., Waters, G., & Olivieri, A. (2000). Activation of Broca's area by syntactic processing under conditions of concurrent articulation. *Human Brain Mapping, 9*(2), 65–71.

Caplan, D., Dede, G., Waters, G., Michaud, J., & Tripodis, Y. (2011). Effects of age, speed of processing, and working memory on comprehension of sentences with relative clauses. *Psychology and Aging, 26*(2), 439–450.

Caplan, D., & Waters, G. S. (1999). Verbal working memory and sentence comprehension. *The Behavioral and Brain Sciences, 22*(1), 77–94; discussion 95–126.

Caramazza, A. (1984). The logic of neuropsychological research and the problem of patient classification in aphasia. *Brain and Language, 21*(1), 9–20.

Carpenter, P. A., Just, M. A., & Reichle, E. D. (2000). Working memory and executive function: evidence from neuroimaging. *Current Opinion in Neurobiology, 10*(2):195–199.

Catani, M., Allin, M. P., Husain, M., Pugliese, L., Mesulam, M. M., Murray, R. M., & Jones, D. K. (2007). Symmetries in human brain language pathways correlate with verbal recall. *Proceedings of the National Academy of Sciences of the United States of America, 104*(43), 17163–17168.

Catani, M., Dell'Acqua, F., Bizzi, A., Forkel, S. J., Williams, S. C., Simmons, A., … Thiebaut de Schotten, M. (2012). Beyond cortical localization in clinico-anatomical correlation. *Cortex, 48*(10), 1262–1287. doi: 10.1016/j.cortex.2012.07.001

Catani, M., & ffytche, D. H. (2005). The rises and falls of disconnection syndromes. *Brain, 128*(Pt 10), 2224–2239.

Catani, M., Jones, D. K., & ffytche, D. H. (2005). Perisylvian language networks of the human brain. *Annals of Neurology, 57*(1), 8–16.

Connor, L. T., Spiro, A., Obler, L. K., & Albert, M. L. (2004). Change in object naming ability during adulthood. *The Journals of Gerontology. Series B, Psychological Sciences and Social Sciences, 59*(5), 203–209.

Constable, R. T., Pugh, K. R., Berroya, E., Mencl, W. E., Westerveld, M., Ni, W., & Shankweiler, D. (2004). Sentence complexity and input modality effects in sentence comprehension: an fMRI study. *NeuroImage, 22*(1), 11–21.

Cooke, A., Zurif, E. B., DeVita, C., Alsop, D., Koenig, P., Detre, J., . . . Grossman, M. (2002). Neural basis for sentence comprehension: grammatical and short-term memory components. *Human Brain Mapping, 15*(2), 80–94.

Corbett, F., Jefferies, E., & Lambon Ralph, M. A. (2008). The use of cueing to alleviate recurrent verbal perseverations: evidence from transcortical sensory aphasia. *Aphasiology, 22*(4), 363–382.

Cotelli, M., Manenti, R., Rosini, S., Calabria, M., Brambilla, M., Bisiacchi, P. S., . . . Miniussi, C. (2010). Action and object naming in physiological aging: an rTMS study. *Frontiers in Aging Neuroscience, 2*, 151.

Crinion, J. T., & Leff, A. P. (2007). Recovery and treatment of aphasia after stroke: functional imaging studies. *Current Opinion in Neurology, 20*(6), 667–673.

Cross, E. S., & Burke, D. M. (2004). Do alternative names block young and older adults' retrieval of proper names? *Brain and Language, 89*(1), 174–181.

Crosson, B. (2013). Thalamic mechanisms in language: a reconsideration based on recent findings and concepts. *Brain and Language, 126*(1), 73–88. doi: 10.1016/j.bandl.2012.06.011

Davis, M. H., Di Betta, A. M., Macdonald, M. J., & Gaskell, M. G. (2009). Learning and consolidation of novel spoken words. *Journal of Cognitive Neuroscience, 21*(4), 803–820.

Dede, G., Caplan, D., Kemtes, K., & Waters, G. (2004). The relationship between age, verbal working memory, and language comprehension. *Psychology and Aging, 19*(4), 601–616.

Dronkers, N. F., Wilkins, D. P., Van Valin, R. D. Jr., Redfern, B. B., & Jaeger, J. J. (2004). Lesion analysis of the brain areas involved in language comprehension. *Cognition, 92*(1–2), 145–177.

Druks, J., Masterson, J., Kopelman, M., Clare, L., Rose, A., & Rai, G. (2006). Is action naming better preserved (than object naming) in Alzheimer's disease and why should we ask? *Brain and Language, 98*(3), 332–340.

Duffau, H., Moritz-Gasser, S., & Mandonnet, E. (2014). A re-examination of neural basis of language processing: Proposal of a dynamic hodotopical model from data provided by brain stimulation mapping during picture naming. *Brain and Language, 131*, 1–10.

Eckert, M. A., Keren, N. I., Roberts, D. R., Calhoun, V. D., & Harris, K. C. (2010). Age-related changes in processing speed: unique contributions of cerebellar and prefrontal cortex. *Frontiers in Human Neuroscience, 4*, 10.

Ellis, A. W., Burani, C., Izura, C., Bromiley, A., & Venneri, A. (2006). Traces of vocabulary acquisition in the brain: Evidence from covert object naming. *NeuroImage, 33*(3), 958–968.

Eslinger, P., & Damasio A. (1981). Age and type of aphasia in patients with stroke. *Journal of Neurology, Neurosurgery, and Psychiatry, 44*, 377–381.

Fedorenko, E., Hsieh, P.-J., Nieto-Castañón, A., Whitfield-Gabrieli, S., & Kanwisher, N. (2010). New method for fMRI investigations of language: Defining ROIs functionally in individual subjects. *Journal of Neurophysiology, 104*(2), 1177–1194.

Fedorenko, E., & Kanwisher, N. (2009). Neuroimaging of language: Why hasn't a clearer picture emerged? *Language and Linguistics Compass, 3*(4), 839–865.

Fedorenko, E., Nieto-Castañón, A., & Kanwisher, N. (2012). Syntactic processing in the human brain: what we know, what we don't know, and a suggestion for how to proceed. *Brain and Language, 120*(2), 187–207.

Fodor, J. (1983). *Modularity of mind*. Cambridge, MA: MIT Press.

Friederici, A. D. (2002). Towards a neural basis of auditory sentence processing. *Trends in Cognitive Sciences, 6*(2), 78–84.

Friederici, A. D. (2006). Broca's area and the ventral premotor cortex in language: functional differentiation and specificity. *Cortex, 42*(2), 472–475.

Friederici, A. D. (2011). The brain basis of language processing: from structure to function. *Physiological Reviews, 91*(4), 1357–1392. doi: 10.1152/physrev.00006.2011

Friederici, A. D. (2012). The cortical language circuit: from auditory perception to sentence comprehension. *Trends in Cognitive Sciences, 16*(5), 262–268. doi: 10.1016/j.tics.2012.04.001

Friederici, A. D., & Gierhan, S. M. (2013). The language network. *Current Opinion in Neurobiology, 23*(2), 250–254. doi: 10.1016/j.conb.2012.10.002

Fuster, J. M. (2003). *Cortex and mind—unifying cognition*. Oxford, UK: Oxford University Press.

Geschwind, N. (1965). Disconnexion syndromes in animals and man. I. *Brain, 88*(2), 237–294.

Gierhan, S. M. (2013). Connections for auditory language in the human brain. *Brain and Language, 127*(2), 205–221.

Goffaux, P., Phillips, N. A., Sinai, M., & Pushkar, D. (2008). Neurophysiological measures of task-set switching: effects of working memory and aging. *The Journals of Gerontology. Series B, Psychological Sciences and Social Sciences, 63*(2), 57–66.

Goral, M., Spiro, A., Albert, M. L., Obler, L. K., & Connor, L. T. (2007). Change in lexical retrieval skills in adulthood. *The Mental Lexicon, 2*(2), 215–240.

Goral, M., Clark-Cotton, M., Spiro, A., Obler, L. K., Verkuilen, J., & Albert, M. L. (2011). The contribution of set switching and working memory to sentence processing in older adults. *Experimental Aging Research, 37*(5), 516–538.

Gotts, S. J., della Rocchetta, A. I., & Cipolotti, L. (2002). Mechanisms underlying perseveration in aphasia: evidence from a single case study. *Neuropsychologia, 40*(12), 1930–1947.

Graves, W. W., Grabowski, T. J., Mehta, S., & Gupta, P. (2008). The left posterior superior temporal gyrus participates specifically in accessing lexical phonology. *Journal of Cognitive Neuroscience, 20*(9), 1698–1710.

Grimaldi, M. (2012). Toward a neural theory of language: Old issues and new perspectives. *Journal of Neurolinguistics, 25*(5), 304–327.

Grimaldi, M., & Craighero, L. (2012). Future perspectives in neurobiological investigation of language. *Journal of Neurolinguistics, 25*(5), 295–303.

Grodzinsky, Y. (2010). The picture of the linguistic brain: how sharp can it be? reply to Fedorenko and Kanwisher. *Language and Linguistics Compass, 4*(8), 605–622.

Grodzinsky, Y., & Amunts, K. (Eds.). (2006). *Broca's region*. New York: Oxford University Press.

Grodzinsky, Y., & Friederici, A. D. (2006). Neuroimaging of syntax and syntactic processing. *Current Opinion in Neurobiology, 16*(2), 240–246.

Hagoort, P. (2005). On Broca, brain, and binding: A new framework. *Trends in Cognitive Sciences, 9*(9), 416–423.

Hammond, E. J., Meador, K. J., Aung-Din, R., & Wilder, B. J. (1987). Cholinergic modulation of human P3 event-related potentials. *Neurology, 37*(2), 346–350.

Hasson, U., Nusbaum, H. C., & Small, S. L. (2006). Repetition suppression for spoken sentences and the effect of task demands. *Journal of Cognitive Neuroscience, 18*(12), 2013–2029.

Helm-Estabrooks, N., Albert, M. L., & Nicholas, M. (2013). *Manual of Aphasia and Aphasia Therapy* (3rd ed.). Austin, TX: ProEd.

Hickok, G., & Poeppel, D. (2000). Towards a functional neuroanatomy of speech perception. *Trends in Cognitive Sciences, 4*(4), 131–138.

Hickok, G., & Poeppel, D. (2004). Dorsal and ventral streams: A framework for understanding aspects of the functional anatomy of language. *Cognition, 92*(1–2), 67–99.

Hickok, G., & Poeppel, D. (2007). The cortical organization of speech processing. *Nature Reviews Neuroscience, 8*, 393–402. doi:10.1038/nrn2113

Jordan, K., Heinze, H. J., Lutz, K., Kanowski, M., & Jäncke, L. (2001). Cortical activations during the mental rotation of different visual objects. *NeuroImage, 13*(1), 143–152.

Just, M. A., & Carpenter, P. A. (1992). A capacity theory of comprehension: individual differences in working memory. *Psychological Review, 99*(1), 122–149.

Kan, I. P., & Thompson-Schill, S. L. (2004). Selection from perceptual and conceptual representations. *Cognitive, Affective and Behavioral Neuroscience, 4*(4), 466–482.

Kane, M. J., Bleckley, M. K., Conway, A. R., & Engle, R. W. (2001). A controlled-attention view of working-memory capacity. *Journal of Experimental Psychology: General, 130*(2), 169–183.

Kane, M. J., & Engle, R. W. (2002). The role of prefrontal cortex in working-memory capacity, executive attention, and general fluid intelligence: an individual-differences perspective. *Psychonomic Bulletin and Review, 9*(4), 637–671.

Kanwisher, N. (2010). Functional specificity in the human brain: a window into the functional architecture of the mind. *Proceedings of the National Academy of Sciences of the United States of America, 107*(25), 11163–11170.

Kemtes, K. A., & Kemper, S. (1997). Younger and older adults' on-line processing of syntactically ambiguous sentences. *Psychology and Aging, 12*(2), 362–371.

Kertesz, A., & McCabe, P. (1977). Recovery patterns and prognosis in aphasia. *Brain, 100*(Pt1), 1–18.

Kertesz, A. (1982). *Western aphasia battery*. New York: Grune and Stratton.

Kho, K. H., Indefrey, P., Hagoort, P., van Veelen, W. M., van Rijen, P. C., & Ramsey, N. F. (2008). Unimpaired sentence comprehension after anterior temporal cortex resection, *Neuropsychologia, 46*, 1170–1178.

Klein, R. B., & Albert, M. L. (2004). Can drug therapies improve language functions of individuals with aphasia? a review of the evidence. *Seminars in Speech and Language, 25*(2), 193–204.

Koelsch, S., Schulze, K., Sammler, D., Fritz, T., Müller, K., & Gruber, O. (2009). Functional architecture of verbal and tonal working memory: an fMRI study. *Human Brain Mapping*, *30*(3), 859–873.

Kotz, S. A., & Schwartze, M. (2010). Cortical speech processing unplugged: a timely subcortico-cortical framework. *Trends in Cognitive Sciences*, *14*(9), 392–399. doi: 10.1016/j.tics.2010.06.005

Kümmermer, D., Hartwigsen, G., Kellmeyer, P., Glauche, V., Mader, I., Klöppel, S., … Saur, D. (2013). Damage to ventral and dorsal language pathways in acute aphasia. *Brain*, *136*(Pt 2), 619–629. doi: 10.1093/brain/aws354

Luke, K. K., Liu, H. L., Wai, Y. Y., Wan, Y. L., & Tan, L. H. (2002). Functional anatomy of syntactic and semantic processing in language comprehension. *Human Brain Mapping*, *16*(3),133–145.

Lustig, C., May, C. P., & Hasher, L. (2001). Working memory span and the role of proactive interference. *Journal of Experimental Psychology: General*, *130*(2), 199–207.

Mackay, A. J., Connor, L. T., Albert, M. L., & Obler, L. K. (2002). Noun and verb retrieval in healthy aging. *Journal of the International Neuropsychological Society*, *8*(6), 764–770.

Maess, B., Koelsch, S., Gunter, T. C., & Friederici, A. D. (2001). Musical syntax is processed in Broca's area: an MEG study. *Nature Neuroscience*, *4*(5), 540–545.

Makuuchi, M., Bahlmann, J., & Friederici, A. D. (2012). An approach to separating the levels of hierarchical structure building in language and mathematics. *Philosophical Transactions of the Royal Society of London. Series B, Biological Sciences*, *367*(1598), 2033–2045.

Makuuchi, M., Bahlmann, J., Anwander, A., & Friederici, A. D. (2009). Segregating the core computational faculty of human language from working memory. *Proceedings of the National Academy of Sciences of the United States of America*, *106*(20), 8362–8367.

Makuuchi, M., & Friederici, A.D. (2013). Hierarchical functional connectivity between the core language system and the working memory system. *Cortex*, *49*(9), 2416–2423.

McClung, J. S., Gonzalez Rothi, L. J., & Nadeau, S. E. (2010). Ambient experience in restitutive treatment of aphasia. *Frontiers in Human Neuroscience*, *4(183)*, 1–19.

McNamara, P., & Albert, M. L. (2004). Neuropharmacology of verbal perseveration. *Seminars in Speech and Language*, *25*(4), 309–321.

Milner, A. D., & Goodale, M. A. (1995). *The visual brain in action*. Oxford, UK: Oxford University Press.

Mimura, M., Albert. M. L., & McNamara, P. (1995). Toward a pharmacotherapy for aphasia. In H. Kirshner (Ed.), *Handbook of Neurological Speech and Language Disorders* (pp. 465–482). New York: Marcel Dekker.

Morrison, C. M., Hirsh, K. W., & Duggan, G. H. (2003). Age of acquisition, ageing, and verb production: normative and experimental data. *The Quarterly Journal of Experimental Psychology. A, Human Experimental Psychology*, *56*(4), 705–730.

Mortensen, L., Mayer, A. S., & Humphreys, G. W. (2006). Age-related slowing of object naming: A review. *Language and Cognitive Processes*, *21*, 238–290.

Myers, E. B., Blumstein, S. E., Walsh, E., & Eliassen, J. (2009). Inferior frontal regions underlie the perception of phonetic category invariance. *Psychological Science*, *20*(7), 895–903.

Nadeau, S. E. (2012). *The neural architecture of grammar*. Cambridge, MA: MIT Press.

Newman, S. D., Just, M. A., Keller, T. A., Roth, J., & Carpenter, P. A. (2003). Differential effects of syntactic and semantic processing on the subregions of Broca's area. *Brain Research. Cognitive Brain Research*, *16*(2), 297–307.

Nicholas, M., Obler, L. K., Albert, M., & Goodglass, H. (1985). Lexical retrieval in healthy aging. *Cortex, 21*(4), 595–606.

Nissen, M. J., Knopman, D. S., & Schacter, D. L. (1987). Neurochemical dissociation of memory systems. *Neurology, 37*(5), 789–794.

Noppeney, U., Phillips, J., & Price, C. (2004). The neural areas that control the retrieval and selection of semantics. *Neuropsychologia, 42*(9), 1269–1280.

Obler L. K., Albert, M. L., Goodglass, H., & Benson, D. F. (1978). Aphasia type and aging. *Brain and Language, 6*, 318–322.

Obler, L. K., Fein, D., Nicholas, M., & Albert, M. L. (1991). Auditory comprehension and aging: decline in syntactic processing. *Applied Psycholinguistics, 12*(4), 433–452.

Obler, L. K., Nicholas, M., Albert, M. L., & Woodward, S. (1985). On comprehension across the adult lifespan. *Cortex, 21*(2), 273–280.

Obler, L. K., Rykhlevskaia, E., Schnyer, D., Clark-Cotton, M. R., Spiro, A., Hyun, J., … Albert, M. L. (2010). Bilateral brain regions associated with naming in older adults. *Brain and Language, 113*(3), 113–123.

Papagno, C. (2011). Naming and the role of the uncinate fasciculus in language function. *Current Neurology and Neuroscience Reports, 11*(6), 553–559.

Papagno, C., Miracapillo, C., Casarotti, A., Romero Lauro, L., Castellano, A., Falini, A., … Bello, L. (2011). What is the role of the uncinate fasciculus? Surgical removal and proper name retrieval. *Brain, 134*(2), 405–414.

Pashek, G. V., & Holland, A. L. (1988). Evolution of aphasia in the first year post-onset. *Cortex, 24*(3), 411–423.

Podzebenko, K., Egan, G. F., & Watson, J. D. (2002). Widespread dorsal stream activation during a parametric mental rotation task, revealed with functional magnetic resonance imaging. *NeuroImage, 15*(3), 547–558.

Poeppel, D. (2011). Genetics and language: a neurobiological perspective on the missing link (-ing hypotheses). *Journal of Neurodevelopmental Disorders, 3*(4), 381–387. doi: 10.1007/s11689-011-9097-0

Poeppel, D., & Embick, D. (2005). The relation between linguistics and neuroscience. In A. Cutler (Ed.), *Twenty-first century psycholinguistics: four cornerstones.* (pp. 103–120). Hillsdale, NJ: Erlbaum.

Poeppel, D., Emmorey, K., Hickok, G., & Pylkkänen, L. (2012). Towards a new neurobiology of language. *The Journal of Neuroscience, 32*(41), 14125–14131.

Poeppel, D., & Hickok, G. (2004). Towards a new functional anatomy of language. *Cognition, 92*(1–2), 1–12.

Price, C. J. (2010). The anatomy of language: a review of 100 fMRI studies published in 2009. *Annals of the New York Academy of Sciences, 1191*, 62–88.

Price, C. J. (2012). A review and synthesis of the first 20 years of PET and fMRI studies of heard speech, spoken language and reading. *NeuroImage, 62*(2), 816–847. doi: 10.1016/j.neuroimage.2012.04.062

Pulvermüller, F., & Berthier, M. (2008). Aphasia therapy on a neuroscience basis. *Aphasiology, 22*(6), 563–599.

Rammsayer, T. H., Rodewald, S., & Groh, D. (2000). Dopamine-antagonistic, anticholinergic, and GABAergic effects on declarative and procedural memory functions. *Brain Research. Cognitive Brain Research, 9*(1), 61–71.

Rogalsky, C., Matchin, W., & Hickok, G. (2008). Broca's area, sentence comprehension, and working memory: an fMRI study. *Frontiers in Human Neuroscience, 2*, 14. doi: 10.3389/neuro.09.014.2008

Saffran, E. M. (2000). Aphasia and the relationship of language and brain. *Seminars in Neurology, 20*(4), 409–418.

Salthouse, T. A. (1996). The processing-speed theory of adult age differences in cognition. *Psychological Review, 103*(3), 403–428.

Saur, D., & Hartwigsen, G. (2012). Neurobiology of language recovery after stroke: lessons from neuroimaging studies. *Archives of Physical Medicine and Rehabilitation, 93*(1 Suppl), S15–S25. doi: 10.1016/j.apmr.2011.03.036

Saxe, R., & Kanwisher, N. (2003). People thinking about thinking people: the role of the temporo-parietal junction in "theory of mind". *NeuroImage, 19*(4), 1835–1842.

Schneider, B. A., Daneman, M., Murphy, D. R., & See, S. K. (2000). Listening to discourse in distracting settings: the effects of aging. *Psychology and Aging, 15*(1), 110–125.

Schnelle, H. (2010). *Language in the Brain*. Cambridge, UK: Cambridge University Press.

Shafto, M. A., Burke, D. M., Stamatakis, E. A., Tam, P. P., & Tyler, L. K. (2007). On the tip-of-the-tongue: neural correlates of increased word-finding failures in normal aging. *Journal of Cognitive Neuroscience, 19*(12), 2060–2070.

Shafto, M. A., Stamatakis, E. A., Tam, P. P., & Tyler, L. K. (2009). Word retrieval failures in old age: the relationship between structure and function. *Journal of Cognitive Neuroscience, 22*(7), 1530–1540.

Stamatakis, E. A., Shafto, M. A., Williams, G., Tam, P., & Tyler, L. K. (2011). White matter changes and word finding failures with increasing age. *PLoS One, 6*(1), e14496.

Szekely, A., D'Amico, S., Devescovi, A., Federmeier, K., Herron, D., Iyer, G., ... Bates, E. (2005). Timed action and object naming. *Cortex, 41*(1), 7–25.

Thompson, C. K., & den Ouden, D. B. (2008). Neuroimaging and recovery of language in aphasia. *Current Neurology and Neuroscience Reports, 8*(6), 475–483.

Tomasi, D., & Volkow, N. D. (2012). Resting functional connectivity of language networks: characterization and reproducibility. *Molecular Psychiatry, 17*(8), 841–854. doi: 10.1038/mp.2011.177

Turken, A. U., & Dronkers, N. F. (2011). The neural architecture of the language comprehension network: Converging evidence from lesion and connectivity analyses. *Frontiers in Systems Neuroscience, 5*, 1. doi: 10.3389/fnsys.2011.00001

Ullman, M. T. (2004). Contributions of memory circuits to language: The declarative/procedural model. *Cognition, 92*(1–2), 231–270.

Ungerleider, L. G., & Mishkin, M. (1982). Two cortical visual systems. In D. J. Ingle, M. A. Goodale, & R.J.W. Mansfield (Eds.), *Analysis of Visual Behavior* (pp. 549–586). Cambridge, MA: MIT Press.

Waters, G., & Caplan, D. (2005). The relationship between age, processing speed, working memory capacity, and language comprehension. *Memory, 13*(3–4), 403–413.

Wierenga, C. E., Benjamin, M., Gopinath, K., Perlstein, W. M., Leonard, C. M., Rothi, L. J., ... Crosson, B. (2008). Age-related changes in word retrieval: role of bilateral frontal and subcortical networks. *Neurobiology of Aging, 29*(3), 436–451.

Wingfield, A., & Grossman, M. (2006). Language and the aging brain: patterns of neural compensation revealed by functional brain imaging. *Journal of Neurophysiology, 96*(6), 2830–2839.

Wingfield, A., Lindfield, K. C., & Kahana, M. J. (1998). Adult age differences in the temporal characteristics of category free recall. *Psychology and Aging, 13*(2), 256–266.

Wingfield, A., Peelle, J. E., & Grossman, M. (2003). Speech rate and syntactic complexity as multiplicative factors in speech comprehension by young and older adults. *Aging, Neuropsychology, and Cognition, 10*(4), 310–322.

Zheng, Z. Z., Munhall, K. G., & Johnsrude, I. S. (2010). Functional overlap between regions involved in speech perception and in monitoring one's own voice during speech production. *Journal of Cognitive Neuroscience, 22*(8), 1770–1781.

3

Executive Functions and Recovery from Aphasia

Executive Functions and Aphasia: Old Questions, New Light

In this chapter, we review the neurocognitive imprint of executive functions on the process of aphasia recovery. We are interested in how both impaired and spared executive abilities help shape the course of language recovery in aphasia. This exploration is anchored in a long history of neuropsychological inquiry investigating whether language is a necessary component of executive processes, such as planning, self-monitoring, and prospective memory (e.g., Carruthers, 2002; Hurlburt, 1990; Keil & Kaszniak, 2002; Luria, 1973; Sokolov, 1968/1972; Zangwill, 1966). Here, we cast this question in a new light to consider ways in which language and executive functions interact behaviorally and neurally within a multifunctional system that operates adaptively to reorganize the brain in the course of aphasia recovery.

In what follows we provide a brief summary of what is currently known about executive functions and their neural underpinnings in the nonaphasic population, highlighting models elucidating the specific relationship between executive functions and language in the healthy brain (e.g., Badre & Wagner, 2007). We then follow with a description of how these functions are typically measured, focusing on the challenges that some of these measures pose for the evaluation of people with aphasia (e.g., increased linguistic demands of some of these tasks) (e.g., Helm-Estabrooks, 2002). We believe that despite these challenges, data obtained through such evaluations can be used to explain some of the variability observed in patterns of aphasia recovery (see Chapter 1).

We then present behavioral findings from aphasia studies concerning the relation of executive functions to aphasia, showing, for example, how impaired shifting behaviors can interact with aspects of lexical retrieval, leading in some cases to patterns of perseveration (e.g., Helm-Estabrooks & Albert, 2004; Stark, 2007), or how the ability to engage in goal-oriented behavior or to demonstrate cognitive flexibility, two executive skills key to conversational success, can affect the recovery of functional communication (Helm-Estabrooks, 2002). For example, sparing of executive functions can promote conversational abilities, while impairment of executive functions can hinder them (e.g., Fridriksson et al., 2006; Raymer, 2005). We also describe studies that demonstrate how such executive-based changes can contribute to the neural reorganization of language in the brain in the course of recovery (e.g., Crosson et al., 2005).

This chapter, then, should provide the reader with a better understanding of key questions that need to be answered in order to characterize the effects of executive functions on aphasia. These include the following: (1) What neurocognitive mechanisms underlie executive functions in the healthy brain? (2) Are there specific models linking these mechanisms to neural correlates of language abilities? (3) How are executive functions assessed in people with and without aphasia? (4) Do executive abilities interact with language problems in aphasia? (5) Can executive functions be used as a reliable prognostic factor to predict aphasia recovery? (6) Is there evidence for the contribution of executive functions to the neural organization of language function in the aphasic brain?

Our discussion in this chapter will be limited to behavioral and neural findings concerning inhibition and switching behaviors in aphasia, which represent only a subset of possible executive effects on aphasia recovery. For ease of exposition, we defer the discussion of how people with aphasia handle tasks requiring sustained and selective attention and working memory, two other major component factors of executive functions (e.g., Alvarez & Emory, 2006), to subsequent chapters (Chapters 4 and 5), knowing full well that they overlap in important ways with the discussion in the current chapter.

Defining Executive Functions

The notion "executive functions," in the broadest sense, refers to those brain-based capabilities that allow us to adapt to changing circumstances by flexibly shifting from one situation to the next (Jurado & Rosselli, 2007; Lezak, 1995; Phillips, 1997; Ylvisaker & Feeney, 1998), relying on self-regulatory and metacognitive functions (Seniow, 2012). To accomplish this goal, we engage in multiple cognitive processes, such as central executive control (Baddeley & Hitch, 1974), attentional control (Anderson et al., 2001; Norman & Shallice, 1986), cognitive flexibility (Anderson et al., 2001; Lafleche & Albert, 1995; Piguet et al., 2002), abstract thinking/reasoning (Delis et al., 2001; Piguet et al., 2002), concept formation (Delis et al., 2001; Lafleche & Albert, 1995; Piguet et al., 2002), strategizing (Borkowski & Burke, 1996; Elliot, 2003), problem solving (Elliot,

2003), initiation (Hobson & Leeds, 2001), updating and sequencing (Elliot, 2003), monitoring (Borkowski & Burke, 1996), inhibition (Delis et al., 2001), impulse control (Delis et al., 2001), goal setting (Anderson et al., 2001; Hobson & Leeds, 2001), and planning or volitional/purposeful action (Banich, 2004; Delis et al., 2001; Lezak, 1983). These allow us to form, initiate, and sustain a plan through to completion.

The multitude of executive system operations has stirred a major controversy surrounding the question of whether they constitute a unitary construct of "executive functioning" or represent independent components (De Frias et al., 2006; Duncan et al., 1996; Duncan, Johnson, Swales, Freer, 1997; Kimberg et al., 1997; Miyake et al., 2001; Parkin & Java, 1999; Stuss & Alexander, 2000; Teuber, 1972). Some researchers have proposed that all executive functions share a component of executive attention and are therefore inseparable (e.g., Blair, 2006; Duncan et al., 1996; McCabe et al., 2010; Shallice & Burgess, 1993). Similarly, inhibition has been proposed as a unifying mechanism accounting for accuracy of executive responses (Barkley, 1997).

Others have postulated the existence of multiple discrete executive abilities that are loosely related to one another (e.g., Blair, Zelazo, & Greenberg, 2005; Fletcher, 1996; Pennington, Bennetto, McAleer, & Roberts, 1996; Pennington & Ozonoff, 1996; Rapport et al., 2000; Zillmer & Spiers, 2001), based on observed dissociations (e.g., Godefroy et al., 1999) or low statistical intercorrelations among different functions (e.g., Lehto, 1996; Salthouse et al., 2003). Miyake et al. (2000) demonstrated that shifting, updating, and inhibition are dissociable but moderately correlated, leading to a third approach which argues for functional unity alongside diversity (e.g., Banich, 2009; Friedman et al., 2008; Garon, Bryson, & Smith, 2008; Miyake & Friedman, 2012).

Models of Executive Functions

Several models have been proposed to account for the ways in which the brain mediates executive functions, under the assumption that these functions are supported by frontal neural substrates (e.g., Luria, 1973). For example, Baddeley has developed a hierarchical model of a prefrontal-based system consisting of working memory (phonological and visual) with storage capacity (Baddeley, 1986; 1992) and a "central executive" system for more complex attentional control/regulation processes with shifting but no storage capabilities (Baddeley & Logie, 1999; Baddeley, 2002). This model, which we review in more detail in the memory chapter (Chapter 5), has become the most influential framework for understanding executive functions (e.g., Miyake et al., 2000), although how its components allow for more specific neurofunctional relations to be expressed remains unclear.

Another hierarchical model is that of Norman and Shallice (1986), which also depicts a prefrontal-based control system, a "supervisory attentional system," distinguishing the planning and decision making associated with automatic versus nonroutine processes.

The validity of this dichotomous model has been questioned, however, because it does not capture possible additional levels of control mediated by subcortical and prefrontal regions (Slattery et al., 2001), such as awareness of self in relation to the environment (Stuss, 1992).

Other models have focused on temporal aspects of executive functions, implicating more widespread neural substrates. For instance, Fuster (2002) has argued that fronto-subcortical regions work to temporally integrate perception, action, and cognition via processes of attention, working memory, and monitoring. Zelazo et al. (1997), in contrast, has proposed to divide executive functions into four temporally and functionally distinct components—problem representation, planning, execution, and evaluation—the optimal performance of which requires the integrity of the entire brain rather than just that of prefrontal regions.

Neural Correlates of Executive Functions

Luria (1973) was among the first to suggest that the frontal lobes subserve executive behaviors (see also Fuster, 1997; Shallice, 1982), a claim later confirmed by studies of patients with frontal lobe damage, also known as the "dysexecutive syndrome" (Baddeley & Wilson, 1988). Typical difficulties include disorders of planning, organizing, goal setting, problem solving, decision making, abstract reasoning, and attention shifting (e.g., Ardila & Surloff, 2004; Goldberg, 2001; Hobson & Leeds, 2001; Lezak et al., 2004; Norris & Tate, 2000; Stuss & Benson, 1986), with impaired working memory taken by some to be the primary source of these disorders (e.g., Baddeley, 1986). However, dysexecutive problems have been found in patients with lesions affecting posterior as well as anterior brain regions, calling into question this claim (Baddeley et al., 1997; Lezak, 1995; Roussel et al., 2012).

Studies of cognitive changes among older adults have also provided evidence for the involvement of the frontal lobes in mediating executive functions, leading to the development of "the frontal aging hypothesis" (e.g., Moscovitch & Wincour, 1992; Phillips & Della Sala, 1998; Rodriguez-Aranda & Sundet, 2006; West, 1996; West & Schwarb, 2006). According to this hypothesis, neural changes in the frontal lobes brought about with age (e.g., Raz, 2005), especially in the dorsolateral prefrontal cortex (Backman et al., 2000; Li & Lindenberger, 2002), adversely affect cognitive control and therefore lead to cognitive decline.

Neuroimaging studies have greatly contributed to the specification of these neural maps, providing evidence for widespread networks within frontal systems (Koechlin et al., 2000; Stuss & Alexander, 2000; Stuss et al., 2002) as well as subcortical circuits (Kassubek et al., 2005; Lewis et al., 2004; Monchi et al., 2006) mediating various executive functions. Important networks have been identified in the right inferior frontal cortex for the manipulation of information (Wager & Smith, 2003); in the superior frontal cortex for updating (Wager & Smith, 2003); in the right dorsolateral frontal lobe for monitoring; in the left dorsolateral for verbal processing (Stuss et al., 2002); in dorsolateral projections to basal ganglia and thalamus for planning, goal setting, shifting, working memory, and monitoring (Royall et al., 2002); in orbitofrontal areas for risk assessment and inhibition of unwanted behaviors (Royall et al., 2002); and in the anterior cingulate for self-corrections (Royall et al., 2002).

NEURAL CORRELATES OF LANGUAGE-EXECUTIVE FUNCTIONS: LINKS TO SEMANTIC AND DISCOURSE-LEVEL PROCESSES

Because damage to lateral portions of the left prefrontal cortex have been found to lead to several language-related executive control deficits—including impaired verbal fluency (Milner, 1964), poor monitoring of verbal information over short periods (Petrides & Milner, 1982), poor concept shifting (Milner, 1963) and difficulties with complex planning (Shallice, 1998)—attempts have been made, especially over the past two decades, to examine these neurofunctional interdependencies in the healthy brain, evaluating the effects of executive functions on certain aspects of semantic and discourse-level processes.

Executive Functions and Semantic Processing: Semantic Control

Executive functions and semantic processing interact to give rise to what is known in the literature as semantic control. This process activates (as opposed to stores) semantic knowledge through cognitive control processes (e.g., Badre & Wagner, 2007; Buckner, 1996; Gabrieli et al., 1996; 1998; Jefferies & Lambon Ralph, 2006; Petersen et al., 1989; Poldrack et al., 1999; Rokies et al., 2001; Wagner et al., 2001). Specifically semantic control involves a two-step process in which word meaning is retrieved and then selected among several semantically related candidates. Controlled retrieval occurs as we search for potentially relevant information, even if only remotely related to the target, when either (1) the semantic information encoded in the stimulus is incomplete and does not suffice for identifying the target stimulus or (2) task-relevant information is not activated. Controlled selection follows retrieval and supports the selection of the item that has the greatest goal-appropriate properties among several activated target-related competitors (e.g., Badre et al., 2005; Badre and Wagner, 2007; Wagner et al., 2001).

The neural foundation of semantic control has been argued to comprise networks in the left inferior frontal gyrus (LIFG) (Bedny, McGill, & Thompson-Schill, 2008; Novick, Trueswell, & Thompson-Schill, 2010; Thompson-Schill, Bedny, & Goldberg, 2005). These networks are known to mediate retrieval and selection of semantic and other types of knowledge (e.g., Badre & Wagner, 2007; Gold & Buckner, 2002; Snyder, Banich, & Munakata, 2011), as shown by reduced brain activation during the processing of automated semantic associations (Raichle et al., 1994), increased activation during the processing of distant semantic relations (Roskies et al., 2001; Wagner et al., 2001), or during matching of latencies (Demb et al., 1995). Relatedly, induction of a virtual lesion in the LIFG through transcranial magnetic stimulation impairs both word retrieval (identification of weakly associated words) and selection (detecting features in the presence of strong distractors) (Whitney et al., 2012).

It has been assumed that within the LIFG the anterior ventral and the posterior dorsal portions mediate controlled use of semantic and phonological information, respectively (e.g., Bokde et al., 2001; Buckner et al., 1995; Poldrack et al., 1999). However, some have proposed that the LIFG subserves selection, but not retrieval (Thompson-Schill et al., 1997), while others have argued for no such separation (Snyder et al., 2011). Some have also indicated that the recruitment of temporoparietal networks is involved in semantic control (Whitney et al., 2011; 2012) but that the role of these networks is distinct from that of the LIFG networks (Badre et al., 2005). For example, LIFG networks have been shown to suppress previously presented relevant semantic information as compared with temporoparietal networks, which, together with LIFG, retrieve less dominant semantic information to match against task-relevant information (Gardner et al., 2012).

Ventral white matter tracts connecting frontotemporal regions, especially projections of the uncinate fasciculus (UF) and the inferior longitudinal fasciculus (IFG), have also been implicated in semantic control processes, as shown in performance on a homonym meaning decision-making task (Duda, McMillan, Grossman, & Gee, 2010). These projections, however, have been identified during the processing of meaningful speech (e.g., Saur et al., 2008; 2010) and so are likely not specialized to perform semantic control.

Other studies have attested to the involvement of cortical-subcortical circuitry in support of the interdependencies of executive-language functions (e.g., Barbas, Garcia-Cabezas, & Zikopoulos, 2012; Crosson, 2013; Nadeau & Crosson, 1997; Radanovic et al. 2003). For example, executive support for word-level processing has been argued to implicate four corticothalamic and thalamocortical mechanisms: (1) frontal selective engagement of cortical areas in an "attentive" state for task performance through the nucleus reticularis; (2) transfer of information from among cortical areas via corticothalamocortical relays, shifting attention as necessary; (3) optimizing focus on task-relevant information through corticothalamocortical feedback mechanisms to ensure processing accuracy; and (4) increasing the signal-to-noise ratio around a selected word selection during expression of a concept via a basal ganglia loop (Crosson, 2013).

These mechanisms have been argued to be the basis for intentional functions, where *intention* refers to the ability to select and initiate an action among several competing candidates (as opposed to attention that involves selection of a stimulus among several possible stimuli and further processes of that stimulus) (Crosson, 2013). Specifically the neural correlates of intention are thought to implicate the supplementary motor area (SMA), pre-SMA, rostral cingulate area, lateral frontal regions, and basal ganglia loops (Heilman, Watson, & Valenstein, 2003), with pre-SMA, dorsal caudate nucleus, and ventral anterior thalamus being responsible for generating meaningful but not nonsense words (Crosson et al., 2003) or word repetition (Crosson et al., 2001). Within this neural setup, the pre-SMA is assumed to create an automated word selection bias that is then processed by the basal ganglia, affecting top-down processing in the course of word selection (Copland, 2003).

Thus evidence is emerging clearly that executive functions and semantic processing interact intimately within the cognitive domain of semantic control. What about the influence of executive functions on discourse processing?

Executive Functions and Discourse Processing

Discourse processing involves language comprehension in context and so requires abilities that fall under the umbrella of executive functions, including the integration of contextual information or matching interpretation with communicative setting, to mention just two. Discourse processing abilities have been argued to rely on the support of frontotemporal networks (e.g., Ferstl & von Cramon, 2002; Mazoyer et al., 1993; Xu et al., 2005). These involve the left lateral frontal regions and dorsomedial prefrontal regions as well as posterior and superior temporal regions beyond Wernicke's area, with evidence for bilateral activation of the anterior temporal lobe (Ferstl, Neumann, Bogler, & von Cramon, 2008). Processing of text coherence (e.g., processing the overall theme of a narrative) has been linked to dorsomedial (BA10) and ventromedial (BA11) prefrontal regions and the posterior cingulate region and inferior precuneus. These regions were identified on the basis of a meta-analysis of 23 neuroimaging studies of comprehension of higher-level language exceeding sentence-level (processing of texts or metaphors) using activation likelihood estimates and replicator dynamics. As pointed out by Ferstl and colleagues (2008), the analyses performed were based on limited empirical data obtained from studies using vastly different methodologies and therefore may underestimate or misrepresent the regions implicated in discourse processing. Because the studies included in the meta-analysis do not provide data directly comparing brain activation patterns for discourse processing to those that might be associated with tasks of executive functions, it is difficult to establish the nature of the neurocognitive link between the two.

Limitations on Neural Mappings

The elusive nature of executive functions has made the mapping of their functional neuroanatomy somewhat of a challenge, with no clear one-to-one mappings of executive functions to frontal lobe activation (e.g., Alvarez & Emory, 2006; Carpenter, Just, & Reichle, 2000). Jurado & Rosselli (2007) have thus described the neural underpinnings of different functions in relation to particular executive tasks, such as the Tower of London (Shallice, 1982) or the Wisconsin Card Sorting Test (Grant & Berg, 1948; Heaton et al., 1993). For example, in a recent meta-analysis of 41 neuroimaging studies of healthy adults, Yuan and Raz (2014) found that a larger volume and greater thickness of prefrontal cortex is more strongly correlated with better performance on the Wisconsin Card Sorting Test than with tests of backward digit span, Trail Making, and Verbal Fluency.

These and similar findings have resulted in a regional specification for executive functions, such as planning, attentional control, cognitive flexibility, and verbal fluency, as detailed in Table 3.1 (based on Jurado & Rosselli's 2007 review).

It is important to note, though, that performance on these executive tasks has shown inconsistent patterns among brain-damaged individuals (Alvarez & Emory, 2006). In some cases, people with frontal lesions have been reported to perform within normal limits on these tests (e.g., Ahola et al., 1996; Damasio, 1994; Eslinger & Damasio, 1985; Schallice & Burgess, 1991). Conversely, people with more diffuse brain damage have been shown to have difficulties on these tests (e.g., Anderson et al., 1991; Axelrod et al., 1996; Grafman et al., 1990; Heaton, 1981; Robinson et al., 1980).

What Do Executive Tasks Really Tell Us?

Nonetheless, despite these caveats, executive tasks are thought to implicate frontal networks, at the very least to handle demands of task novelty and/or complexity (e.g., Duffy & Campbell, 2001; Duke & Kaszniak, 2000; Filley, 2000; Luria, 1973; Shallice, 1998). However, because these tasks typically tap a myriad of cognitive functions (e.g., Barcelo, 2001; Godefroy et al., 2010; Kafer & Hunter, 1997; Phillips, 1997; Rabbitt, 1997; Reitan & Wolfson, 1994), it is not clear whether they measure a unitary or diverse construct with distinct neural underpinnings. For example, the Wisconsin Card Sorting Test (WCST) (Grant & Berg, 1948; Heaton, 1993) is usually considered a measure of set-shifting/flexibility (Ashendorf & McCaffrey, 2008; Rhodes, 2004), but it can also be taken to measure functions such as inhibitory control of previously presented sets (Salthouse et al., 2003), problem solving (Greve et al., 2002), and strategizing/updating (Bishara et al., 2010).

Moreover, impaired performance on a given executive test can be attributed to rather different neural sources (Keil & Kaszniak, 2002). Poor performance on the Rey-Osterreith Complex Figure Test, for example, could result from a parietal-occipital-based visual impairment and/or frontally mediated organizational deficit (Lezak, 1995).

ASSESSING EXECUTIVE FUNCTIONS IN PEOPLE WITH APHASIA

Most executive tasks have not been developed with clinical populations in mind (Miyake, Emerson, & Friedman, 2000), making the assessment of people with aphasia challenging. For instance, many of the most common executive tasks include verbal components, where executive skills can be masked by language impairment, thus reducing their diagnostic validity and level of specificity (Beeson et al., 1993; Glosser & Goodglass, 1990; Helm-Estabrooks, 2002; Keil & Kaszniak, 2002; Murray & Ramage, 2000; Purdy,

TABLE 3.1
NEURAL NETWORKS OF EXECUTIVE FUNCTIONS

Executive Function	Task(s) Used	Brain Region Identified
Planning (Dagher et al., 1999; Goethals et al., Lazeron et al., 2000; Morris et al., 1993; Owen et al., 1996; 2004; Wagner et al., 2006)	Tower of London	Left prefrontal cortex (PFC); Middle dorsolateral prefrontal cortex (DLPFC) and head of caudate; DLPFC and lateral premotor cortex; DLPFC, anterior cingulated cortex (ACC), cuneus and precuneus, supramarginal gyrus (SMG), and angular gyrus; Right PFC; Rostrolateral PFC
Attention control (Collette et al., 2001; Fassbender et al., 2004; Gerton et al., 2004; Kaufmann et al., 2005; Lie et al., 2006; Naghama et al., 2001; Siegel et al., 1995)	Continuous Performance Test Haylings Test Wisconsin Card Sorting Test Digit Span Sustained Attention Response Task Stroop	Medial superior frontal gyrus, lateral inferior temporal gyrus; Left PFC, middle and inferior frontal lobe; Anterodorsal PFC; Right DLPFC, bilateral inferior parietal lobe (IPL); Right ventral PFC, right IPL, left putamen, left DLPFC; Caudal ACC and DLPFC
Cognitive Flexibility (Berman et al., 1995; Catafau et al., 1998; Hirshorn & Thompson-Schill, 2006; Lombardi et al., 1999; Naghama et al., 2001; Perianez et al., 2004)	Wisconsin Card Sorting Test Verbal Fluency	DLPFC, parietal, temporal cortices; left posterior frontal region, inferior cingulate; right dorsolateral fronto-subcortical circuit; posteroventral pfc; inferior frontal gyrus (IFG), ACC, SMG; left IFG
Verbal/Nonverbal Fluency (Audenaert et al., 2000; Frith et al., 1991; Jahanshahi et al., 2000; Paulesu et al., 1997; Phelps et al., 1997; Pihlajamaki et al., 2000)	Verbal Fluency Random Number Generation Controlled Oral Word Association	Left DLPFC; Left IFG, left thalamus; Left IFG, ACC, superior frontal sulcus; Left DLPFC, ACC, superior parietal cortex; Left medial temporal lobe, Restrosplenial area, left superior parietal lobe; left inferior PFC, right inferior PFC

1992). The Stroop test (Stroop, 1935), for example, requires reading aloud. More appropriate might be nonverbal tasks (e.g., Basso et al., 1973; Helm-Estabrooks et al., 1995; van Mourik et al., 1992; Ramsberger & Rende, 2002), such as Raven's Colored Progressive Matrices (Raven, 1981), which measure visual analogical thinking (selecting a missing piece that best completes a specific design out of six options).

Even performance on nonverbal tasks, however, might rely to a certain degree on basic comprehension skills that could interfere with executive task performance (Basso et al., 1981; Borod, Carper, & Goodglass, 1982; Borod, Carper, Goodglass, & Naeser, 1984; Keil & Kaszniak, 2002; van Mourik et al., 1992). This is particularly true in cases in which brain damage extends over a large area, where more severe language and cognitive impairments might be predicted, with the cognitive deficit potentially being a manifestation of the aphasia (Fucetola, Connor, Strube, & Corbetta, 2009).

Moreover, the administration of nonverbal tasks can involve problems with following instructions, even in the face of preserved comprehension, reflecting difficulties processing task novelty and complexity (Keil & Kaszniak, 2002). Although these barriers can be circumvented by appropriate adaptations, such as lifting time constraints, simplifying instructions, and using gestures to complement verbal instructions (e.g., Glosser & Goodglass, 1990; Ramsberger & Rende, 2002), the administration of executive tests to people with aphasia, even nonverbal tests, remains challenging.

Nonetheless, Keil and Kaszniak (2002) have identified specific tests of executive functions that could be highly useful in testing aphasic people's abilities to (1) plan, schedule, strategize, and follow rules; (2) generate, initiate, and be fluent; and (3) engage in abstract thinking (form concepts and reason). These are detailed in Table 3.2. Tests of shifting and inhibition, such as Stroop (Spreen & Straus, 1998; Stroop, 1935) and Trail Making B (Reitan, 1960), have been ranked by the authors as only moderately appropriate for testing in aphasia and so were not included in the table.

Another appropriate task is the clock drawing test (where participants are asked to draw a clock and set it to 10 minutes past 11), included in Helm-Estabrooks's (2001) Cognitive Linguistic Quick Test (CLQT). It can give a good sense of an aphasic person's executive abilities to plan and execute the task (e.g., sequencing the steps necessary to draw the circle, place of numbers, and adjust the hands) (Helm-Estabrooks & Albert, 2004). This test, however, taps additional nonexecutive skills (e.g., visuospatial skills) and so may not be specific enough to tease apart executive behaviors. A task that more specifically targets executive abilities is the coin switch, in which participants are asked to guess the hand in which the examiner is hiding a coin, with the examiner changing his or her hand every few trials (for a recent description, see Albert & Knoefel, 2011). Impaired performance on this task can reflect, for example, poor inhibitory control of previous responses, a hallmark of many aphasic responses on language testing, as discussed below.

The tests described above do not include real-life tasks, which might be more ecologically valid (Brandimonte et al., 1996; Burgess et al., 1998; Eslinger & Damasio, 1985; Kliegel et al., 2008; Mesulam, 1986; Murray & Ramage, 2000) but are subject to extreme variability and therefore are difficult to tabulate (Keil & Kaszniak, 2002). However, a recent review of executive performance-based tasks appropriate for the functional assessment of stroke patients can be found in Poulin, Korner-Bitensky, and Dawson (2013), who created a large table of different assessment tools such as the Activities of Daily

TABLE 3.2
EXECUTIVE MEASURES USEFUL FOR PEOPLE WITH APHASIA

Functions Assessed	Test Name	Description	Score
Planning, scheduling, strategizing, and ability to follow rules	Porteus Mazes (Porteus, 1965)	Tracing a path through drawn mazes of increasing complexity	Efficiency, impulsivity
	Rey-Osterrieth Complex Figure (Duley, Wilkins, Hamby, Hopkins, Burwell, Barry, 1993)	Drawing and reproducing a complex geometrical figure	Number of correct elements, strategy
	Tower of London (Shallice, 1982)	Moving three rings from starting point to target position, using a minimal number of moves	Number of moves, time to complete task
	Tower of Hanoi (Goel & Grafman, 1995)	Moving three discs of varying sizes from starting point to target position, using a minimal number of moves, adhering to a stacking rule based on size	Number of moves, time to complete task
	Virtual Planning Test (Miotto & Morris, 1998)	Organizing time-specific and time-nonspecific events into a period of time	Omitted items, misordering
	Visual Search Test (Trenerry, Crosson, DeBoe, & Leber, 1990)	Finding a token hidden beneath one of several blue boxes presented on a computer screen	Strategy, between and within search errors
Generating, initiating, and fluency	Graphic Pattern Generation (Glosser & Goodglass, 1990)	Generating novel designs to a stimulus consisting of five dots	Number of designs produced; number of perseverations
	Sequence Generating Test (Glosser & Goodglass, 1990)	Generating random sequences of three numbers using a computer keypad	Number of perseverations, perseveration distance, and response to feedback
Abstract thinking	Category Test (DeFilippis & McCampbell, 1979)	Sorting six distinct sets of items by a certain abstract principle	Accuracy
	Raven's Colored Progressive Matrices (Raven, 1981)	Choice of best-fitting missing piece to complete given design	Accuracy
	Wisconsin Card Sorting Test (Grant & Berg, 1948)	Sorting of cards by color, form, number; change in sorting principle occurs without warning	Number of categories achieved, number of perseverations

Source: Adapted from Keil, K., & Kaszniak, A. W. (2002). Examining executive function in individuals with brain injury: a review. *Aphasiology, 16,* 305–335.

Living Profile (Dutil et al., 2005), Execution of a Cooking Task (Chevignard et al., 2000, 2008), and others, which more closely resemble actual situations patients might encounter. In that table, task descriptions are given, the executive domains tested are listed, and data about test reliability (test-retest, interrater, and internal consistency) and validity (e.g., factorial, predictive) are provided.

Executive Dysfunction in Aphasia: Dissociable from Language Impairment?

Persons with aphasia can experience poststroke executive dysfunction both in the acute stage (e.g., Zinn, Bosworth, Hoenig, & Swartzwelder, 2007) and chronically (e.g., Glosser & Goodglass, 1990; van Mourik et al., 1992; Purdy, 1992; Rende, 2000). Some studies of executive abilities among people with chronic aphasia have used scores on intelligence tests (Archibald, Wepman, & Jones, 1967; Borod, Carper, & Goodglass, 1982; De Renzi, Faglioni, Savoiardo, & Vignolo, 1966; Edwards, Ellams, & Thompson, 1976; Hjelmquist, 1989; Kertesz & McCabe, 1975; Larrabee & Haley, 1986), both verbal (Reitan, 1960) and nonverbal (e.g., Ellis & Young, 1996), to determine the presence of an executive disorder. In these studies, people with aphasia have been found to perform significantly lower on intelligence tests (e.g., Basso et al., 1981), compared to normal controls and/or brain-damaged individuals without aphasia. To the extent that intelligence is a measure of executive function (e.g., "fluid intelligence" in Duncan, Burgess, & Emslie, 1995; Salthouse, 2005; Salthouse et al., 2003, 2006), these findings suggest possible executive dysfunction in aphasia but do not specify explicit patterns of impairment.

Some researchers (e.g., Basso et al., 1973; Hamsher, 1991) have argued that such executive dysfunction in aphasia is simply a coincidence deriving from the neuroanatomical proximity of the neural substrates mediating language functions and executive abilities (they receive their blood supply from the same source—the middle cerebral artery—which is commonly damaged in aphasia (e.g., Albert et al., 1981; Nolte, 1993). In contrast, however, we argue that changes in executive functions in aphasia, when present, interact systematically with language changes to affect the process of recovery.

A specific and extremely common behavioral manifestation of executive dysfunction in aphasia is impaired switching/cognitive flexibility (e.g., Rende, 2000; Purdy, 2002), which reduces the ability to regulate responses from previous tasks so as to avoid interference effects (Rogers & Monsell, 1995). This results in a "switching cost," where increased reaction times and reduced performance accuracy are observed, reflecting a dysfunction in the mechanisms of reconfiguration (initiation of a new rule) and interference that brings about omissions or substitutions (e.g., Chiou & Kennedy, 2009). Switching costs (the difference between the reaction times and error rates on a switch vs. a nonswitch task) have been found to be especially great among people with left hemisphere damage

(Mecklinger et al., 1999), including persons with aphasia, in whom the ability to switch between go/no-go tasks by inhibiting the "go" or "no-go" stimulus (Drewe, 1975) has been reported to be diminished, leading to inefficient reconfiguration and interference (Chiou & Kennedy, 2009). Reduced executive efficiency—as measured by speed (rate), accuracy (correctness), and efficiency (number of moves to complete task) responses to standard executive tasks, such as those listed in Table 3.2—have also been reported by Purdy (2002).

In some cases of aphasia, such shifting deficits have been dissociated from patterns of language impairment (Caspari, Parkinson, LaPointe, & Katz, 1998; Glosser & Goodglass, 1990; Goldenberg, Dettmers, Grothe, & Spatt, 1994; Gutbrod, Cohen, Mager, & Meier, 1989; Murray, Ramage, & Hopper, 2001). Glosser & Goodglass (1990), for example, found that while all of their aphasic participants of course showed linguistic deficits, those with frontal lesions exhibited greater executive problems than those with retrorolandic or mixed lesions, as measured by performance (e.g., accuracy or number of perseverations) on nonverbal tasks, such as the Graphic Pattern Generation, Sequence Generation Task, and the Tower of Hanoi Test (for descriptions of these tasks, see Table 3.2).

Other cases of aphasia have demonstrated a significant correlation between executive abilities, as measured by tests such as the WCST and Raven's Colored Progressive Matrices, and language measures of comprehension and naming (e.g., Baldo et al., 2005; Baldo, Bunge, Wilson, & Dronkers, 2010; Jefferies & Lambon Ralph, 2006). Because this pattern was also observed among healthy adults under conditions of articulatory suppression (comparison of performance with concurrent verbal shadowing, nonverbal shadowing, or no shadowing), the authors of these studies concluded that language and executive skills involving problem solving are tightly linked via processes of covert language.

PERSEVERATION IN APHASIA

Switching impairment in aphasia can result in what is known as perseveration (e.g., Allison & Hurwitz, 1967; Helmick & Berg, 1976; Santo-Pietro & Rigrodsky, 1982), typically defined as an involuntary continuation or recurrence of ideas, experiences, or behavior, in the absence of an appropriate stimulus, which can appear in many neurological conditions (Albert, 1990; Albert & Sandson, 1986; Sandson & Albert, 1984, 1987). Patterns of perseveration can be divided into three broad categories: (1) stuck-in-set, which refers to an inability to shift to a different category or framework of response in the face of a new task, (2) continuous perseveration, which involves the continuation of a behavior in the absence of an intervening response/stimulus, and (3) recurrent perseveration, which is the recurrence of a previous response after a new stimulus is presented and an intervening response has been provided (Helm-Estabrooks & Albert, 2004).

BEHAVIORAL FINDINGS RELATED TO LANGUAGE PERFORMANCE

Certain subtypes of perseveration are more tightly linked to language performance than others, specifically affecting people with aphasia as opposed to other brain-damaged individuals (e.g., Sandson & Albert, 1987). These include, in particular, recurrent perseveration of whole or parts of words, as in (1) semantic perseveration, when a previous word is repeated after a semantically related word is elicited; (2) lexical perseveration, where no straightforward semantic relation between the previous and new responses holds; (3) program-of-action perseveration, when the new response provided includes the initial sound of the previous response; and (4) phonemic perseveration, when part of the phonemic structure of the previous response is included in the new response.

These types of perseveration can adversely affect lexical retrieval, especially on tasks of confrontation naming (e.g., Emery & Helm-Estabrooks, 1989) regardless of aphasia type (Helm-Estabrooks et al., 1998). Indeed, Albert and Sandson (1986) found a strong relationship between perseveration and anomia and proposed that, in patients with lesions in the posterior left hemisphere, recurrences occur by disrupted naming as a result of failed searches for a target in semantic memory. This finding argues against the claim that executive dysfunction in aphasia is observed exclusively in Broca-type aphasias, where linguistic and executive dysfluency are thought to mirror one another (e.g., Filley, 1995, 2000). Instead, a more specific mechanism has been proposed to explain the interaction between executive functions with language problems, irrespective of output fluency, whereby difficulties accessing information in semantic memory allow for the involuntary release of previously primed information resulting in perseverative errors (e.g., Albert & Sandson, 1986; Helm-Estabrooks & Albert, 2004; Shindler, Caplan, & Hier, 1984). In people with posterior lesions, this problem has been linked to their demonstrated poor self-monitoring (Buckingham, 1985).

SEMANTIC CONTROL IN APHASIA

More recent studies have tied deficits of semantic processing in aphasia to impaired semantic control, which, as pointed out earlier in the chapter, is an executive-based function (e.g., Corbett, Jefferies, Ehsan, & Lambon Ralph, 2009; Jefferies & Lambon Ralph, 2006; Jefferies, Patterson, & Lambon Ralph, 2008). For example, studies have contrasted performance on semantic processing tasks comprising varying task demands between people with semantic dementia (SD) and those with stroke-based aphasia (e.g., Corbett, Jefferies, Ehsan, & Lambon Ralph, 2009; Jefferies & Lambon Ralph, 2006; Jefferies, Patterson, & Lambon Ralph, 2008). Findings indicate that both patient groups performed poorly on tasks of semantic memory in which the processing of semantically related competitors was required, but they differed in their ability to control changing task demands. People with SD showed little variability in performance across task demands, while persons with aphasia performed consistently only when task demands were kept constant (e.g., Jefferies & Lambon Ralph, 2006). This lack of flexibility in manipulating semantic knowledge across variable task demands was reduced among the aphasic participants in the presence of phonemic cueing, which emphasizes the dissociation between their control deficit and intact semantic knowledge (Jefferies, Patterson, & Lambon Ralph, 2008). The vulnerability of persons with aphasia to changes in executive task demands has also been shown for nonverbal tasks, including impairments in nonroutine usages of everyday objects and improved performance under more structured task conditions that provided verbal and visual cues (e.g., Corbett, Jefferies, & Lambon Ralph, 2009; 2011).

Impaired semantic control in aphasia has been reported for people with lesions in left prefrontal cortical circuits. Thompson-Schill and colleagues (1998), for example, showed that aphasic participants with left inferior prefrontal lesions implicating neural substrates in Brodmann's BA 44 but not those with prefrontal lesions excluding this region or those with right hemisphere damage performed poorly on noun selection tasks with high competing demands. However, aphasic participants with lesions in temporoparietal networks have also been shown to have difficulties with semantic control (e.g., Berthier, 2001; Jefferies & Lambon Ralph, 2006; Noonan, Jefferis, Corbett, & Lambon Ralph, 2010), although their deficits were not as severe as in those with anterior brain damage (Gardner et al., 2012; Schnur et al., 2009).

The executive-based deficits produced by prefrontal lesions among persons with aphasia can affect their performance on tasks involving cumulative competition across cycles, also known as refractory effects, because stimuli serve both as targets and distractors on different trials (Gardner et al., 2012). The ability to perform such tasks has been argued to depend on whether the control network can generate timely task-appropriate responses that activate semantic information within the semantic store, which becomes more challenging with increased competition and/or open-ended task demands (e.g., Badre et al., 2005; Thompson-Schill et al., 1997; Whitney et al., 2011) and leads to reduced accuracy in both verbal and nonverbal responses (Gardner et al., 2012). Based on these and similar findings, some have proposed that that the neural networks of the LIFG specifically mediate selection among already retrieved items (e.g., Robinson, Shallice, & Cipolotti, 2005) and can even impair sentence production in tasks where the probe refers to several propositions (Robinson, Shallice, Bozzali, & Cipolotti, 2010).

In another semantic control study using diffusion tensor imaging and resting-state functional magnetic resonance imaging data, Harvey et al. (2013) found involvement of white matter tracts connecting frontotemporoparietal regions in aphasic word comprehension deficits. Specifically participants in whom compromised structural integrity and weaker connectivity of the uncinate fasciculus (UF) but limited damage to the anterior temporal and inferior frontal pathways was observed were also those who performed poorly on word comprehension tasks (as measured by the ability to reject semantic foils and the ability to retrieve semantic information about an item while ignoring other semantic relationships).

Subcortical circuitry has also been identified as an intersection for the convergence of language and executive deficits in aphasia, although most studies of thalamic aphasia did not conduct behavioral assessments of executive functions. An exception is Radanovic et al.'s (2003) study, which found that left but not right thalamic lesions implicating corticothalamiccortical reciprocal connections can lead to anomia or paraphasic misselections associated with low scores on tasks of executive functions such as trail making and the WCST. The authors interpreted this finding as a formulation deficit, which impairs language organization and conceptual association. These deficits were different from those they observed in their participants with right thalamic lesions, who had problems with visuospatial perception and discourse-related impairments, especially in temporal-sequential ordering (Radanovic et al., 2003), reflecting more of a "thought" disorder (Chatterjee et al., 1997). Other studies of aphasic people with thalamic lesions (e.g., Raymer et al., 1997) have relied on sophisticated experimental designs meant to differentiate levels of word processing deficits—lexical, semantic, and lexicosemantic. The behavioral patterns and their neural correlates have been discussed in detail by Crosson (2013).

EXECUTIVE FUNCTIONS AND FUNCTIONAL COMMUNICATION IN APHASIA

Executive functioning among people with aphasia has also been linked to their level of functional communication, affecting macro-level conversational organization rather than word- or phrasal-level structures (e.g., Ramsberger, 1994, 2005). A similar relationship between executive functions and discourse skills has also been demonstrated for persons with traumatic brain injury, in whom narrative abilities were associated with set-shifting skills (Coelho, Liles & Duffy, 1995). Specifically, poor scores on the WCST were correlated with low scores on measures of story structure, but not with poor performance on measures of sentence production and local cohesion. The contribution of executive functions to functional communication among people with aphasia accounts perhaps for the weak link reported between extent of their language deficit and their degree of conversational success (e.g., spared executive functions can positively affect the well-formedness of an conversational exchange even in the face of extreme word-finding difficulties) (Irwin, Wertz, & Avent, 2002; Ramsberger & Rende, 2002).

Aphasia studies exploring the relationship between executive function and conversational abilities (e.g., Fridriksson et al., 2006) have often defined functional communication operationally as an ability to communicate a message effectively in a natural setting using modalities that could include grammatical structures or other modes of communication, such as appropriate gestures (definitions based on the works of Holland [1980] and Frattali et al., [1995]). Impaired executive shifting has been found to limit the extent to which people with aphasia can use alternative nonlinguistic modes of communication in conversation, because people with aphasia trained to use alternative gestural and pictorial symbols did not shift to those modalities even in instances of failed verbal communication (Purdy, Duffy, & Coelho, 1994). Such executive problems—measured by poor performance on tests of shifting attention, working memory, and concept formation—have been found to constrain the ability of the aphasic person to shift focus, resulting in patterns of linguistic perseveration and difficulties in choosing a conversational strategy, especially to repair an ineffectual one, most notably in settings with multiple participants (Frankel, Penn, & Ormond-Brown, 2007).

Transactional success with an aphasic interlocutor largely depends on six executive functions: monitoring, self-regulation, planning, attending to input, switching, and regulation of cognitive resources (Ramsberger, 2005). In the absence of these, a person with aphasia might fail to take into account questions directed at him or her, ignore requests for clarification, confirm shared knowledge, establish a strategy for a dialogue (e.g., yes/no questions), keep track of what has been and still needs to be said, inhibit an inappropriate response, and form/understand new concepts/ideas (Fridriksson et al., 2006). In a study of 20 aphasic participants, Ramsberger and Rende (2002) found that 8 of 9 executive measures were significantly associated with variables of conversational success.

Comparable findings were reported by Fridriksson et al. (2006), who noted significant correlations among executive measures of sequencing, inhibition, planning, cognitive flexibility, working memory, attention, perception, and motor skills. The tests they used included executive tasks such as the WCST and the Color Trails Tests (D'Elia, Satz, Uchiyama, & White, 1996) and the four assessment batteries of the American Speech-Language Hearing Association Functional Assessment of Communication Skills for Adults (Frattali et al., 1995). Results indicated that those participants with a greater number of prompts and errors on the executive tests were also those with lower conversational independence and quality.

Importantly, spared executive skills have also been reported to have a remedial effect on conversational skills (e.g., Ramsberger, 2005). Using a neuropsychological battery testing attention, verbal and nonverbal working memory, memory, planning, and concept formation, and methods of conversational analysis, Frankel and colleagues found, for example, that preserved interference control and planning accompanied good concentration and tracking of content in conversation, and that memory for previously mentioned information went along with planned conversational strategies, turn taking, and topic management (Frankel, Penn, & Ormond-Brown, 2007).

NEURAL CORRELATES OF DISCOURSE AND EXECUTIVE
FUNCTIONS IN APHASIA

The study of the biological bases of executive functions and conversational skills among people with aphasia is relatively underexplored, as most such neuroimaging studies on this topic focus on discourse problems observed in adults following traumatic brain injury (e.g., Ferstl, Guthke, & von Cramon, 2002). A double dissociation has been found between discourse-level and syntactic sequencing among nonaphasic people with prefrontal cortex (PFC) lesions, who were unable to perform temporal sequencing at the script level but were capable of forming grammatical sequences, compared to people with agrammatic aphasia with lesions in Broca's areas, who showed the opposite pattern (Sirigu et al., 1998).

Deficits in spontaneous discourse have been identified more systematically in patients with frontal lesions in both hemispheres (Barbizet, Duizabo, & Flavigny, 1975). In addition, narratives produced by patients with PFC lesions contained syntactically simplified sentences and perseverative opening segments, while patients with orbitofrontal lesions produced syntactically complex stories with a thematic focus that was less well regulated (Kaczmarek, 1984). A more recent study by Coelho, Lê, Mozeiko, Krueger, and Grafman (2012), however, has revealed persistent impairment of discourse production alongside executive deficits following brain injury to the dorsolateral prefrontal cortex (DLPFC). These researchers found that people with a damaged left DLPFC had particular problems producing narratives, in terms of measures of coherence and story components, and that these measures were associated with nonverbal measures of poor working memory.

Alexander (2006) proposed a functional neuroanatomy linking narrative production to executive goal-directed behavior, arguing that the communication of complex verbal messages is more closely related to difficulties with action planning rather than with aphasia per se. In his model he assumes three hierarchically organized levels of language-based procedures—basic grammar/syntax, complex syntax, and narrative discourse—which rely on interconnected but somewhat separable frontal-subcortical networks that support differing attention demands. The assumption is that the more complex and more open-ended the language procedure is, the less automatized and more attention-dependent it becomes, implicating medial frontal regions (bilaterally).

Damage to these language-related networks, Alexander contends, can result in independent patterns of impairments, each representing a prototypical clinical form of language communication impairment. He describes a progression of language communication deficits following a posterior frontal-to-polar and/or lateral-to-medial frontal neural path, mapping onto impairments from basic morphosyntactic linguistic operations through more complex grammatical structures to narrative discourse. This progression reflects a clinical axis moving from typical agrammatical nonfluent aphasia through less aphasic patterns—as in transcortical motor aphasia or dynamic aphasia—to a nonaphasic, more executive-based deficit of complex narrative discourse disorder. The discourse deficits are related to impaired attentional processes resulting from lesioned superior medial and left ventrolateral frontal networks. Although this proposal directly links executive functions to discourse ability in aphasia, it is based on two case studies and tacitly relies on clinical aphasia classifications, which, as mentioned in Chapter 2, have been found to be empirically problematic.

Prognostic Value of Executive Functions in Aphasia

Because scores on language communication measures (e.g., the Communication Abilities in Daily Living; Holland, 1980), have been found to be strongly correlated with scores on tests of executive functions (e.g., the WCST), it has been argued that executive abilities such as set shifting can be used to predict aphasic person's ability to enhance his or her conversational success (e.g., Purdy & Koch, 2006). For example, executive functions have been shown to predict the extent to which a person with aphasia might be able benefit from training in alternative methods of communication (e.g., Purdy & Koch, 2006). In a study examining whether people with severe aphasia could benefit from training on a computer program (C-Speak Aphasia) to enhance their functional communication, participants who were able to provide more information on selected probe tasks following treatment were also those with more preserved executive functions at baseline, as measured by Helm-Estabrooks' (2001) scores on their Cognitive Linguistic Quick Test (Nicholas, Sinotte, & Helm-Estabrooks, 2005).

Although the exact role of executive skills in the treatment of aphasia has yet to be clarified (e.g., Seniow, Litwin, & Lesniak, 2009), executive functions have been found to be predictive of an aphasic person's ability to engage in certain aspects of aphasia therapy (Helm-Estabrooks, 2002). Indeed, generating responses, selecting among options, and applying strategies are important skills that might affect the course of aphasia treatment (Lawson & Rice, 1989; Purdy, 1992). One goal of therapy is to have a patient generalize learned strategies to real-life situations, a goal that might not be attained in the presence of a strategy-forming deficit (e.g., Purdy, 1992) or problems with abstract reasoning (e.g., Reitan, 1988). Or, conversely, preserved executive abilities could presumably enhance treatment effects. Put differently, "the process of post-stroke rehabilitation requires the involvement of all cognitive and emotional abilities of the patient. Deficits in any of these domains can impede not only the process of language function restoration, but also the compensation for the patients' disability and their regaining of independence" (Seniow, Litwin, & Lesniak, 2009, p. 91).

High performance on Raven's Colored Progressive Matrices task and the WCST has been found to predict good context-based learning abilities among people with aphasia (i.e., quicker attainment of performance criterion and maintenance of long-term generalizations post-intervention) (Hinckley, Carr, & Patterson, 2001). In a series of studies comparing the efficacy of errorless and errorful learning in anomia treatment, where examiner feedback was manipulated, higher performance on the WCST and self-ratings of response accuracy but not language scores were positively correlated with long-term naming gains (Fillingham et al., 2005, 2006). Comparable results were reported in a series of studies exploring anomia treatment among Cantonese-speaking people with aphasia (Law et al., 2006, 2008; Yeung, Law, & Yau, 2009, 2010), with best naming outcomes (successful phonological generalization on untrained items) observed among those with the highest scores on the Test of Nonverbal Intelligence

(Brown et al., 1997), a test of concept formation and abstract reasoning. However, in a larger scale study (*n* = 30), Lambon Ralph et al. (2010) found that the best predictors of anomia therapy outcome were both language performance as measured by naming scores and cognitive factors as measured by executive functions, attention, and visual recall tests.

Such findings are reminiscent of the earlier observation that higher poststroke IQ is associated with better executive skills, paving the way for speedier aphasia recovery (Bailey, Powell, & Clark, 1981). Of course general intellectual abilities are considered to be distinct from executive functions (e.g., Ardila et al., 2006; Crinella & Yu, 2000; Friedman et al., 2006), especially from inhibition and shifting abilities (Miyake et al., 2000), so their prognostic value for aphasia recovery would likely be independent of that of executive functions.

Interestingly, executive functioning and abstract reasoning, assessed via many of the tests described throughout this chapter, have been shown to have excellent prognostic value, independently predicting long-term cognitive and functional outcome among first-ever stroke survivors (Nys et al., 2005) as well as in the general stroke population (Barker-Collo et al., 2012). Patients with executive dysfunction immediately following a first-time stroke were found to be seven times more likely to exhibit persistent cognitive problems at 6 months postevaluation as opposed to those with spared executive skills. However, because the assessment of cerebral atrophy in that study was performed using a very basic analysis of computed tomography/magnetic resonance imaging scans, it is difficult to determine whether lesion characteristics may have also contributed to the reported long-term cognitive impairment (Nys et al., 2005). Although hemispheric lateralization has not been shown to reliably predict poststroke cognitive outcomes, those with anterior lesions following both left- and right-sided ischemic stroke have been found to demonstrate more persistent executive and linguistic dysfunction 5 years postonset than those whose lesions were more posterior (Barker-Collo et al., 2012).

The extent to which cognitive rehabilitation, which targets specific impaired cognitive functions in a patient, is efficacious for people with aphasia is not known (e.g., Chapey, 2008). The benefits of such treatments are typically focused on the efficacy for stroke survivors in general (e.g., Cicerone et al., 2011; Cumming, Marshall, & Lazar, 2013; Poulin, Korner-Bitensky, Dawson, & Behrer, 2012; Rholing, Faust, Beverly, & Demakis, 2009). It has been argued, for example, that the treatment of executive functions can enhance the ability to learn compensatory strategies, reducing the burden of poststroke executive dysfunction, although the superiority of such a cognitive intervention has not been demonstrated (Poulin, Korner-Bitensky, Dawson, & Behrer, 2012). Also, it is not clear whether techniques designed to stimulate neural plasticity in disorders with focal brain damage, such as aphasia, can be used to promote functional recovery when nonfocal cognitive deficits are observed (Cumming, Marshall, & Lazar, 2013).

EFFECTS ON NEURAL REORGANIZATION IN THE APHASIC BRAIN

Attempts have been made to target language support systems in aphasia in the treatment of naming deficit, exploring their effects on brain reorganization in chronic aphasia. These include, for example, studies of the effects of incorporating intention treatment, which targets mechanisms responsible for action initiation, on improving naming performance (Crosson et al., 2005, 2007, 2009).

In an fMRI study of two people with mild anomic nonfluent aphasia who received intention treatment and attention treatment without an intention component, Crosson et al. (2005) found treatment-induced neural changes in posterior persylvian regions. Because intention refers to the ability to select and initiate an action and because nonfluent aphasia often manifests as a deficit in selection and initiation of verbal output, the authors defined aphasia as a disorder of intention and predicted therapy gains for the intention but not the attention protocol. This prediction was supported by behavioral findings that demonstrated picture-naming benefits following intention treatment as compared with baseline performance (Richards et al., 2002).

In this protocol, initiation of the word finding trial was marked by performance of a left-hand motion on the left side (lifting a lid to press a button in a box, or repeating the target stimulus after the examiner using a nonsymbolic circular left-hand gesture if performance was incorrect). This initiation sequence was designed to stimulate brain activity in the right medial frontal intention mechanisms, on the assumption that following stroke, the right hemisphere subsumes some language functions. The authors further assumed that activation of left-medial structures—the presupplementary motor cortex—could interfere with this right hemisphere activation via the right basal ganglia and so reduce the processing efficiency of the linguistic information. Their treatment program was thus aimed at minimizing this inefficiency by shifting brain activity to the right pre-SMA and right lateral frontal region.

However, the aphasic participants showed differential responses to these interventions, one benefiting from both treatments and the other responding only to the intention protocol. The authors attributed these differences to neuroanatomical distinctions between the lesions of the two participants. The participant who gained from both treatments had a lesion that spared the left basal ganglia and thalamus, which enabled natural pretreatment right hemisphere reorganization of language functions, in which the left basal ganglia continued to suppress the tendency to activate the left frontal mechanisms. In the participant who responded only to the intention intervention, these subcortical structures were damaged, interfering with the natural between hemisphere transfer of word production abilities, enabled by intention intervention (triggered by left-hand movements). Because of this subcortical damage, continued left hemisphere activation could not be suppressed, leading to increased activation of right hemisphere frontal mechanisms to accomplish this inhibition. As a result, Crosson et al. (2005) suggested that assessing the extent of the basal ganglia damage can be used as a guide to the incorporation or exclusion of an intention component into the aphasia therapy program.

In a subsequent study, rapid picture relearning following intention treatment, generalizable to untrained items, was replicated by Crosson and colleagues, who found intervention effects in 89% of 23 people with moderate aphasia (Crosson et al., 2007). Neural correlates of these treatment effects involved reduced activity in left frontal networks, with concomitant increased right hemisphere activation in motor and premotor cortices and pars opercularis, in response to category-member generation tasks (Crosson et al., 2009). Although this reduced activation speaks to increased processing efficiency in service of word production, language abilities that continue to be subserved by the damaged left hemisphere are also critical for regaining word production abilities (Crosson, 2008; Naeser et al., 2005).

We have discussed these findings in the context of potential beneficial effects of treating aspects of executive functions to enhance functional recovery of language in aphasia. However, it is difficult to determine whether the treatment effects just reviewed are in fact a result of targeting executive functions. They are perhaps more strongly linked to the motor component of initiation (Picard & Strick, 1996), which we revisit in Chapter 7. Nonetheless, the encouraging results from these studies suggest that incorporating nonlinguistic executive components into therapy could perhaps enhance language performance and directly contribute to the neural reorganization of language functions in the course of aphasia recovery.

A recent functional neuroimaging study by Brownsett and colleagues (Brownsett, Warren, Geranmayeh, Woodehead, Leech, & Wise, 2014) set out to explore the neural effects of cognitive control on language performance in aphasia and to determine whether these neural patterns are related to recovery from aphasia. They examined domain-general brain activation in the midline frontal cortex, known as the salience network, which was spared among their 16 participants, as related to performance on standardized test before and after a 4-week home computer-based treatment protocol. In addition, during scanning, they asked the participants to complete a sentence-repetition task of simple sentences, which was designed to induce brain activation in language-based regions subserving speech perception, comprehension, verbal working memory, and prearticulatory rehearsal as well as regions mediating task-performance skills, such as attention, conflict resolution, and response suppression. To mimic the perceptual difficulties in the aphasic group, healthy controls were administered perceptually challenging sentences that were noise vocoded (to create distorted speech) and received a 2-week program training them to process such sentences.

Using regions of interest obtained from the healthy controls, the authors found three patterns of brain activation in both groups. The first was in the expected language perception areas, specifically the superior temporal gyri. The second was in premotor, primary sensorimotor, basal ganglia, thalami, and paravermal cerebellum, which reflect anticipation and planning of motor response—repetition—during speech perception.

The third was increased activation in the salience and executive networks and decreased activation in the default mode network. Activation of the dorsal anterior cingulate cortex and superior frontal gyrus predicted the participants' language performance on picture naming regardless of extent of lesion and age, suggesting a relationship between general cognitive control and residual language processing in aphasia. Once again, there is evidence for neural multifunctionality in the service of recovery of language functions in aphasia.

References

Ahola, K., Vilkki, J., & Servo, A. (1996). Frontal tests do not detect frontal infarctions after ruptured intracranial aneurysm. *Brain and Cognition*, *31*(1), 1–16.

Albert, M. & Knoefel, J. (2011). *Clinical Neurology of Aging*. New York: Oxford University Press.

Albert, M. L. (1990). The role of perseveration in language disorders. *Journal of Neurolinguistics*, *4*(3–4), 471–478.

Albert, M. L., Goodglass, H., Helm, N., Rubens, A., & Alexander, M. (1981). *Clinical aspects of dysphasia*. New York: Springer-Verlag.

Albert, M. L., & Sandson, J. (1986). Perseveration in aphasia. *Cortex*, *22*(1), 103–115.

Alexander, M. P. (2006). Impairments of procedures for implementing complex language are due to disruption of frontal attention processes. *Journal of the International Neuropsychological Society*, *12*(2), 236–247.

Allison, R. S., & Hurwitz, L. J. (1967). On perseveration in aphasics. *Brain*, *90*(2), 429–448.

Alvarez, J. A., & Emory, E. (2006). Executive function and the frontal lobes: a meta-analytic review. *Neuropsychological Review*, *16*(1), 17–42.

Anderson, S. W., Damasio, H., Jones, R. D., & Tranel, D. (1991). Wisconsin card sorting test performance as a measure of frontal lobe damage. *Journal of Clinical and Experimental Neuropsychology*, *13*(6), 909–922.

Anderson, V., Northam, E., Hendy, J., & Wrenall, J. (2001). *Developmental neuropsychology: a clinical approach*. New York: Psychology Press.

Archibald, Y., Wepman, J. M., & Jones, L. V. (1967). Nonverbal cognitive performance in aphasic and nonaphasic brain-damaged patients. *Cortex*, *3*(3), 275–294.

Ardila, A., Pineda, D., & Rosselli, M. (2006). Correlation between intelligence test scores and executive function measures. *Archives of Clinical Neuropsychology*, *15*, 31–36.

Ardila, A., & Surloff, C. (2004). *Dysexecutive Syndromes*. San Diego, CA: Medlink: Neurology.

Ashendorf, L., & McCaffrey, R. J. (2008). Exploring age-related decline on the Wisconsin card sorting test. *Clinical Neuropsychology*, *22*(2), 262–272.

Axelrod, B. N., Goldman, R. S., Heaton R. K., Curtiss, G., Thompson, L. T., Chelune, G. J., & Kay, G. G. (1996). Discriminability of the Wisconsin card sorting test using the standardization sample. *Journal of Clinical and Experimental Neuropsychology*, *18*, 338–342.

Bäckman, L., Ginovart, N., Dixon, R. A., Wahlin, T. B., Wahlin, A., Halldin, C., & Farde, L. (2000). Age-related cognitive deficits mediated by changes in the striatal dopamine system. *American Journal of Psychiatry*, *157*(4), 635–637.

Baddeley, A. (1986). *Working memory*. Oxford, UK: Oxford University Press.

Baddeley, A. (1992). Working memory. *Science, 225*, 556–559.

Baddeley, A. (2002). Fractionating the central executive. In D. T. Stuss & R. T. Knight (Eds.), *Principles of frontal lobe function* (pp. 246–260). New York: Oxford University Press.

Baddeley, A., Della Sala, S., Papagno, C., & Spinnler, H. (1997). Dual-task performance in dysexecutive and nondysexecutive patients with a frontal lesion. *Neuropsychology, 11*(2), 187–194.

Baddeley, A., & Hitch, G. (1974). Working memory. In G. A. Bower (Ed.), *The psychology of learning and motivation* (pp. 47–89). New York: Academic Press.

Baddeley, A., & Logie, R. (1999). Working memory: The multiple-component model. In A. Miyake & P. Shah (Eds.), *Models of working memory: mechanisms of active maintenance and executive control* (pp. 28–61). New York: Cambridge University Press.

Baddeley, A., & Wilson, B. (1988). Frontal amnesia and the dysexecutive syndrome. *Brain and Cognition, 7*, 212–230.

Badre, D., Poldrack, R. A., Paré-Blagoev, E. J., Insler, R., & Wagner, A. D. (2005). Dissociable controlled retrieval and generalized selection mechanisms in ventrolateral prefrontal cortex. *Neuron, 47*, 907–918.

Badre, D., & Wagner, A. D. (2007). Left ventrolateral prefrontal cortex and the cognitive control of memory. *Neuropsychologia, 45*, 2883–2901.

Bailey, S., Powell, G. E., & Clark, E. (1981). A note on intelligence and recovery from aphasia: the relationship between Raven's matrices scores and change on the Schuell aphasia test. *International Journal of Language & Communication Disorders, 16*(3), 193–203.

Baldo, J. V., Bunge S. A., Wilson S. M., & Dronkers N. F. (2010). Is relational reasoning dependent on language? A voxel-based lesion symptom mapping study. *Brain and Language, 113*, 59–64.

Baldo, J. V., Dronkers, N. F., Wilkins, D., Ludy, C., Raskin, P., & Kim, J. (2005). Is problem solving dependent on language? *Brain and Language, 92*, 240–250.

Banich, M. T. (2004). *Cognitive neuroscience and neuropsychology*. Boston: Houghton Mifflin.

Banich, M.T. (2009). Executive function. The search for an integrated account. *Current Directions in Psychological Science, 18*(2), 89–94.

Barbas, H., Garcia-Cabezas, M. A., & Zikopoulos, B. (2013). Frontal-thalamic circuits associated with language. *Brain and Language, 126*(1), 49–61.

Barbizet, J., Duizabo, P., & Flavigny, R. (1975). Role of the frontal lobes in language. *Revue Neurologique, 131*(8), 525–544.

Barcelo, F. (2001). Does the Wisconsin card sorting test measure pre-frontal function? *Spanish Journal of Psychology, 4*, 79–100.

Barker-Collo, S., Starkey, N., Lawes, C. M., Feigin, V., Senior, H., & Parag, V. (2012). Neuropsychological profiles of 5-year ischemic stroke survivors by Oxfordshire stroke classification and hemisphere of lesion. *Stroke, 43*(1), 50–55.

Barkley, R. (1997). Behavioral inhibition, sustained attention, and executive functions: Constructing a unifying theory. *Psychological Bulletin, 121*, 65–94.

Basso A., Capitani, E., Luzzatti, C., & Spinnler, H. (1981). Intelligence and left hemisphere disease: the role of aphasia, apraxia, and size of lesion. *Brain, 104*, 721–734.

Basso, A., De Renzi, E., Faglioni, P., Scotti, G., & Spinnler, H. (1973). Neuropsychological evidence for the existence of cerebral areas critical to the performance of intelligence tests. *Brain, 96*, 715–728.

Bedny, M., McGill, M., & Thompson-Schill, S. L. (2008). Semantic adaptation and competition during word comprehension. *Cerebral Cortex, 18*(11), 2574–2585.

Beeson, P. M., Bayles, K. A., Rubens, A. B., & Kaszniak, A. W. (1993). Memory impairment and executive control in individuals with stroke-induced aphasia. *Brain and Language, 45,* 253–275.

Berthier, M. L. (2001).Unexpected brain-language relationships in aphasia: evidence from transcortical sensory aphasia associated with frontal lobe lesions. *Aphasiology, 15*(2), 99–130.

Bishara, A. J., Kruschke, J. K., Stout, J. C., Bechara, A., McCabe, D. P., & Busemeyer, J. R. (2010). Sequential learning models for the Wisconsin card sort task: assessing processes in substance dependent individuals. *Journal of Mathematical Psychology, 54,* 5–13.

Blair, C. (2006). How similar are fluid cognition and general intelligence? A developmental neuroscience perspective on fluid cognition as an aspect of human cognitive ability. *Behavioral and Brain Sciences, 29,* 109–125.

Blair, C., Zelazo, P. D., & Greenberg, M. T. (2005). The measurement of executive function in early childhood. *Developmental Neuropsychology, 28*(2), 561–571.

Bokde, A. L., Tagamets, M. A., Friedmann, R. B., & Horwitz, B. (2001). Functional interactions of the inferior frontal cortex during the processing of words and word-like stimuli. *Neuron, 30*(2), 609–617.

Borkowski, J. G., & Burke, J. E. (1996). Theories, models, and measurements of executive functioning: an information processing perspective. In G. R. Lyon & N. A. Krasnegor (Eds.), *Attention, memory, and executive function* (pp. 235–261). Baltimore, MD: Paul Brookes.

Borod, J. C., Carper, M., & Goodglass, H. (1982). WAIS performance IQ in aphasia as a function of auditory comprehension and constructional apraxia. *Cortex, 18*(2), 199–201.

Borod, J.C., Carper, M., Goodglass, H., & Naeser, M. (1984). Aphasic performance on a battery of constructional, visuospatial, and quantitative tasks: factorial structure and CT scan localization. *Journal of Clinical Neuropsychology, 6*(2), 189–204.

Brandimonte, M., Einstein, G. O., & McDaniel, M. A. (1996). *Prospective memory: theory and applications*. Mahwah, NJ: Erlbaum.

Brown, L., Sherbenou, R. J., & Johnsen, S. K. (1997). *Test of nonverbal intelligence* (3rd ed.). Austin, TX: Pro-Ed.

Brownsett, S.L.E. Warren, J. E., Geranmayeh, F., Woodhead, Z., Leech, R., & Wise, R.J.S. (2014). Cognitive control and its impact on recovery from aphasic stroke. *Brain, 137,* 242–254.

Buckingham, H. (1985). Perseveration in aphasia. In S. Newman & R. Epstein (Eds.), *Current perspectives in dysphasia*. Edinburgh: Churchill Livingstone.

Buckner, R. L. (1996). Beyond HERA: Contributions of specific prefrontal brain areas to long-term memory retrieval. *Psychonomic Bulletin & Review, 3*(2), 149–158.

Buckner, R. L., Raichle, M. E., & Petersen, S. E. (1995). Dissociation of human prefrontal cortical areas across different speech production tasks and gender groups. *Journal of Neurophysiology, 74*(5), 2163–2173.

Burgess P. W., Alderman N., Evans J., Emslie H., & Wilson B. A. (1998). The ecological validity of tests of executive function. *Journal of the International Neuropsychological Society, 4*(6), 547–558.

Carpenter, P. A., Just, M. A., & Reichle, E. D. (2000). Working memory and executive function: Evidence from neuroimaging. *Current Opinion in Neurobiology, 10*(2), 195–199.

Carruthers, P. (2002). The cognitive functions of language. *Behavioral and Brain Sciences, 25*(6), 657–674.

Caspari, I., Parkinson, S. R., LaPointe, L. L., & Katz, R. C. (1998). Working memory and aphasia. *Brain and Cognition, 37*, 205–223.

Chapey, R. (2008). *Language intervention strategies in aphasia and related neurogenic communication disorders* (5th ed.). Baltimore, MD: Wolters Kluwer/Lippincott Williams & Wilkins.

Chatterjee, A., Yapundich, R., Mennemeier, M., Mountz, J. M., Inampudi, C., Pan, J. W., & Mitchell, G.W. (1997). Thalamic thought disorder: on being "a bit addled." *Cortex, 33*(3), 419–440.

Chevignard, M., Pillon, B., Pradat-Diehl, P., Taillefer, C., Rousseau, S., Le Bras, C., & Dubois, B. (2000). An ecological approach to planning dysfunction: script execution. *Cortex, 36*(5), 649–669.

Chevignard, M. P., Taillefer, C., Picq, C., Poncet, F., Noulhiane, M., & Pradat-Diehl, P. (2008). Ecological assessment of the dysexecutive syndrome using execution of a cooking task. *Neuropsychological Rehabilitation, 18*(4), 461–485.

Chiou, H. S., & Kennedy, M.R.T. (2009). Switching in adults with aphasia. *Aphasiology, 23*(7–8), 1065–1075.

Cicerone, K. D., Langenbahn, D. M., Braden, C., Malec, J. F., Kalmar, K., Fraas, M., ... Ashman, T. (2011). Evidence-based cognitive rehabilitation: Updated review of the literature from 2003 through 2008. *Archives of Physical Medicine and Rehabilitation, 92*(4), 519–530.

Coelho, C., Lê, K., Mozeiko, J., Krueger, F., & Grafman, J. (2012). Discourse production following injury to the dorsolateral prefrontal cortex. *Neuropsychologia, 50*(14), 3564–3572.

Coelho, C. A., Liles, B. Z., & Duffy, R. J. (1995). Impairments of discourse abilities and executive functions in traumatically brain-injured adults. *Brain Injury, 9*(5), 471–477.

Copland, D. (2003). The basal ganglia and semantic engagement: potential insights from semantic priming in individuals with subcortical vascular lesions, Parkinson's disease, and cortical lesions. *Journal of the International Neuropsychological Society, 9*(7), 1041–1052.

Corbett, F., Jefferies, E., Ehsan, S., & Lambon Ralph, M. A. (2009). Different impairments of semantic cognition in semantic dementia and semantic aphasia: evidence from the non-verbal domain. *Brain, 132*(Pt9), 2593–2608.

Corbett, F., Jefferies, E., & Lambon Ralph, M. A. (2009). Exploring multimodal semantic control impairments in semantic aphasia: evidence from naturalistic object use. *Neuropsychologia, 47*(13), 2721–2731.

Corbett, F., Jefferies, E., & Lambon Ralph, M. A. (2011) Deregulated semantic cognition follows prefrontal and temporo-parietal damage: evidence from the impact of task constraint on nonverbal object use. *Journal of Cognitive Neuroscience, 23*(5), 1125–1135.

Crinella, F. M., & Yu, J. (2000). Brain mechanisms and intelligence. Psychometric g and executive function. *Intelligence, 27*(4), 299–327.

Crosson, B. (2008). An intention manipulation to change lateralization of word production in nonfluent aphasia: current status. *Seminars in Speech and Language, 29*(3), 188–200.

Crosson, B. (2013). Thalamic mechanisms in language: A reconsideration based on recent findings and concepts. *Brain and Language, 126*(1), 73–88.

Crosson, B., Benefield, H., Cato, M. A., Sadek, J. R., Moore, A. B., Wierenga, C. E., ... Briggs, R. W. (2003). Left and right basal ganglia and frontal activity during language generation: contributions to lexical, semantic, and phonological processes. *Journal of the International Neuropsychological Society, 9*(7), 1061–1077.

Crosson, B., Fabrizio, K. S., Singletary, F., Cato, M. A., Wierenga, C. E., Parkinson, R. B., ... Rothi, L.J. (2007). Treatment of naming in nonfluent aphasia through manipulation of intention and attention: a phase 1 comparison of two novel treatments. *Journal of the International Neuropsychological Society, 13*(4), 582–594.

Crosson, B., Moore, A. B., Gopinath, K., White, K. D., Wierenga, C. E., & Gaiefsky, M.E., ... Gonzalez Rothi, L. J. (2005). Role of the right and left hemispheres in recovery of function during treatment of intention in aphasia. *Journal of Cognitive Neuroscience, 17*(3), 392–406.

Crosson, B., Moore, A. B., McGregor, K. M., Chang, Y. L., Benjamin, M., Gopinath, K., ... White, K. D. (2009). Regional changes in word-production laterality after a naming treatment designed to produce a rightward shift in frontal activity. *Brain and Language, 111*(2), 73–85.

Crosson, B., Sadek, J. R., Maron, L., Gökçay, D., Mohr, C. M., Auerbach, E. J., ... Briggs, R. W. (2001). Relative shift in activity from medial to lateral frontal cortex during internally versus externally guided word generation. *Journal of Cognitive Neuroscience, 13*(2), 272–283.

Cumming, T. B., Marshall, R. S., & Lazar, R. M. (2013). Stroke, cognitive deficits, and rehabilitation: still an incomplete picture. *International Journal of Stroke, 8*(1), 38–45.

Damasio, A. R. (1994). *Descartes' error: emotion, reason, and the human brain.* New York: Grosset/Putnam.

De Frias, C., Dixon, R., & Strauss, E. (2006). Structure of four executive functioning tests in healthy older adults. *Neuropsychology, 20*(2), 206–214.

De Renzi, E., Faglioni, P., Savoiardo, M., & Vignolo, L. A. (1966). The influence of aphasia and of the hemispheric side of the cerebral lesion on abstract thinking. *Cortex, 2*(4), 399–420.

Delis, D. C., Kaplan, E., & Kramer, J. H. (2001). *Delis-Kaplan executive function system.* San Antonio, TX: Psychological Corporation.

Demb, J. B., Desmond, J. E., Wagner, A. D., Vaidya, C. J., Glover, G. H., & Gabrieli, J. D. (1995). Semantic encoding and retrieval in the left inferior prefrontal cortex: a functional MRI study of task difficulty and process specificity. *Journal of Neuroscience, 15*(9), 5870–5878.

Drewe, E. A. (1975). Go no-go learning after frontal lobe lesions in humans. *Cortex, 11*, 8–16.

Duda, J. T., McMillan, C., Grossman, M., & Gee, J. C. (2010). Relating structural and functional connectivity to performance in a communication task. *Medical Image Computing and Computer-Assisted Intervention, 13*(Pt2), 282–289.

Duffy, J. D., & Campbell, J. J. (2001). Regional prefrontal syndromes. In D. P. Salloway, P. F. Malloy, & J. D. Duffy (Eds.), *The frontal lobes and psychiatric illness,* (pp. 113–123). Washington, DC: American Psychiatric Publishing.

Duke, L. M., & Kaszniak, A. W. (2000). Executive control functions in degenerative dementias: a comparative review. *Neuropsychogical Review, 10*(2), 75–99.

Duncan, J., Burgess, P., & Emslie, H. (1995). Fluid intelligence after frontal lobe lesions. *Neuropsychologia, 33*(3), 261–268.

Duncan, J., Emslie, H., Williams, P., Johnson, R., & Freer, C. (1996). Intelligence and the frontal lobe: the organization of goal-directed behavior. *Cognitive Psychology, 30*(3), 257–303.

Duncan, J., Johnson, R., Swales, M., & Freer, C. (1997). Frontal lobe deficits after head injury: Unity and diversity of function. *Cognitive Neuropsychology, 14*, 713–741.

Dutil, E., Bottari, C., Vanier, M., & Gaudreault, C. (2005). *Activities of daily living profile, (Profil des AVQ: Description de l'outil)* (4th ed.). Montréal: Les Éditions Émerion.

Edwards, S., Ellams, J., & Thompson, J. (1976). Language and intelligence in dysphasia: are they related? *International Journal of Language & Communication Disorders, 11*(2), 83–94.

Elliot, R. (2003). Executive functions and their disorders. *British Medical Bulletin, 65*, 49–59.

Ellis, A. W., & Young, A. W. (1996). *Human cognitive neuropsychology.* East Sussex, UK: Psychology Press.

Emery, P., & Helm-Estabrooks, N. (1989). The role of perseveration in aphasic confrontation naming performance. *Proceedings of Clinical Aphasiology Conference, 18*, 64–83.

Eslinger, P. J., & Damasio, A. R. (1985). Severe disturbance of higher cognition after bilateral frontal lobe ablation: patient EVR. *Neurology, 35*(12), 1731–1741.

Ferstl, E. C., Guthke, T., & von Cramon, D. Y. (2002). Text comprehension after brain injury: left prefrontal lesions affect inference processes. *Neuropsychology, 16*(3), 292–308.

Ferstl, E. C., Neumann, J., Bogler, C., & von Cramon, D. Y. (2008). The extended language network: a meta-analysis of neuroimaging studies on text comprehension. *Human Brain Mapping, 29*(5), 581–593.

Ferstl, E. C., & von Cramon, D. Y. (2002). What does the frontomedian cortex contribute to language processing: coherence or theory of mind? *NeuroImage, 17*(3), 1599–1612.

Filley, C.M. (1995). *Neurobehavioral anatomy.* Niwot: University Press of Colorado.

Filley, C. (2000). Clinical neurology and executive dysfunction. *Seminars in Speech and Language, 21*(2), 95–108.

Fillingham, J. K., Sage, K., & Lambon Ralph, M.A. (2005). Treatment of anomia using errorless versus errorful learning: are frontal executive skills and feedback important? *International Journal of Language and Communication Disorders, 40*(4), 505–523.

Fillingham, J. K., Sage, K., & Lambon Ralph, M. A. (2006). The treatment of anomia using errorless learning. *Neuropsychological Rehabilitation, 16*(2), 129–154.

Fletcher, J. (1996). Executive functions in children: Introduction to the special series. *Developmental Neuropsychology, 12*, 1–3.

Frankel, T., Penn, C., & Ormond-Brown, D. (2007). Executive dysfunction as an explanatory basis for conversation symptoms of aphasia: A pilot study. *Aphasiology, 21*, 814–828.

Frattali, C. M., Thompson, C. M., Holland, A.L., Wohl, C. B., & Ferketic, M. M. (1995). The FACS of life: ASHA facs—a functional outcome measure for adults. *American Speech-Language-Hearing Association, 37*(4), 40–46.

Fridriksson, J., Nettles, C., Davis, M., Morrow, L., & Montgomery, A. (2006). Functional communication and executive function in aphasia. *Clinical Linguistics and Phonetics, 20*, 401–410.

Friedman, N. P., Miyake, A., Corley, R. P., Young, S. E., Defries, J. C., & Hewitt, J. K. (2006). Not all executive functions are related to intelligence. *Psychological Science, 17*(2), 172–179.

Friedman, N. P., Miyake, A., Young, S. E., Defries, J. C., Corley R. P., & Hewitt, J. K. (2008). Individual differences in executive functions are almost entirely genetic in origin. *Journal of Experimental Psychology: General, 137*(2), 201–225.

Fucetola, R., Connor, L. T., Strube, M. J., & Corbetta, M. (2009). Unraveling nonverbal cognitive performance in acquired aphasia, *Aphasiology, 23*(12), 1418–1426.

Fuster, J. M. (1997). *The prefrontal cortex—anatomy, physiology, and neuropsychology of the frontal lobe* (3rd ed). Philadelphia: Lippincott-Raven.

Fuster, J. M. (2002). Physiology of executive functions: the perception-action cycle. In D. T. Stuss & R. T. Knight (Eds.), *Principles of frontal lobe function* (pp. 96–108). Oxford, UK: Oxford University Press.

Gabrieli, J. D., Desmond, J. E., Demb, J. B., Wagner, A. D., Stone, M. V., Vaidya, C. H., & Glover, G. H. (1996). Functional magnetic resonance imaging of semantic memory processes in the frontal lobes. *Psychological Science, 7*(5), 278–283.

Gabrieli, J. D., Poldrack, R. A., & Desmond, J. E. (1998). The role of left prefrontal cortex in language and memory. *Proceedings of the National Academy of Sciences of the United States of America, 95*(3), 906–913.

Gardner, H. E., Lambon Ralph,.M. A., Dodds, N., Jones, T., Ehsan, S., & Jefferies, E. (2012). The differential contributions of pFC and temporo-parietal cortex to multimodal semantic control: exploring refractory effects in semantic aphasia. *Journal of Cognitive Neuroscience, 24*(4), 778–793.

Garon, N., Bryson, S. E., & Smith, I. M. (2008). Executive function in preschoolers: a review using an integrative framework. *Psychological Bulletin, 134*(1), 31–60.

Glosser, G., & Goodglass, H. (1990). Disorders in executive control functions among aphasic and other brain-damaged patients. *Journal of Clinical and Experimental Neuropsychology, 12*(4), 485–501.

Godefroy, O., Azouvi, P., Robert, P., Roussel, M., LeGall, D., & Meulemans, T. (2010). On the behalf of the GREFEX study group dysexecutive syndrome. Diagnostic criteria and validation study. *Annals of Neurology, 68*, 855–864.

Godefroy, O., Cabaret, M., Petit-Chenal, V., Pruvo, V. P., & Rousseaux, M. (1999). Control functions of the frontal lobes: modularity of the central-supervisory system? *Cortex, 35*, 1–20.

Gold, B. T., & Buckner, R. L. (2002). Common prefrontal regions coactivate with dissociable posterior regions during controlled semantic and phonological tasks. *Neuron, 35*(4), 803–812.

Goldberg, E. (2001). *The executive brain: frontal lobes and the civilized mind*. New York: Oxford University Press.

Goldenberg, G., Dettmers, H., Grothe, C., & Spatt, J. (1994). Influence of linguistic and nonlinguistic capacities on spontaneous recovery of aphasia and on success of language therapy. *Aphasiology, 8*, 443–456.

Grafman, J., Litvan, I., Gomez, C., & Chase, T. N. (1990). Frontal lobe function in progressive supranuclear palsy. *Archives of Neurology, 47*(5), 553–558.

Grant, D. A., & Berg, E. A. (1948). A behavioral analysis of degree of reinforcement and ease of shifting to new responses in a Weigl-type card-sorting problem. *Journal of Experimental Psychology, 38*, 404–411.

Greve, K. W., Love, J. M., Sherwin, E., Mathias, C. W., Ramzinski, P., & Levy, J. (2002). Wisconsin card sorting test in chronic severe traumatic brain injury: factor structure and performance subgroups. *Brain Injury, 16*, 29–40.

Gutbrod, K., Cohen, R., Mager, B., & Meier, E. (1989). Coding and recall of categorized material in aphasics. *Journal of Clinical and Experimental Neuropsychology, 11*(6), 821–841.

Hamsher, K. (1991). Intelligence and aphasia. In M. Sarno (Ed.), *Acquired Aphasia* (2nd ed.). San Diego, CA: Academic Press.

Heaton, R. K. (1981). *A manual for the Wisconsin card sorting test*. Odessa, FL: Psychological Assessment Resources.

Heaton, R. K., Chelune, G. J., Talley, J. L., Kay, G. G., & Curtis, G. (1993). *Wisconsin card sorting test (WCST) manual revised and expanded*. Odessa, FL: Psychological Assessment Resources.

Heilman, K., Watson, R., & Valenstein, E. (2003). Neglect and related disorders. In K. Heilman & E. Valenstein (Eds.), *Clinical Neuropsychology* (pp. 296–346). New York: Oxford University Press.

Helm-Estabrooks, N. (2001). *Cognitive linguistic quick test (CLQT)*. San Antonio, TX: The Psychological Corporation.

Helm-Estabrooks, N. (2002). Cognition and aphasia: a discussion and a study. *Journal of Communication Disorders, 35*(2), 171–186.

Helm-Estabrooks, N., & Albert, M. L. (2004). *Manual of aphasia and aphasia therapy* (2nd ed.). Austin, TX: ProEd.

Helm-Estabrooks, N., Bayles, K., Ramage, A., & Bryant, S. (1995). The relationship between cognitive performance and aphasia severity, age and education: females versus males. *Brain and Language, 51*(1), 139–141.

Helm-Estabrooks, N., Ramage, A., Bayles, K. A., & Cruz, R. (1998). Perseverative behavior in fluent and non-fluent aphasic adults. *Aphasiology, 12*(7/8), 689–698.

Helmick, J. W., & Berg, C. B. (1976). Perseveration in brain-injured adults. *Journal of Communication Disorders, 9*(2), 143–156.

Hinckley, J. J., Patterson, J., & Carr, T. H. (2001). Differential effects of context- and skill-based treatment approaches: Preliminary findings. *Aphasiology, 15*, 463–476.

Hjelmquist, E. K. (1989). Concept formation in non-verbal categorization tasks in brain-damaged patients with and without aphasia. *Scandinavian Journal of Psychology, 30*(4), 243–254.

Hobson, P., & Leeds, L. (2001). Executive functioning in older people. *Reviews in Clinical Gerontology, 11*, 361–372.

Holland, A. (1980). *CADL communicative abilities in daily living: a test of functional communication for aphasic patients*. Baltimore, MD: University Park Press.

Hurlburt, R. T. (1990). *Sampling normal and schizophrenic inner experience*. New York: Plenum Press.

Irwin, W. H., Wertz, R. T., & Avent, J. R. (2002). Relationships among language impairment, functional communication, and pragmatic performance in aphasia. *Aphasiology, 16*(8), 823–835.

Jefferies, E., & Lambon Ralph, M. A. (2006). Semantic impairment in stroke aphasia versus semantic dementia: a case-series comparison. *Brain, 129*(8), 2132–2147.

Jefferies, E., Patterson, K., & Lambon Ralph, M. A. (2008). Deficits of knowledge versus executive control in semantic cognition: insights from cued naming. *Neuropsychologia, 46*(2), 649–658.

Jurado, M. B., & Rosselli, M. (2007). The elusive nature of executive functions: a review of our current understanding. *Neuropsychology Review, 17*(3), 213–233.

Kaczmarek, B.L.J. (1984). Neurolinguistic analysis of verbal utterances in patients with focal lesions of frontal lobes. *Brain and Language, 21*(1), 52–58.

Kafer, K. L., & Hunter, M. (1997). On testing the face validity of planning/problem-solving tasks in a normal population. *Journal of the International Neuropsychological Society, 3*(2), 108–119.

Kassubek, J., Unrath, A., Huppertz, H. J., Lulé, D., Ethofer, T., Sperfeld, A. D., & Ludolph, A. C. (2005). Global brain atrophy and corticospinal tract alterations in ALS, as investigated by voxel-based morphometry of 3-D MRI. *Amyotrophic Lateral Sclerosis and Other Motor Neuron Disorders, 6*(4), 213–220.

Keil, K., & Kaszniak, A. W. (2002). Examining executive function in individuals with brain injury: a review. *Aphasiology, 16*, 305–335.

Kertesz, A., & McCabe, P. (1975). Intelligence and aphasia: performance of aphasics on Raven's coloured progressive matrices (RCPM). *Brain and Language, 2*, 387–395.

Kimberg, D.Y., D'Esposito, M., & Farah, M.J. (1997). Cognitive functions in the prefrontal cortex: working memory and executive control. *Current Directions in Psychological Science, 6*(6), 185–192.

Kliegel, M., Mackinlay, R., & Jäger, T. (2008). Complex prospective memory: development across the lifespan and the role of task interruption. *Developmental Psychology, 44*, 612–617.

Koechlin, E., Corrado, G., Pietrini, P., & Grafman, J. (2000). Dissociating the role of the medial and lateral anterior prefrontal cortex in human planning. *Proceedings of the National Academy of Sciences of the United States of America, 97*(13), 7651–7656.

Lafleche, G., & Albert, M. (1995). Executive function deficits in mild Alzheimer's disease. *Neuropsychology, 9*, 313–320.

Lambon Ralph, M. A., Snell, C., Fillingham, J. K., Conroy, P., & Sage, K. (2010). Predicting the outcome of anomia therapy for people with aphasia post CVA: both language and cognitive status are key predictors. *Neuropsychological Rehabilitation, 20*(2), 289–305.

Larrabee, G., & Haley, J. (1986). Another look at VIQ-PIQ scores and unilateral brain damage. *International Journal of Neuroscience, 29*, 141–148.

Law, S.-P., Wong, W., Sung, F., & Hon, J. (2006). A study of semantic treatment of three Chinese anomic patients. *Neuropsychological Rehabilitation, 16*, 601–609.

Law, S.-P., Yeung, O., & Chiu, K. (2008). Treatment for anomia in Chinese using an ortho phonological cueing method. *Aphasiology, 22*, 139–163.

Lawson, M., & Rice, D. (1989). Effects of training in use of executive strategies on a verbal memory problem resulting from closed head injury. *Journal of Clinical and Experimental Neuropsychology, 11*, 842–854.

Lehto, J. (1996). Are executive function tests dependent on working memory capacity? *Quarterly Journal of Experimental Psychology, 49*(1), 29–50.

Lewis, S. J., Dove, A., Robbins, T. W., Barker, R. A., & Owen, A. M. (2004). Striatal contributions to working memory: a functional magnetic resonance imaging study in humans. *European Journal of Neuroscience, 19*(3), 755–760.

Lezak, M. D. (1983). *Neuropsychological Assessment* (2nd ed.). New York: Oxford University Press.

Lezak, M. D. (1995). *Neuropsychological Assessment* (3rd ed.). New York: Oxford University Press.

Lezak, M. D., Howieson, D. B., & Loring, D. W. (2004). *Neuropsychological assessment* (4th ed.). New York: Oxford University Press.

Li, K.Z.H., & Lindenberger, U. (2002). Relations between aging sensory/sensorineuromotor and cognitive functions. *Neuroscience & Biobehavioral Reviews, 26*(7), 777–783.

Luria, A. R. (1973). *The working brain: an introduction to neuropsychology.* New York: Basic Books.

Mazoyer, B. M., Tzourio, N., Frak, V., Syrota, A., Murayama, N., & Levrier, O. (1993). The cortical representation of speech. *Journal of Cognitive Neuroscience, 5,* 467–479.

McCabe, D. P., Roediger, H. L., McDaniel, M. A., Balota, D. A., & Hambrick, D. Z. (2010). The relationship between working memory capacity and executive functioning: evidence for a common executive attention construct. *Neuropsychology, 24*(2), 222–243.

Mecklinger, A. D., von Cramon, D. Y., Springer, A., & Matthes-von Cramon, G. (1999). Executive control functions in task switching: Evidence from brain injured patients. *Journal of Clinical and Experimental Neuropsychology, 21*(5), 606–619.

Mesulam, M. M. (1986). Frontal cortex and behavior. *Annals of Neurology, 19*(4), 320–325.

Milner, B. (1963). Effects of different brain lesions on card sorting: the role of the frontal lobes. *Archives of Neurology, 9,* 100–110.

Milner, B. (1964). Some effects of frontal lobectomy in man. In J. M. Warren & K. Akert (Eds.), *The frontal granular cortex and behavior* (pp. 313–334). New York: McGraw-Hill.

Miyake, A., & Friedman, N. P. (2012). The nature and organization of individual differences in executive functions: four general conclusions. *Current Directions in Psychological Science, 21*(1), 8–14.

Miyake, A., Emerson, M. J., & Friedman, N. P. (2000). Assessment of executive functions in clinical settings: problems and recommendations. *Seminars in Speech and Language, 21,* 169–183.

Miyake, A., Friedman, N. P., Emerson, M. J., Witzki, A. H., Howeter, A., & Wager, T. D. (2000). The unity and diversity of executive functions and their contributions to complex frontal lobe tasks: a latent variable analysis. *Cognitive Psychology, 41*(1), 49–100.

Miyake, A., Friedman, N. P., Rettinger, D. A., Shah, P., & Hegarty, M. (2001). How are visuospatial working memory, executive functioning, and spatial abilities related? A latent-variable analysis. *Journal of Experimental Psychology: General, 130*(4), 621–640.

Monchi, O., Petrides, M., Strafella, A. P., Worsley, K. J., & Doyon, J. (2006). Functional role of the basal ganglia in the planning and execution of actions. *Annals of Neurology, 59*(2), 257–264.

Moscovitch, M., & Winocur, G. (1992). Frontal lobes and memory. In L. R. Squire (Ed.), *The encyclopedia of learning and memory: neuropsychology.* Hillsdale, NJ: Erlbaum.

Murray, L. L., & Ramage, A. E. (2000). Assessing the executive function abilities of adults with neurogenic communication disorders. *Seminars in Speech and Language, 21*(2), 153–167.

Murray, L. L., Ramage, A. E., & Hopper, A. (2001). Memory impairments in adults with neurogenic communication disorders. *Seminars in Speech and Language, 22*(2), 127–136.

Nadeau, S. E., Crosson, B. (1997). Subcortical aphasia. *Brain and Language, 58*(3), 355–402.

Naeser, M. A., Martin, P. I., Nicholas, M., Baker, E. H., Seekins, H., Kobayashi, M., ... Pascual-Leone, A. (2005). Improved picture naming in chronic aphasia after TMS to part of right Broca's area, an open-protocol study. *Brain and Language, 93(1),* 95–105.

Nicholas, M., Sinotte, M. P., & Helm-Estabrooks, N. (2005). Using a computer to communicate: Effect of executive function impairments in people with severe aphasia. *Aphasiology, 19,* 1052–1065.

Nolte, J. (1993). *The human brain: an introduction to its functional anatomy* (3rd ed.). St Louis, MO: Mosby Year Book.

Noonan, K. A., Jefferies, E., Corbett, F., & Lambon Ralph, M. A. (2010). Elucidating the nature of deregulated semantic cognition in semantic aphasia: evidence for the roles of prefrontal and tempoparietal cortices. *Journal of Cognitive Neuroscience, 22*(7), 1597–1613.

Norman, D. A., & Shallice, T. (1986). Attention to action: willed and automatic control of behavior. In R. J. Davidson, G. E. Schwartz, & D. Shapiro (Eds.), *Consciousness and self-regulation: advances in research and theory*. New York: Plenum.

Norris, G., & Tate, R. L. (2000). The behavioral assessment of the dysexecutive syndrome (BADS): ecological, concurrent, and construct validity. *Neuropsychological Rehabilitation, 10*(1), 33–45.

Novick, J. M., Trueswell, J. C., & Thompson-Schill, S. L. (2010). Broca's area and language processing: evidence for the cognitive control connection. *Language and Linguistics Compass, 4*(10), 906–924.

Nys, G. M., Van Zandvoort, M. J., De Kort, P. L., Jansen, B. P., Van der Worp, H. B., Kappelle, L. J., & De Haan, E. H. (2005). Domain-specific cognitive recovery after first-ever stroke: a follow-up study of 111 cases. *Journal of the International Neuropsychological Society, 11*(7), 795–806.

Parkin, A., & Java, R. (1999). Deterioration of frontal lobe function in normal aging: influences of fluid intelligence versus perceptual speed. *Neuropsychology, 9*, 304–312.

Pennington, B. F., Bennetto, L., McAleer, O., & Roberts, R. J. (1996). Executive functions and working memory: Theoretical and measurement issues. In R. G. Lyon and N. A. Krasnegor (Eds.), *Attention, memory, and executive function* (pp. 327–348). Baltimore, MD: Paul H. Brookes.

Pennington, B. F., & Ozonoff, S. (1996). Executive functions and developmental psychopathology. *Journal of Child Psychology and Psychiatry, 37*(1), 51–87.

Petersen, S. E., Fox, P. T., Posner, M. I., Mintun, M., & Raichle, M. E. (1989). Positron emission topographic studies of the processing of single words. *Journal of Cognitive Neuroscience, 1*(2), 153–170.

Petrides, M., & Milner, B. (1982). Deficits on subject-ordered tasks after frontal- and temporal-lobe lesions in man. *Neuropsychologia, 20*(3), 249–262.

Phillips, L. H. (1997). Do "frontal tests" measure executive function? Issues of assessment and evidence from fluency tests. In P. Rabbitt (Ed.), *Methodology of frontal and executive function* (pp. 191–213). Hove, UK: Psychology Press.

Phillips, L. H., & Della Sala, S. (1998). Aging, intelligence, and anatomical segregation in the frontal lobes. *Learning and Individual Differences, 10*(3), 217–243.

Picard, N., & Strick, P. L. (1996). Motor areas of the medial wall: a review of their location and functional activation. *Cerebral Cortex, 6*(3), 342–353.

Piguet, O., Grayson, D. A., Broe, G. A., Tate, R. L., Bennett, H. P., Lye T. C., ... Ridley, L. (2002). Normal aging and executive functions in "old-old" community dwellers: poor performance is not an inevitable outcome. *International Psychogeriatrics, 14*(2), 139–159.

Poldrack, R. A., Wagner, A. D., Prull, M. W., Desmond, J. E., Glover, G. H., & Gabrieli, J. D. (1999). Functional specialization for semantic and phonological processing in the left inferior prefrontal cortex. *NeuroImage, 10*(1), 15–35.

Poulin, V., Korner-Bitensky, N., & Dawson, D. R. (2013). Stroke-specific executive function assessment: a literature review of performance-based tools. *Australian Occupational Therapy Journal*, *60*(1), 3–19.

Poulin, V., Korner-Bitensky, N., Dawson, D. R., & Bherer, L. (2012). Efficacy of executive function interventions after stroke: a systematic review. *Topics in Stroke Rehabilitation*, *19*(2), 158–171.

Purdy, M. (1992). *The relationship between executive functioning ability and communication success in aphasic adults*. Ann Arbor, MI: University Microfilms International.

Purdy, M., Duffy, R., & Coelho, C. (1994). An investigation of the communicative use of trained symbols in aphasic adults following multimodality training. In P. Lemme (Ed.), *Clinical aphasiology* (Vol. 22, pp. 345–356). Austin, TX: Pro-Ed.

Purdy, M., & Koch, A. (2006). Prediction of strategy usage by adults with aphasia. *Aphasiology*, *20*(2/3/4), 337–348.

Rabbitt, P. (1997). Methodologies and models in the study of executive function. In P. Rabbitt (Ed.), *Methodology of frontal and executive function* (pp. 1–38). East Sussex, UK: Psychology Press.

Radanovic, M., Azambuja, M., Mansur, L. L., Porto, C. S., & Scaff, M. (2003). Thalamus and language: interface with attention, memory and executive functions. *Arquivos de Neuro-psiquiatria*, *61*(1), 34–42.

Raichle, M. E., Fiez, J. A., Videen, T. O., MacLeod, A. K., Pardo, J. V., Fox, P. T., & Peterson, S. E. (1994). Practice-related changes in human brain functional anatomy during nonmotor learning. *Cerebral Cortex*, *4*(1), 8–26.

Ramsberger, G. (1994). Functional perspective for assessment and rehabilitation of persons with severe aphasia. *Seminars in Speech & Language*, *15*(1), 1–16

Ramsberger, G. (2005). Achieving conversational success in aphasia by focusing on non-linguistic cognitive skills: A potentially promising new approach. *Aphasiology*, *19*, 1066–1073.

Ramsberger, G., & Rende, B. (2002). Measuring transactional success in the conversation of people with aphasia. *Aphasiology*, *16*(3), 337–353.

Rapport, M. D., Chung, K. M., Shore, G., Denney, C. B., & Isaacs, P. (2000). Upgrading the science and technology of assessment and diagnosis: laboratory and clinic-based assessment of children with ADHD. *Journal of Clinical Child and Adolescent Psychology*, *29*(4), 555–568.

Raven, J. (1981). *Manual for Raven's progressive matrices and vocabulary scales. Research supplement no. 1: the 1979 British standardisation of the standard progressive matrices and Mill Hill Vocabulary Scales, together with comparative data from earlier studies in the UK, US, Canada, Germany, and Ireland*. Oxford, UK: Oxford Psychologists Press/San Antonio, TX: The Psychological Corporation.

Raymer, A.M. (2005). Naming and word-retrieval problems. In L. LaPointe (Ed.), *Aphasia and related neurogenic language disorders* (3rd ed.). New York: Thieme.

Raymer, A. M., Moberg, P., Crosson, B., Nadeau, S., & Rothi, L. J. (1997). Lexical-semantic deficits in two patients with dominant thalamic infarction. *Neuropsychologia*, *35*(2), 211–219.

Raz, N. (2005). The aging brain observed in vivo: differential changes and their modifiers. In R. Cabeza, L. Nyberg, & D. Park (Eds.), *Cognitive neuroscience of aging* (pp. 19–57). New York: Oxford University Press.

Reitan, R. (1988). Integration of neuropsychological theory, assessment, and application. *The Clinical Neuropsychologist, 2*(4), 331–349.

Reitan, R. M. (1960). The validity of the trail making test as an indicator of organic brain damage. *Perceptual and Motor Skills, 8*, 271–276.

Reitan, R. M., & Wolfson, D. (1994). A selective and critical review of neuropsychological deficits and the frontal lobes. *Neuropsychology Review, 4*(3), 161–198.

Rende, B. (2000). Cognitive flexibility: theory, assessment, and treatment. *Seminars in Speech and Language, 21*(2), 121–132.

Rhodes, M. G. (2004). Age-related difference in performance on the Wisconsin card sorting test: A meta-analytic review. *Psychology and Aging, 19*, 482–494.

Rholing, M. L., Faust, M. E., Beverly, B., & Demakis, G. (2009). Effectiveness of cognitive rehabilitation following acquired brain injury: a meta-analytic re-examination of Cicerone et al.'s (2000, 2005) systematic reviews. *Neuropsychology, 23*(1), 20–39.

Richards, K., Singletary, F., Rothi, L. J., Koehler, S., & Crosson, B. (2002). Activation of intentional mechanisms through utilization of nonsymbolic movements in aphasia rehabilitation. *Journal of Rehabilitation Research and Development, 39*(4), 445–454.

Robinson, A. L., Heaton, R. K., Lehman, R.A.W., & Stilson, D. W. (1980). The utility of the Wisconsin card sorting test in detecting and localizing frontal lobe lesions. *Journal of Consulting and Clinical Psychology, 48*, 605–614.

Robinson, G., Shallice, T., Bozzali, M., & Cipolotti, L. (2010). Conceptual proposition selection and the LIFG: neuropsychological evidence from a focal frontal group. *Neuropsychologia, 48*(6), 1652–1663.

Robinson, G., Shallice, T., & Cipolotti, L. (2005). A failure of high level verbal response selection in progressive dynamic aphasia. *Cognitive Neuropsychology, 22*(6), 661–694.

Rodríguez-Aranda, C., & Sundet, K. (2006). The frontal hypothesis of cognitive aging: factor structure and age effects on four "frontal tests" among healthy individuals. *Journal of Genetic Psychology, 167*(3), 269–287.

Rogers, R. D., & Monsell, S. (1995). The costs of a predictable switch between simple cognitive tasks. *Journal of Experimental Psychology: General, 124*, 207–231.

Roskies, A. L., Fiez, J. A., Balota, D. A., Raichle, M. E., & Petersen, S. E. (2001). Task-dependent modulation of regions in the left inferior frontal cortex during semantic processing. *Journal of Cognitive Neuroscience, 13*(6), 829–843.

Roussel, M., Dujardin, K., Henon, H., & Godefroy, O. (2012). Is the frontal dysexecutive syndrome due to a working memory deficit? Evidence from patients with stroke. *Brain, 135*, 2192–2201.

Royall, D. R., Lauterbach, E. C., Cummings, J. L., Reeve, A., Rummans, T. A., Kaufer, D. I., ... Coffey, C. E. (2002). Executive control function: a review of its promise and challenges for clinical research: a report from the Committee on Research of the American Neuropsychiatric Association. *Journal of Neuropsychiatry and Clinical Neurosciences, 14*(4), 377–405.

Salthouse, T. A. (2005). Relations between cognitive abilities and measures of executive functioning. *Neuropsychology, 19*(4), 532–545.

Salthouse, T. A., Atkinson, T. M., & Berish, D. E. (2003). Executive functioning as a potential mediator of age-related cognitive decline in normal adults. *Journal of Experimental Psychology: General, 132*(4), 566–594.

Salthouse, T. A., Siedlecki, K. L., & Krueger, L. E. (2006). An individual differences analysis of memory control. *Journal of Memory and Language, 55*, 102–125.

Sandson, J., & Albert, M. L. (1984). Varieties of perseveration. *Neuropsychologia, 22*, 715–732.

Sandson, J., & Albert, M. L. (1987). Perseveration in behavioral neurology. *Neurology, 37*(11), 1736–1741.

Santo-Pietro, M. J., & Rigrodsky, S. (1982). The effects of temporal and semantic conditions on the occurrence of the error response of perseveration in adult aphasics. *Journal of Speech and Hearing Research, 25*(2), 184–192.

Saur, D., Kreher, B. W., Schnell, S., Kümmermer, D., Kellmeyere, P., Vry, M. S., ... Weiller, C. (2008). Ventral and dorsal pathways for language. *Proceedings of the National Academy of Sciences of the United States of America, 105*(46), 18035–18040.

Saur, D., Schelter, B., Schnell, S., Kratochvil, D., Küpper, H., Kellmeyer, P., ... Weiller, C. (2010). Combining functional and anatomical connectivity reveals brain networks for auditory language comprehension. *NeuroImage, 49*(4), 2187–2197.

Schnur, T. T., Schwartz, M. F., Yimberg, D. Y., Hirshorn, E., Coslett, H. B., & Thompson-Schill, S. L. (2009). Localizing interference during naming: convergent neuroimaging and neuropsychological evidence for the function of Broca's area. *Proceedings of the National Academy of Sciences of the United States of America, 106*(1), 322–327.

Seniów, J. (2012) Executive dysfunctions and frontal syndromes. *Frontiers in Neurology and Neuroscience, 30*, 50–53.

Seniów, J., Litwin, M., & Lesniak, M. (2009). The relationship between non-linguistic cognitive deficits and language recovery in patients with aphasia. *Journal of the Neurological Sciences, 283*(1–2), 91–94.

Shallice, T. (1982). Specific impairments of planning. *Philosophical Transactions of the Royal Society, Series B, 298*, 199–209.

Shallice, T. (1998). *From neuropsychology to mental structure*. London: Cambridge University Press.

Shallice, T., & Burgess, P. W. (1991). Deficits in strategy application following frontal lobe damage in man. *Brain, 114*(Pt 2), 727–741.

Shallice, T., & Burgess, P. (1993). Supervisory control of action and thought selection. In A. D. Baddeley & L. Weiskrantz (Eds.), *Attention: selection, awareness, and control* (pp. 171–187). Oxford, UK: Oxford University Press.

Shindler, A. G., Caplan, L. R., & Hier, D. B. (1984). Intrusions and perseverations. *Brain and Language, 23*, 148–158.

Sirigu, A., Cohen, L., Zalla, T., Pradat-Diehl, P., Van Eeckhout, P., Grafman, J., & Agid, Y. (1998). Distinct frontal regions for processing sentence syntax and story grammar. *Cortex, 34*, 771–778.

Slattery, M., Garvey, M., & Swedo, S. (2001). Frontal-subcortical circuits: a functional developmental approach. In D. G. Lichter & J. L. Cummings (Eds.), *Frontal subcortical circuits in psychiatric and neurological disorders* (pp. 314–333). New York: Guilford Press.

Snyder, H. R., Banich, M. T., & Munakata, Y. (2011). Choosing our words: selection and retrieval processes recruit shared neural substrates in left ventrolateral prefrontal cortex. *Journal of Cognitive Neuroscience, 23*(11), 3470–3482.

Sokolov, A. N. (1972). *Inner speech and thought* (G.T. Onischenko, Trans.). New York: Plenum Press. (Original work published 1968).

Stark, J. (2007). A review of classical accounts of verbal perseveration and their modern-day relevance. *Aphasiology, 21*(10–11), 928–959.

Stroop, J. R. (1935). Studies of interference in serial verbal reactions. *Journal of Experimental Psychology, 18*, 643–662.

Stuss, D. T. (1992). Biological and psychological development of executive functions. *Brain and Cognition, 20*(1), 8–23.

Stuss, D. T., & Alexander, M. P. (2000). Executive functions and the frontal lobes: A conceptual review. *Psychological Research, 63*(3–4), 289–298.

Stuss, D. T., & Benson, D. F. (1986). *The frontal lobes*. New York: Raven Press.

Stuss, D. T., Binns, M. A., Murphy, K. J., & Alexander, M. P. (2002). Dissociations within the anterior attentional system: effects of task complexity and irrelevant information on reaction time speed and accuracy. *Neuropsychology, 16*(4), 500–513.

Teuber, H. L. (1972). Unity and diversity of frontal lobe functions. *Acta Neurobiologiae Experimentalis (Warsaw), 132*(2), 615–656.

Thompson-Schill, S. L., Bedny, M., & Goldberg, R. F. (2005). The frontal lobes and the regulation of mental activity. *Current Opinion in Neurobiology, 15*(2), 219–224.

Thompson-Schill, S. L., D'Esposito, M., Aguirre, G. K., & Farah, M. J. (1997). Role of left inferior prefrontal cortex in retrieval of semantic knowledge: a reevaluation. *Proceedings of the National Academy of Sciences of the United States of America, 94*(26), 14792–14797.

Thompson-Schill, S. L., Swick, D., Farah, M. J., D'Esposito, M., Kan, I. P., & Knight, R. T. (1998). Verb generation in patients with focal frontal lesions: a neuropsychological test of neuroimaging findings. *Proceedings of the National Academy of Sciences of the United States of America, 95*(26), 15855–15860.

van Mourik, M., Verschaeve, M., Boon, P., Paquier, P., & van Harskamp, F. (1992). Cognition in global aphasia: indicators for therapy. *Aphasiology, 6*(5), 491–499.

Wager, T. D., & Smith, E. E. (2003). Neuroimaging studies of working memory: a meta-analysis. *Cognitive, Affective & Behavioral Neuroscience, 3*(4), 255–274.

Wagner, A. D., Paré-Blagoev, E. J., Clark, J., & Poldrack, R. A. (2001). Recovering meaning: left prefrontal cortex guides controlled semantic retrieval. *Neuron, 31*(2), 329–338.

West, R., & Schwarb, H. (2006). The influence of aging and frontal function on the neural correlates of regulative and evaluative aspects of cognitive control. *Neuropsychology, 20*(4), 468–481.

West, R. L. (1996). An application of prefrontal cortex function theory to cognitive aging. *Psychological Bulletin, 120*(2), 272–292.

Whitney, C., Kirk, M., O'Sullivan, J., Lambon Ralph, M. A., & Jefferies, E. (2011). The neural organization of semantic control: TMS evidence for a distributed network in left inferior frontal and posterior middle temporal gyrus. *Cerebral Cortex, 21*(5), 1066–1075.

Whitney, C., Kirk, M., O'Sullivan, J., Lambon Ralph, M. A., & Jefferies, E. (2012). Executive semantic processing is underpinned by a large-scale neural network: revealing the contribution of left prefrontal, posterior temporal, and parietal cortex to controlled retrieval and selection using TMS. *Journal of Cognitive Neuroscience, 24*(1), 133–147.

Xu, J., Kemeny, S., Park, G., Frattali, C., & Braun, A. (2005). Language in context: emergent features of word, sentence, and narrative comprehension. *Neuroimage, 25*, 1002–1015.

Yeung, O., Law, S. P., & Yau, M. (2010). Executive functions and aphasia treatment outcomes: data from an ortho-phonological cueing therapy for anomia in Chinese. *International Journal of Speech-Language Pathology, 12*(6), 529–544.

Yeung, O., Law, S. P., & Yau, M. (2009). Treatment generalization and executive control processes: Preliminary data from Chinese anomic individuals. *International Journal of Language and Communication Disorders, 44*(5), 784–794.

Ylvisaker, M., & Feeney, T. J. (1998). *Collaborative Brain Injury Intervention: Positive Everyday Routines.* San Diego, CA: Singular Publishing.

Yuan, P., & Raz, N. (2014). Prefrontal cortex and executive functions in healthy adults: a meta-analysis of structural imaging studies. *Neuroscience & Behavioral Reviews, 42,* 180–192.

Zangwill, O. (1966). Psychological deficits associated with frontal lobe lesions. *International Journal of Neurology, 5,* 395–401.

Zelazo, P. D., Carter, A., Reznick, J., & Frye, D. (1997). Early development of executive functions: A problem-solving framework. *Review of General Psychology, 1,* 198–226.

Zillmer, E. A., & Spiers, M. V. (2001). *Principles of neuropsychology.* Belmont, CA: Wadsworth.

Zinn, S., Bosworth, H. B., Hoenig, H. M., & Swartzwelder, H. S. (2007). Executive function deficits in acute stroke. *Archives of Physical Medicine and Rehabilitation, 88*(2), 173–180.

4

Attention Systems and Recovery from Aphasia

Introduction

This chapter considers evidence describing how attention systems interact with changes in language abilities at both behavioral and neural levels, so as to affect brain reorganization and functional recovery among people with aphasia. Attention deficits are commonly recognized as a consequence of traumatic brain injury or right hemisphere strokes (Barker-Collo et al., 2009; Corbetta, Kincade, Lewis, Snyder, & Sapir, 2005; Murray, 2002; Tatemichi et al., 1994), but there is increasing evidence that many people with aphasia, too, suffer from attention deficits (e.g., Kalbe et al., 2005; Korda & Douglas, 1997; Kurland, 2011; Murray, 2004, 2012; Sturm et al., 1997; Tseng, et al., 1993). Kreindler and Fradis (1968), for example, found impaired performance among persons with aphasia but not among healthy controls on verbal and nonverbal tasks involving focused attention in response to stimuli presented both visually and auditorily. Several aphasiologists have thus suggested that a complete understanding of aphasic syndromes cannot be obtained without considering attentional deficiencies as a potential factor affecting language performance in this population (e.g., Erickson, Goldinger, and LaPointe, 1996; Hula & McNeil, 2008; Murray, 2000; Silkes, McNeil, & Drton, 2004).

Findings that attest to the tight link between attention systems and linguistic processes date back to early studies of auditory attention. These include studies of dichotic listening (e.g., Kimura, 1967), which examined a person's ability to ignore auditory information presented in one ear while stimuli were presented in both ears, as well as studies which explored the famously known "cocktail party effect" (Cherry, 1953), where a person's capacity to override competing speech noise was analyzed. Other examples include more recent studies of naming performance among persons with no neurological disorder under increasingly more challenging task demands, which indicate that word retrieval can be temporarily degraded, if attention systems are sufficiently taxed (e.g., Silkes, McNeil, & Drton, 2004).

However, much of what is currently known about the ways in which attention and language systems work in concert to yield a correct and timely linguistic response is based on studies of attention in persons with aphasia (e.g., Kurland, 2011). In this chapter, then, we clarify basic concepts associated with attention systems and focus on their particular relationship to language processes as evidenced in behavioral studies exploring the effects of attention on language performance among persons with aphasia (e.g., Hula & McNeil, 2008). We review how these concepts have been implemented in studies of aphasia assessment and therapy (e.g., Connor & Fucetola, 2011), summarizing the main findings, while indicating important conceptual and methodological limitations (e.g., Murray, 2012). To the extent possible, we also discuss the neural underpinnings of these attention-language interdependencies, which are only now emerging from neuroimaging studies exploring patterns of neural plasticity in both systems in response to aphasia treatment (e.g., Marcotte et al., 2013).

Some of our discussion inevitably iterates issues already considered in Chapter 3, as certain attention systems explicitly overlap with specific executive functions (e.g., set shifting and alternating attention). In other cases we foreshadow topics to be discussed in subsequent chapters (e.g., the intersection between attention and memory, which rests on the well-known argument that information better attended to is more easily encoded, stored, and retrieved [Craik & Lockhart, 1972]). Indeed, most attention models recognize the intersection among attention systems and higher cognitive systems such as working memory (e.g., Mirsky et al., 1991; Sohlberg et al., 2003; Sohlberg & Mateer, 2001). In spite of these overlaps, we will reserve the discussion of working memory to the "memory" chapter of the book (Chapter 5), a choice that highlights the challenges associated with dividing the brain into neat, functionally discrete units in a system that is inherently multifunctional.

Components of Attention

Attention has long been recognized as a multidimensional, complex, cognitive construct, implicating multiple cortical, subcortical, and brain stem structures (e.g., Fan et al., 2002; Filley, 2002; Mirsky et al., 1991; Murray, 2002; 2012; Posner & Petersen, 1990; Shallice et al., 2008; Styles, 1997; van Zomeren & Brouer, 1994). However, decades of research have yet to yield a formal characterization of attention and its components or to identify their neural underpinnings clearly (e.g., Filley, 2002). This lack of clarity derives in part from long-standing disagreements about whether attention is a causal factor controlling behavior or an emergent product of cognitive processing, whether it functions as a limited capacity resource system or a regulator of information flow, and whether the temporal features of attentional processes necessarily reflect serial processing (e.g., Kurland, 2011).

At the most basic level, the brain engages attentional processes in order to stop us from being overwhelmed by the highly stimulating environment in which we live (Filley, 2002; Petry et al., 1994). To this end, attentional processes enable us to select a stimulus among several sources for a brief instance or a longer period, in service of effective goal-directed behavior (e.g., Murray, 2002). This notion reiterates James's (1890) original claim that attention serves to alternate focus among several simultaneous stimuli, withdrawing from one stimulus in order to be able to handle other(s) more effectively. Such effective behavior can be accomplished if one is sufficiently "attentive" to react to a stimulus, stays on task, and switches one's focus to meet the demands of the environment. Our ability to assign a stimulus priority processing status has indeed been argued to depend on task novelty, sufficient levels of arousal, attentional engagement, and availability of processing resources during task performance (Kahneman, 1973).

Aspects of attention thus involve, at the very least, selectivity, orientation, arousal, vigilance, and motivation (e.g., Kurland, 2011). Most models of attention include four main components: *sustained attention*, which keeps us on task; *selective attention*, which helps with response selection; *alternating attention*, which allows us to switch our focus; and *divided attention*, which involves simultaneous attention to several stimuli. For ease of exposition, we divide the different attention components into two groups—*basic and complex attention functions*—following O'Donnell (2002). This division implies a hierarchical organization of attention systems, a view adopted by many clinicians, in order to capture patterns of functional recovery from a state of coma (e.g., Sohlberg & Mateer, 2001). We are not making the claim that this particular hierarchy, even if clinically valid, should be proposed for understanding the interaction among attention components and language systems, although some basic functions are clearly a prerequisite for more complex linguistic operations (e.g., McNeil, Odell, & Tseng, 1991).

BASIC ATTENTION: SUSTAINED ATTENTION, VIGILANCE, AND AROUSAL

Sustained attention, also termed *vigilance,* is assumed to support the ability to stay on task over the duration of an activity (Erickson, Goldinger, & LaPointe, 1996; Filley, 2002; Korda & Douglas, 1997; Laures, 2005; Laures, Odell, & Coe, 2003; Sohlberg & Mateer, 2001). This ability is expressed as a consistent behavior in response to the occasional presentation of stimuli during a continuous and/or repetitive task—for example, monitoring the appearance of a target, such as a cross, on a computer screen for several minutes, as other nontarget shapes, such as circles and squares, are randomly appear on the screen (e.g., Murray, 2002).

Vigilance is correlated with certain physiological biomarkers—including heart rate, blood pressure, and cortisol levels—which together constitute an *arousal* system that reflects the level of wakefulness of a person (Filley, 2002; Posner, Saper, Schiff, & Plum, 1982) and fuels the attention resources necessary for subsequent cognitive processing (e.g., Laures, Odell, & Coe, 2003; Murray, 2002). This claim is supported by the observation that changes in levels of arousal can affect perceptual discrimination of stimuli and that, clinically, impaired arousal is comorbid with deficits in attention (Laures, Odell, & Coe, 2003). However, it is possible to have impaired attention with intact arousal (e.g., persons in an acute confusional state who are both wakeful but highly distractible), suggesting that, neuroanatomically, there is a dissociation between these two systems (Filley, 2002).

The neuroanatomy of the arousal system (Gitelman, 2003) encompasses the mesencephalic reticular formation and parts of the thalamus, known as the ascending reticular activating system, as well as the brainstem and basal forebrain nuclei. Together, these components modulate neuronal responsivity and thus necessarily affect cortical and subcortical areas subserving attention functions (Kinomura et al., 1996). Physiological measures of arousal reflect the activation of the sympathetic nervous system (SNS) and the hypothalamic-pituitary-adrenal (HPA) axis, which are triggered at different time points in arousing situations to support immediate and prolonged responses to stimuli (Laures, Odell, & Coe, 2003). Specific biomarkers associated with these systems (e.g., heart rate variability with SNS and levels of salivary cortisol with HPA axis) are also known to be biomarkers of stress reactivity (e.g., Piazza et al., 2010), induced, for example, by the stress of anticipating or performing a language task (e.g., Cahana-Amitay et al., 2011; Laures-Gore et al., 2007, 2010). We return to this point in Chapter 6, where we discuss the interplay among emotional state (e.g., depression and anxiety), attention resources, and language performance in persons with aphasia (see also Cahana-Amitay et al., 2011).

COMPLEX ATTENTION: SELECTIVE, FOCUSED, ALTERNATING, DIVIDED ATTENTION

The ability to select a particular source of information among several for the purpose of cognitive processing is known as *selective attention* (e.g., Petry et al., 1994). This process is a prerequisite for any cognitive task as it allows the determination of which aspects of the stimulus are task-relevant and need to be attended to; it can be thought of as a filter (Kurland, 2011).

Selective attention also involves the rejection of distractors via inhibition of irrelevant information and is, therefore, often regarded as a process of *focused attention* (e.g., Murray, 1999; Murray, Holland, & Beeson, 1997). By focusing attention, interference associated with the automatic processing of a given distractor is minimized, based on perceptual and cognitive information used to identify task-relevant information (e.g.,

Lavie et al., 2004). To determine what constitutes task-relevant information, we rely on analyses of bottom-up elements, such as object features (e.g., Lupyan & Mirman, 2013; Treisman, 1993), as well as top-down components, such as establishing set (Desimone & Duncan, 1995; Kastner & Ungerleider, 2000).

To better understand these processes, consider performance on the Stroop task (Stroop, 1935), which is designed to test the ability to inhibit automatic responses (e.g., Murray, 2002). In this task, stimuli are presented in two conditions: low and high interference. In the low-interference condition, participants are asked to name words printed in different colors, as in "red," "blue," "tan," "green," "blue," "red," "tan," etc. In the high-interference condition, they are to name the color of print (the ink in which the words are printed) but to ignore the word itself. Thus if the word 'green' appears in red print, the target word is "red," not "green." Failure to ignore nontarget interfering words in the high-interference condition or slowness in reaction time to targets in the low-interference condition (which should be rapid, as both target word and ink color are the same), can be indicative of an inhibitory problem.

Indeed, in our day-to-day lives we are required, more often than not, to attend to several stimuli simultaneously—a process involving more than just inhibition of a competing stimulus. Such attention is termed *divided attention* (e.g., Kahneman, 1973; Murray, Holland, & Beeson, 1997; Wickens, 1984, 1989) and ties in with other complex attention processes that allow us to switch between tasks with different processing demands or among features within a given task. Such switching, known as *alternating attention,* is cognitively demanding and has been found to adversely affect task performance as measured in terms of accuracy and/or reaction time (Kurland, 2011). This type of attention also involves executive control processes of the sort already described in Chapter 3.

Mechanisms of "Complex" Attention

The mechanisms underlying complex attention systems are commonly argued to involve the allocation of processing resources, from a limited available pool, to meet the specific processing demands associated with a given task (e.g., Erickson, Goldinger, & LaPointe, 1996; Kahneman, 1973; McNeil, 1997). Hula and McNeil (2008) described this *resource allocation* function as a "power supply," consisting of a single pool of resources with several reservoirs, in which resources can be allocated flexibly to support the computational demands of tasks in variable domains. These domains include but are not limited to language, math, art, and music. In this context, attention is construed as "capacity" or "effort" per time unit, the function of which is to "energize" task-specific machinery. Tasks that demand little processing effort are assumed to involve *automatic* attention processing, whereas those that require greater effort are considered to be *controlled,* implicating conscious attention allocation (e.g., Schneider & Shiffrin, 1977). The distinction between these two types of processing are sometimes referred to as *reflexive* and *voluntary,* respectively (Baars, 2007).

A good example of tasks with increased processing demands are *dual tasks*, in which concurrent processing of information from multiple sources is required for successful task completion (e.g., Murray, Holland, & Beeson, 1998). The synthesis of these inputs is assumed to implicate "competition" (e.g., Erickson, Goldinger, & LaPointe, 1996; Murray, 1999), whereby several neural mechanisms compete for the same processing resources (Kurland, 2011). The extraction of task-relevant information under these conditions becomes most challenging when the competing tasks share certain properties and pose similar demands on related processing systems (e.g., when both target and distractor consist of verbal components) (Duncan, 2006). Such resource sharing can result in delayed processing of the primary task at hand, thus hindering performance (Hula & McNeil, 2008).

Attention allocation toward a task may be negatively affected by several other factors (e.g., McNeil, 1983; McNeil et al., 1991). For example, the task performer's view of the task goals can lead to overemphasis of certain aspects of the task at hand, to which more resources would be unevenly directed. Another contributor is inappropriate evaluation of task demands, where underestimation can result in insufficient resource allocation and subsequent inefficient processing. Under such circumstances, the attention allotted to the task may fail to achieve a minimal threshold of activation to allow for its completion, especially if task demands overload the processing system, as is the case with the performance of dual tasks.

Breakdown of performance on dual tasks has also been explained in terms of *bottleneck* processing, according to which simultaneous activation of a specific operation yields a bottleneck that forces the attention system into *serial* rather than *parallel* processing (e.g., Pashler, 1984, 1990, 1994). Within this framework, attention processing is assumed to proceed in three stages, involving (1) precentral perceptual encoding of the stimulus, (2) central response selection, and (3) postcentral response initiation/execution. It is assumed that the second, or central processing stage, can engage only one process at a time, leading to bottlenecks primarily during response selection. As a result, reaction time to the second task is slowed down, as the central processing modulating of that task cannot begin until the processing of the first one is completed. The closer the temporal gap between the tasks (which is sometimes termed the "psychological refractory period"), the greater the delay in reaction time of the second task. Because most dual-task experiments bias participants to perform tasks sequentially rather than simultaneously, it is difficult to compare the empirical validity of the two attention processing approaches.

THE RELATIONSHIP BETWEEN ATTENTION AND LANGUAGE

Attention modulation of language functions is assumed to involve arousal, which allows for the generation and allocation of mental attention and more complex attention systems that activate language-related computations (e.g., McNeil et al., 1991). This claim is based largely on patterns observed in studies of language performance among persons with aphasia, which demonstrate how a compromised attention system can result in unequal distribution and inefficient allocation of resources in service of language performance, thus hindering linguistic functions at all levels, from phoneme discrimination to discourse processing (Connor & Fucetola, 2011).

Interestingly, though, "aphasic-like" language performance, in the form of impaired lexical retrieval, for example, can also be induced in neurologically healthy adults when their attention system is strained by adverse processing conditions, such as dual-task paradigms, speeded stimulus presentation, or decreased perceptual salience of linguistic stimuli (e.g., Hula & McNeil, 2008; Murray, 1999; Silkes, McNeil, & Drton, 2004). This normal-to-aphasic language deficit continuum is suggestive of a general association between attention systems and some aspects of language performance inherent to the neurocognitive system (Hula & McNeil, 2008; Murray, 2000; Silkes, McNeil, & Drton, 2004).

The Neural Basis of Attention

The right hemisphere is claimed to be the primary player in mediating attention processes in the brain (for a recent review, see Bartolomeo, de Schotten, & Chica, 2012). Roughly speaking, these brain structures are dedicated to the selection of salient components of the stimuli; for example, spatial features, from the environment (Baars, 2007; Filley, 2002; Posner, 1992). This argument is based in part on the observation that damage to the right but not the left hemisphere results in persistent visual neglect, which impairs one's ability to visually attend to stimuli located in one's contralateral hemispace (e.g., Filley, 2002). Contralateral neglect, sometimes observed among people with left hemisphere damage, is usually less severe and transient.

However, beyond this gross hemispheric differentiation, the specific neural underpinnings of attention systems are still poorly understood. Most researchers would agree that attention systems rely on the activation of neural networks encompassing cortical, subcortical, and brain stem structures (Murray, 2002, 2004). Some have suggested dividing these networks into posterior and anterior systems. The former is assumed to mediate orientation via parietal cortices and the latter complex attention functions, such as focused and divided attention, through the dorsolateral prefrontal cortex and anterior cingulate gyri (e.g., Murray, Holland, Beeson, 1997).

Others have argued that attention networks can be grouped into two categories: (1) a diffuse attention network that functions to support arousal and sustained attention via white matter pathways connecting the thalamus to cortical regions in both hemispheres and (2) specialized anatomically segregated attention networks that subserve domain-specific attentional capacities in particular brain regions, such as the activation of visual cortices in response to tasks that require visual attention (e.g., Filley, 2002).

Weintraub (2000) described such an attention system with two neuroanatomically distinct main functions—*state* and *channel*. The state function was presumed to be mediated by frontosubcortical structures and largely subserving rapid modulation of information processing. The channel function, in contrast, was thought to rely on corticocortical monosynaptic connections consisting of a number of overlapping distributed neural networks.

Posner and colleagues have proposed a three-component *interactive* attentional system consisting of orienting, executive, and alertness systems, with distinct neural supports (e.g., Fan et al., 2002; Posner & Petersen, 1990), as follows: (1) The orienting system determines the direction of attention in space toward a critical stimulus in a top-down fashion via the parietal lobes, superior colliculi, and pulvinar structures; damage to these structures can lead to deficits in focus shifting. (2) The executive system is responsible for response selection among several options (resolving conflict) using the anterior cingulate, dorsolateral prefrontal, and posterior parietal cortices, where sensory input is processed and made available for further cognitive manipulation. (3) The alertness system maintains a state of vigilance in service of higher cognitive functions (Parasuraman, 2000), especially when the environment is understimulating, through the right lateral prefrontal regions. These regions have also been argued to house attention networks with frontal and prefrontal projections in which the orienting system is subserved by parietofrontal networks particularly in the right hemisphere; the executive system is supported by lateral prefrontal portions, and the alertness system is mediated by frontoparietal regions and some thalamic projections (e.g., Corbetta & Shulman, 2002; Driver et al., 2004; Fan et al., 2003, 2005; Mort et al., 2003). The neural networks subserving attention functions are shown in Figure 4.1.

An alternative approach has been proposed by Stuss and colleagues (Alexander et al., 2005; Stuss et al., 1995, 2002, 2005), where the more frontal attentional systems are viewed as clusters of processes roughly corresponding to Posner's executive component. These include action initiation and maintenance through response (which can be viewed as "cognitive effort") for actions that are not overlearned, mediated by superior medial frontal cortex, and action monitoring against task goals to allow corrective action, if necessary, implicating the right lateral frontal cortex (Shallice, 2006) (see also Chapter 3).

Current neuroanatomical models of attention explore the interplay between brain regions, such as the posteroparietal and cingulate cortices, which modulate *top-down* attention processes, and *bottom-up* "competition" among the neuronal representations of stimuli which occurs primarily in sensory association cortices (e.g., Kastner & Ungerleider, 2001). Under such a view, visual attention is a product of feed-forward signals from visual cortices and feed-back signals from parietofrontolimbic networks, which together positively bias the "survival" of the neuronal representation of the attended target (Gitelman, 2003). Some have argued that at a neurobiological level, this "attentional effort" implicates the cholinergic system (e.g., Sarter, Gehring, & Kozak, 2005).

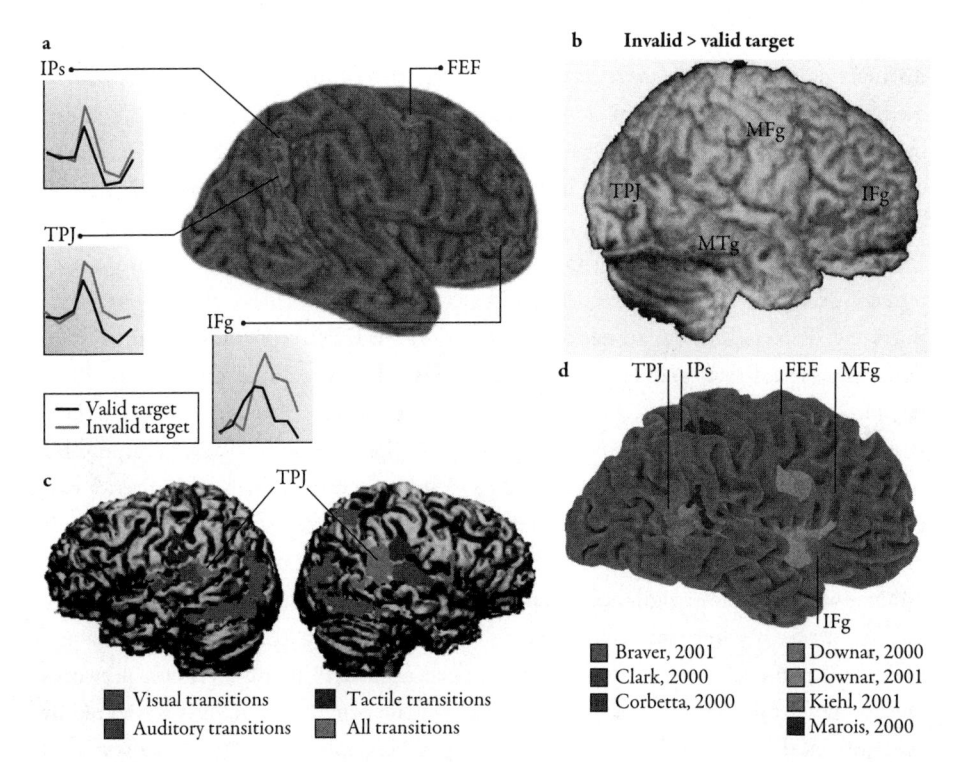

FIGURE 4.1 The functional neuroanatomy of attention systems (See color insert.)
Reprinted by permission from Macmillan Publishers Ltd [Nature Review Neuroscience], Corbetta, M. & Shulman, G.L. (2002). Control of goal-directed and stimulus-driven attention in the brain. *Nature Review Neuroscience, 3*(3), 1602–1610, copyright 2002.

(a) Human brain activity produced by attending to a location. Subjects see an arrow that cues one of two locations and covertly attend to the location indicated in preparation for a target at that location. The functional magnetic resonance imaging (fMRI) response is averaged over 13 subjects. The graphs show the time course of the fMRI signal after the cue. Signals are transient in occipital regions but sustained (gray arrow) in the parietal cortex and frontal eye field (FEF). (b) Human brain activity produced by attending to a direction of motion. Subjects see an arrow that cues a direction of motion and prepare for a subsequent target moving in that direction. The response is averaged over 14 subjects. The graphs contrast the response seen when the arrow cues a direction of motion with that observed when a cue instructs the subject to view the display passively. Directional cues produce sustained signals in frontal (FEF) and parietal (aIPs, pIPs) areas but transient signals in occipital areas (MT+). (c) Left: meta-analysis of studies of visual attention. Subjects expected a simple visual attribute, such as location or direction of motion, or a more complex array. Foci of activation from the expectation period are smoothed and projected onto the visible human brain. The area of maximal overlap between studies is in the pIPs. The figure shows regions that are activated by attending to and detecting visual stimuli (preparatory activity has been averaged with visual- and motor-detection activity). (d) Anticipatory activity in a macaque V3A neuron during a memory-guided task. (adapted with permission from Ref. 27 © 2000 The American Physiological Society). The graph shows the single-unit activity as the monkey performs two tasks while fixating the center of the screen. In the fixation task, a small stimulus is presented peripherally and the monkey is rewarded for maintaining fixation. In the memory-guided task, the monkey has to remember the location of the stimulus and after a variable delay make a saccade to that location. Activity is increased in the memory-guided task before stimulus onset, perhaps reflecting attention to the stimulus location.

aIPs, anterior intraparietal sulcus; Fus, fusiform cortex; MT+, middle temporal complex; pIPs, posterior IPs; vIPs, ventral IPs (junction of the vIPs and transverse occipital sulcus); PoCes, postcentral sulcus; PrCes, precentral sulcus; SFs, superior frontal sulcus; SPL, superior parietal lobule. Right: meta-analysis of imaging studies of visual attention and detection.

Source: Corbetta, M., & Shulman, G. L. (2002). Control of goal-directed and stimulus-driven attention in the brain. *Nature Reviews Neuroscience, 3*(3), 201–215, Figure 6. Reprinted by permission from Macmillan Publishers Ltd [Nature Review Neuroscience], copyright 2002.

Specific claims about the neural bases of "competition" in attention systems have been made by Duncan (2006), who proposed that biased competition toward a stimulus that best fits task demands reaches its peak in a "multiple-demand" pattern. In this pattern, target-related information from multiple tasks is processed globally via frontoparietal cortices. These regions are assumed to contain highly flexible neurons that adapt in order to engage in this integrative process and are crucial for attention focusing when processing of common cognitive material is called for. This view of "neural flexibility" is similar to the "neural multifunctionality" perspective espoused throughout this book.

The functional neuroanatomy of the attention networks is often attributed to brain activation observed in tasks measuring reaction times (e.g., Fan et al., 2002). Shallice et al. (2008), for example, analyzed the performance of four groups of brain-damaged participants on two sustained counting judgment tasks (estimating the number of auditory stimuli presented) that varied in speed of stimulus presentation (and therefore in degree of vigilance required) to further isolate the functional properties of the attention neural networks. They demonstrated that patients with damage in superior medial regions involving Brodmann's areas 24, 32, and 9 were worse at correctly estimating the number of stimuli presented in both conditions compared with the other patient groups, who were primarily impaired on the faster condition, suggesting that these medial regions are activated via a process they term *energizing*, which is called for when the rate of stimulus is suboptimal (either too low, when the operating systems are underaroused, or too high, in the face of excessive cognitive effort). In the course of "energizing, the current task schema is activated but no motor response is instigated.

In a recent meta-analysis of neuroimaging studies of sustained attention, Langner and Eickhoff (2012) showed that the ability to stay focused on a task, especially if it is cognitively undemanding or repetitive, implicates right-lateralized dorsomedial, mid- and ventrolateral prefrontal areas, the anterior insula, parietal cortices, and subcortical circuits. This architecture represents a complex interplay between top-down task maintenance over time and bottom-up processes involving target-based reorientation of attention.

Neural Underpinnings of Attention—Language Interlinks

As pointed out in the introduction to this chapter, the notion that attention and language are interdependent has been around for more than half a century. Evidence for the neurobiological basis of this relationship has been accumulating over the past 20 years, with neuroimaging studies showing the involvement of attention networks in different language tasks, including novel verb generation (Petersen & Fiez, 1993) and self-monitoring, error detection, and self-correction in verb generation tasks (Myachykov & Posner, 2005).

However, specific neurobiological models explicating the details of this attention-language relationship continue to remain underspecified. Much of the relevant research has focused on identifying the neural substrates implicated in response selection associated with lexical retrieval tasks, where stimuli with competing linguistic features are presented (e.g., Badre & Wagner, 2007; Gold & Buckner, 2002; Synder, Banich, & Munakata, 2011; Thompson-Schill et al., 1997, 1998; Wagner et al., 2001). Performance on such tasks has been argued to involve what is known as *semantic control*, mediated, by and large, by left-prefrontal neural architectures. The reader is referred to Chapter 3 for further details.

Attention modulation has also been found to play a role in sentence processing mediated by the anterior temporal lobe (ATL), contributing to the processing of both compositional semantic features and syntactic properties of sentences (Rogalsky & Hickok, 2009). Participants were asked to track occasional semantic anomalies or syntactic errors, focusing their attention either on semantic integration or on syntactic aspects of the stimuli. The experimental runs involved analyses of brain activation only in response to the error free stimuli, because the purpose of the study was to tease apart the neural underpinning of semantic and syntactic integration functions in sentence processing. The authors assumed that focused attention on specific features of sentence presentation—semantic or syntactic—would increase blood oxygenation level-dependent responses in the regions recruited for these distinct functions. Although this study was not designed to determine whether this attention modulation reflects enhanced signal-to-noise or a generalized attention effect unrelated to language processing, the hemodynamic responses identified in the region of interest—ATL—were left-lateralized, reducing the likelihood of a generalized attention effect.

In a different recent functional neuroimaging study, Fedorenko, Duncan, and Kanwisher (2012) explored whether language and domain-general networks supporting cognitive functions such as attention are represented independently in the brain. The study was designed to explicitly tease apart brain mechanisms specifically associated with language functions from those that are more domain general, mediating functions, such as inhibition of task-irrelevant information. All the tasks used in the study have been found to activate frontal brain regions implicating BA44 and BA45 (language tasks—reading of sentences and lists of nonwords; cognitive tasks—arithmetic addition, spatial and verbal working memory; multisource interference task; and Stroop). Each task had two conditions that differed in terms of level of difficulty, and this contrast was used to characterize brain activation patterns. Findings indicate that the language and domain-general architectures reside side by side in BA44 and BA45, with domain-general neural structures enveloping the language structures posteriorly (toward the inferior precentral sulcus), dorsally (toward the inferior frontal sulcus), and ventrally. This intricate functional neuroanaomical architecture is shown in Figure 4.2.

Under a neural multifunctionality approach, one could imagine how such a structural configuration would allow for an interaction between a strained language system, as is the case with aphasia, and surrounding domain-general neural circuits. In what follows we review evidence in support of this idea.

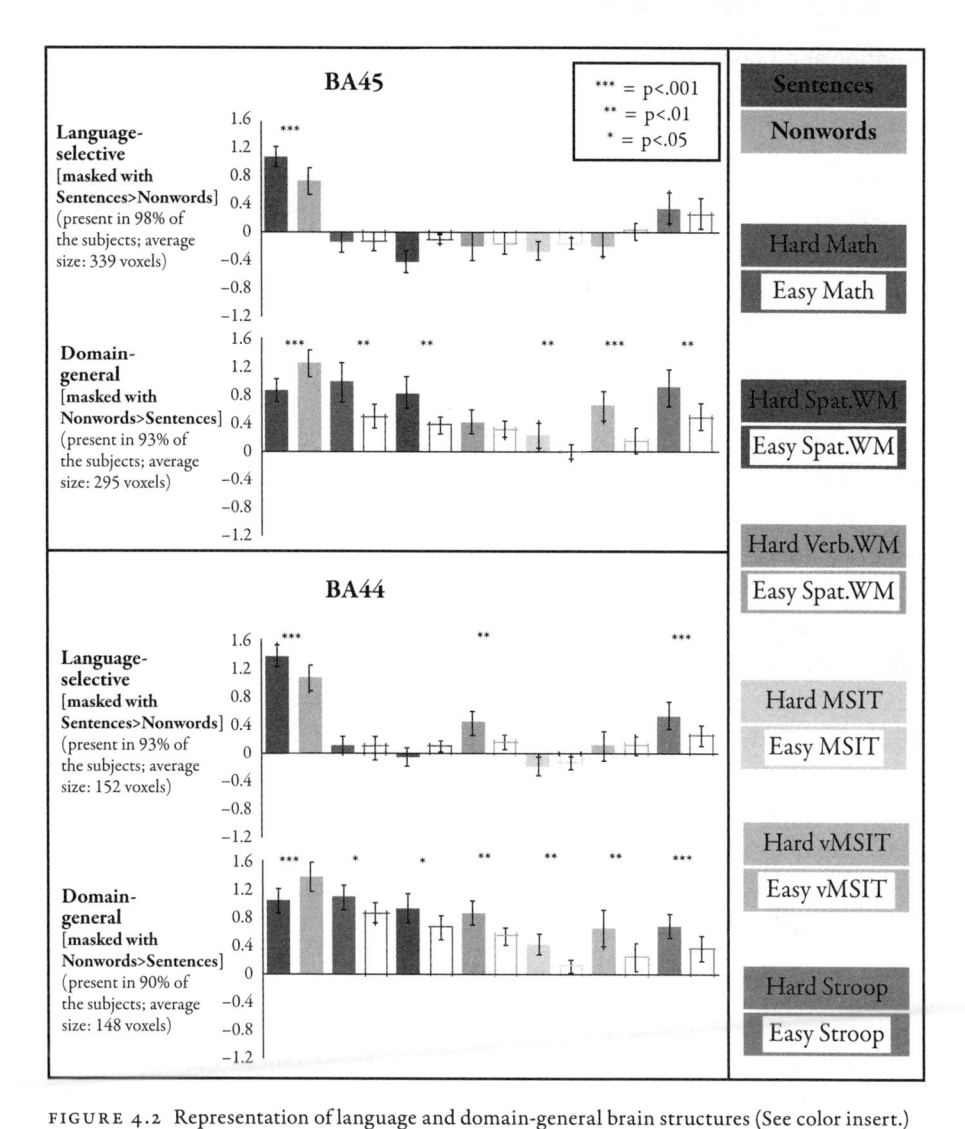

FIGURE 4.2 Representation of language and domain-general brain structures (See color insert.)
Functional profiles of language-selective and domain-general functional ROIs. Magnitude of response (in percent signal change from the fixation baseline) of language-selective and domain-general regions within BA45 (top box) and BA44 (bottom box) to each of the two conditions in each of the seven tasks. Language-selective regions are defined by intersecting BA45/44 with sentences > nonwords activation, and domain-general regions are defined by intersecting BA45/44 with nonwords > sentences activation. All magnitudes shown are estimated from data independent of those used to define the regions; responses to the sentences and nonwords are estimated using a left-out run. Error bars represent SEM by participants. *$P < .05$; **$P < .01$; ***$P < .001$. In the math task, participants added smaller versus larger numbers; in the spatial and verbal working memory (WM) tasks, participants kept in memory fewer versus more locations or digits, respectively; and in the three cognitive control tasks (MSIT, vMSIT, Stroop), participants had to inhibit a prepotent but task-irrelevant response and choose instead the task-relevant response.

Source: Reprinted under the Creative Commons Attribution License from Fedorenko, E., Duncan, J., & Kanwisher, N. (2012). Language-selective and domain-general regions lie side by side within Broca's area. Current Biology, 22, 2059–2062, Figure 2.

Attention and Aphasia: Neurobehavioral Evidence

NEURAL UNDERPINNINGS

Attention deficits in persons with aphasia are often observed among those with damage to brain structures in the left frontal lobe and subcortical structures, including the thalamus, anterior cingulate gyrus, and caudate nucleus (e.g., Murray, 2004; Sinotte & Coelho, 2007). Persons with right hemisphere damage can also present with "language" problems, but these are less severe and qualitatively different from those that persons with aphasia exhibit. For example, some word-finding difficulties in right hemisphere patients are associated with visuoperceptual problems rather than lexical-semantic deficits (Murray, 2000).

The neural implications of such attention-related changes for the aphasic brain are also manifested as reduced physiological brain activation, measured in event-related potential studies (e.g., Peach, Newhoff, & Rubin, 1992, 1994). In such studies, waveforms obtained in response to tasks demanding attention to a concurrent presentation of visual and auditory stimuli were found to be different between persons with and without aphasia, with the aphasic participants showing increased latency and decreased amplitudes (termed mismatch negativity), associated with automatic attention processing. Other physiological changes reported for persons with aphasia involve altered cardiovascular and neuroendocrine reactivity measured in response to auditory attention vigilance tasks (e.g., Laures, Odell, & Coe, 2003). These have been found to implicate a reduction in blood pressure and an increase in cortisol levels along with a decrease in task performance accuracy that has not been observed in persons free of brain damage.

BEHAVIORAL PATTERNS

It is difficult to establish whether the attention deficits that persons with aphasia exhibit are independent of or intertwined with their primary language disorder (Connor & Fucetola, 2011). However, at the most intuitive level, it is clear that successful completion of a language task involving, for example, auditory comprehension depends in some crucial (even if undefined) way on directing attention toward incoming linguistic stimuli, which, more often than not, involves ignoring other distracting input (McNeil et al., 2004).

Indeed, attention deficits among persons with aphasia have been found to negatively influence language functions in multiple domains, including production (e.g., Crosson, 2000; Murray, Holland, & Beason, 1998), reading comprehension (e.g., Coelho, 2005; Sinotte & Coelho, 2007), and auditory comprehension (e.g., Albert & Bear, 1974; Blumstein et al., 1985; Carpenter, Miyake & Just, 1994; McNeil, Odell, & Tseng, 1991). Impaired complex attention skills have been reported to be most detrimental to auditory comprehension, lexical retrieval, and communication independence, whereas deficient basic attention skills have been more directly linked to communicative difficulties (Murray, 2012).

Attention deficits demonstrated by persons with aphasia encompass most attention types, impairing language performance on tasks involving orienting, sustaining, focusing, and dividing attention (e.g., Erickson, Goldinger, & LaPointe, 1996; Hoffman et al., 2009; Kalbe et al., 2005; Korda & Douglas, 1997; Lambon Ralph et al., 2010; Laures, 2005; Laures, Odell, & Coe, 2003; Marien et al., 2009; McNeil, Odell, Tseng, 1991; Murray, Holland, & Beeson, 1998; Murray, 1999; 2000; Oksala et al., 2009; Robertson et al., 1994; Sturm et al., 1997). These adverse effects manifest primarily as increased number of errors and slower reaction times, which further exacerbate existing language deficits (e.g., Martin & Allen, 2008; McNeil, 1997; Murray, 2004; 2006, 2012).

For example, some persons with aphasia have been shown to respond more slowly to stimuli presented in their right versus their left visual field after being cued to the opposite side of the visual space or to a central fixation point (Petry et al., 1994). These poor spatial attention skills were correlated with six of the seven language measures used in that study to assess language performance, suggesting that degree of attention deficits in persons with aphasia (including even neglect) can be used as an indicator of disease severity. We revisit related findings in Chapter 8, where we discuss the relationship between attention, language, and visual processing.

Similarly, declines in reaction times and/or accuracy have also been observed in aphasic performance on tasks that place demands on sustained attention, as measured by performance on auditory and/or visual vigilance tasks (e.g., Erickson, Goldinger, & LaPointe, 1996; Korda & Douglas, 1997; Laures, Odell, & Coe, 2003). Poorest performance in these studies was reported for tasks with greater attention demands. LaPointe and Erickson (1991), for instance, found that persons with aphasia showed poorer word-identification abilities compared with healthy controls; however, this occurred only when they were asked to detect target words interspersed among nontargets while performing a competing task but not under a focused attention condition.

Indeed, most of the insights regarding adverse effects of attention problems on aphasic language performance are based on studies of *selective attention* in aphasia using *dual-task* paradigms. In these studies participants are typically asked to complete low- and high-attention-demand tasks that involve either completing a language task alone or performing a language task—such as phoneme monitoring, semantic judgment, lexical decision, grammaticality judgment, or lexical retrieval—with a concurrently administered additional task (e.g., Hula, McNeil, & Sung, 2007; King & Hux, 1996; Murray, 1997; 2000; Murray, Holland & Beeson, 1997; Tseng, McNeil, & Milenkovic, 1993). The language task remains the same across the conditions, to allow for the detection of attention effects on language performance (as measured by the difference scores between the two conditions).

Results from these studies indicate that compromised auditory comprehension (lexical and syntactic aspects) or impaired spoken language abilities (lexical, syntactic, and pragmatic aspects) are related to increased attention demands among persons with and without aphasia, with greater decrements observed among the aphasic participants (e.g., Murray, 2002). Because these studies did not involve evaluation of other cognitive abilities, it is difficult to attribute the impairments observed to attention rather than other cognitive domains. In other studies that did include additional cognitive measures (e.g., Helm-Estabrooks, 2002; Nicholas et al., 2011), scores were collapsed across tasks, making it difficult to tease apart specific effects of attention on patterns of impaired language performance (e.g., Connor & Fucetola, 2011; Murray, 2012).

Other attempts to determine whether attention and language problems are interlinked in persons with aphasia include the examination of statistical associations between performances on both task types (e.g., Hinckley & Nash, 2007; Kalbe et al., 2005). The utility of this approach has yet to be determined, since the findings are limited and mixed and focus only on the relationship between language scores and visual scanning as a measure of attention.

In a recent study, Murray (2012) attempted to address these different methodological pitfalls by exploring the effects of attention functions, as measured mostly by nonverbal tests in both auditory and visual modalities on different aspects of language and communication among persons with and without aphasia. She found that most of her aphasic participants demonstrated visual and auditory attention problems as well as other cognitive deficits affecting executive functions and memory compared with nonaphasic controls but that these deficits were quite variable, including scores in the unimpaired range. These findings highlight once again what appears to be a hallmark of aphasic performance—variability—which has guided much of the study of cognitive contributions to language performance in aphasia and has served as an inspiration to the writing of this book.

MECHANISMS OF ATTENTION ALLOCATION IN APHASIA

To explain the role of attention processes in shaping language performance in aphasia, some researchers have postulated a *resource allocation deficit* in the aphasic brain, which affects *access* to linguistic knowledge but does not involve *loss* of language functions (e.g., Hula & McNeil, 2008; McNeil, Odell, & Tseng, 1991; Tseng, McNeil, and Milenkovic, 1993). In its strongest form, this view assumes that the neural damage incurred in aphasia spares linguistic representations but impairs the particular mechanisms that activate, select, and inhibit linguistic elements (e.g., Erickson, Goldinger, & LaPointe, 1996; Murray, Holland, & Beeson, 1997; Silkes, McNeil, & Drton, 2004). Clearly not all patterns of aphasic language impairment can be reduced to attention deficits, but they point to those aspects of language performance that are more vulnerable to these problems (e.g., Murray, 2002).

This approach to language impairment in aphasia rests on two key assumptions: first, that attention is a limited-capacity processing resource that is flexibly activated to support different aspects of linguistic performance—such as response selection, sustained behavior, or inhibition of irrelevant responses—and second, that impaired selection of the correct route to linguistic information in the aphasic brain necessarily involves a breakdown in the cognitive machinery that regulates such selection. Within such a resource allocation approach to aphasia, persons with aphasia are assumed to be challenged by the *performance* of language tasks and that this challenge arises when (1) task demands exceed the available processing resources, (2) resources misdirected due to poor evaluation of task demands, and/or (3) resources are mobilized inefficiently (slowly) (e.g., Murray, 1999; Murray, Holland, & Beeson, 1997, 1998; Tseng, McNeil, & Milenkovic, 1993).

Support for some of these ideas can be found in studies of *automatic* and *controlled* processing in persons with and without aphasia, which explored differences in priming effects between these populations in response to presentation of stimuli at variable intervals (Copland et al., 2002; Hagoort, 1993; Hunting-Pompon, Kendall, & Bacon Moore, 2011; Petry et al., 1994). Findings from these studies are somewhat mixed. Some indicate that persons with aphasia have problems with both automatic and controlled processing compared with healthy controls—as measured, for example, by slow lexicosemantic activation and poor inhibition of alternately activated items in response to short and long interstimulus intervals (presentation of target after the prime at 100 and 800 ms, respectively) (e.g., Copland et al., 2002). Others report differences between the two populations only in terms of automatic processing capacities, with differential performances at 100 ms but comparable patterns at 800 ms (e.g., Hunting-Pompon, Kendall, & Bacon Moore, 2011). These divergent findings do not allow us to draw explicit conclusions about which aspects of the attention machinery are "broken" in aphasia, but they are suggestive of a deficit.

Indeed, the view of aphasia as a resource-allocation problem was developed in light of several observations about aphasic performance, including priming effects such as those described above, preserved metalinguistic awareness, and highly variable language patterns within and across subjects (e.g., Kurland, 2011). Moreover, persons with aphasia have been shown to be stimulated to perform correctly when exposed to a myriad of nonlinguistic factors, such as visual properties of stimuli (size, shape, or color), loudness, or speed of stimulus presentation (e.g., Kurland, 2011). Decreasing the rate of stimulus presentation, for example, has been found to enhance auditory comprehension (e.g., Connor, Albert, Helm-Estabrooks, & Obler, 2000). Together, these observations suggest that response selection in aphasia can be molded into highly flexible compensatory strategies (e.g., Hula & McNeil, 2008).

Treatment of Attention in Aphasia

The presumed relationship between the malleability of aphasic language performance and attention systems has inspired intervention studies designed to tease apart the effects of attention deficits on aphasia treatment outcomes (e.g., Coelho, 2005; Murray, 1999; 2004; Sinotte & Coelho, 2007). Such studies have explored whether focusing on attention skills in therapy would result in language performance gains (e.g., Connor, Albert, Helm-Estabrooks, & Obler, 2000; Helm-Estabrooks, 2011). For example, Hardin & Ramsberger (2004, 2011) used a computer program targeting specific visual and auditory attention systems in an attempt to improve aphasic conversational performance. Communicative success is a function of multiple complex cognitive processes (see also Chapter 3), which, in terms of attention, may include the simultaneous interpretation of verbal and nonverbal stimuli, attention shifts among topics, prolonged sustained effort, and filtering of potential distractors, to mention a few.

An underlying assumption in many such attention training studies is that useful targets of intervention are not linguistic representations in and of themselves, but rather nonlinguistic functions that could affect the access to those representations (e.g., Hula & McNeil, 2008; Murray, Holland, & Beeson, 1997). Unfortunately the evidence emerging from these studies is mixed and provides only a limited picture of the exact nature of attention deficits in aphasia, as studies have focused on a subset of attention systems (e.g., selective attention) and modalities (primarily visual), failing to rule out the potential contributions of other cognitive impairments to aphasic performance, such as deficient inhibition or self-monitoring (also discussed in Chapter 3) (Murray, 2012).

Many of these attention training studies also suffer from common methodological problems that plague aphasia treatment studies in general, including small sample sizes, variable dosages of duration and frequency of treatment, different definitions for what constitutes performance criteria, inconsistency in measures used to assess attention and/or language, to mention a few. Nonetheless, because the extent to which persons with aphasia carry over treatment effects from the clinic to different functional settings has been shown to depend on the status of their cognitive abilities (e.g., Helm-Estabrooks, 2011; Nicholas, Sinotte, & Helm-Estabrooks, 2005, 2011), it is important to examine the relative contribution of attention training to aphasic performance.

Helm-Estabrooks and colleagues (Helm-Estabrooks & Albert, 1991; Helm-Estabrooks, Connor, & Albert, 2000) developed an attention training program comprising several nonverbal tasks (e.g., symbol cancellation, repeated graphomotor patterns) that progress hierarchically from targeting simpler sustained attention abilities to complex alternating attention tasks. Participants who partook in the program for 32 to 34 treatment sessions, showed postintervention improvements on measures of auditory comprehension as well as visual analytic reasoning, suggesting generalization of treatment effects to both non-linguistic and linguistic materials (Ramsberger, 2005). However, not all attention training interventions have resulted in such generalization (e.g., Sturm & Willmes, 1991). It appears that the most efficacious results are obtained when multitask situations are targeted as a whole rather than being broken down to subtasks, an approach that has been shown to reduce the time required to learn tasks that rely on complex attention abilities and increase generalization to untrained items (Murray, 2004).

Another well-known attention training intervention is attention process training (APT) (Sohlberg & Mateer, 1986; Sohlberg et al., 2001; 2003), which in its newer version (APT II) also includes a hierarchical set of attention tasks originally designed to treat both auditory and visual attention problems in individuals with traumatic brain injury. The treatment has been found to be efficacious for persons with stroke as well (Barker-Collo et al., 2009) and has thus been administered to persons with stroke-based aphasia (e.g., Coelho, 2005; Murray, 2004; Murray et al., 2006; Sinotte & Coelho, 2007).

Use of APT II to treat reading difficulties in a person with aphasia, for example, has resulted in greater reading speed over time, associated with improved sustained attention, increased ability to concentrate, and better coping with distractions (Coelho, 2005). However, treatment outcomes associated with the APT program have not always been encouraging, demonstrating great variability in treatment effects. These include, for example, minimal to modest gains in standardized attention measures (e.g., the test of everyday attention developed by Robertson et al., 1994) and language measures (e.g., the Aphasia Diagnostic Profiles, Helm-Estabrooks, 1992), along with no change in daily attention and communication skills (Murray, Keeton, & Karcher, 2006). This observation has led to the claim that direct attention training enhances only discrete attention abilities and does not promote cognitive functioning per se (e.g., Barker-Collo et al., 2009; Murray, 2004; Murray, Keeton, & Karcher, 2006).

Failure to attain measurable functional changes through attention training programs has been attributed to different methodological shortcomings, such as the use of attention stimuli consisting of verbal components. As a result, only persons with relatively mild aphasia may be able to complete the treatment (Murray, 2002; Sohlberg et al., 2003), and gains in their language performance may be too difficult to capture in standardized language tests targeting variable levels of aphasia severity (Helm-Estabrooks, 2011).

Another major methodological factor masking the impact of attention deficits on aphasic language performance is the ecological validity of the attention training tasks (e.g., Murray, 2004). Most laboratory-contrived tasks targeting attention do not simulate real-world attention challenges, where multiple distractions—such as television, street noise, and multitalker environments (e.g., restaurants)—may interfere with successful language use (e.g., Erickson, Goldinger, & LaPointe, 1996). Thus it has been argued that quiet lab environments can stand in the way of enhancing treatment generalizations necessary for handling real-life burdens on attention and language functioning (Murray, Holland, & Beeson, 1997, 1998). In addition, clinical settings may not be as motivating as everyday situations, thus undercutting the attention abilities that the treated clients may exhibit in treatment (Korda & Douglas, 1997; Murray, 2002).

Ideally, aphasia therapy programs should try to incorporate both cognitive and psycholinguistic features into the interventions so as to maximize the efficacy of the treatment administered (e.g., Cahana-Amitay, Albert, & Oveis, 2014). In a recent study of naming therapy for persons with anomic aphasia, Conroy et al. (2012) took exactly such an approach by tying together cognitive aspects of item responsiveness, (i.e., cue duration to the psycholinguistic features the items to be named, including age of acquisition, frequency, and imageability). Their purpose was to determine whether the relationship between these factors affects treatment outcomes (i.e., naming accuracy). They found that correct naming of items following therapy was linked to shortest pretreatment cueing duration and word imageability and that this relationship was sustained throughout therapy, although there was a consistent reduction in cue duration over the first 6 of 10 therapy sessions. The finding that least cueable items pretreatment are also those that are best named following treatment is unsurprising. Given the putative relationship between item responsiveness and attention abilities, it would have been informative to consider whether differences in the performances of the participants were linked to their neuropsychological profiles.

NEURAL APPROACHES TO THE ROLE OF ATTENTION IN APHASIA TREATMENT

Some aphasia treatment studies have focused on engaging preserved right-hemisphere attention mechanisms to improve language performance (e.g., Anderson, 1996; Coslett, 1999), even though our understanding of the neural bases of the effects of impaired attention on language performance in aphasia is still rather incomplete. Dotson et al. (2007), for example, demonstrated that placing stimuli in participants' left hemispace (ipsilateral to their stroke) activates intact attention systems in the right hemisphere and, in doing so, enhances naming performance in persons with fluent aphasia. However, their findings are based on three participants only, with only two of the three showing improvement, making the characterization of the exact contribution of the right-hemisphere attention functions somewhat challenging.

In a much larger study, though, Crosson and colleagues (2007) were able to demonstrate that participants with profound language impairment showed improvement following attention treatment that also generalized to untrained items, in which picture placement in the participants' left hemispace constituted the attention manipulation. Again, the rationale was that this placement would activate attention mechanisms that would stimulate the right posterior perisylvian cortex and enhance mechanisms crucial for word processing. The effects of this treatment, however, were less noticeable among participants with moderate-to-severe aphasia, who responded better to an intention training program focused primarily on the action planning and initiation aspects of response selection. The details of this intervention are provided in Chapter 3.

Coslett (1999), however, was able to provide some insight into the neuroanatomical correlates underlying this behavioral observation, as he found that directing attention to his participants' left hemispace improved naming exclusively among aphasic persons with parietal brain damage (see also Borod et al., 1984). Gonzalez-Rothi (1995) suggested that gradual shifting of linguistic stimuli back to the patients' right hemispace would likely stimulate the automatic activation of attention processes whenever language processing is called for.

Other neurally driven treatment programs have been designed to reduce the adverse effects of attention deficits on aphasic performance through pharmacotherapy targeting the dopaminergic and noradrenergic systems (recently reviewed in Cahana-Amitay, Albert, & Oveis, 2014). The underlying assumption in many of these studies was that targeting these deficient neurotransmission systems in damaged prefrontal, motor, and association areas would enhance impaired linguistic functions mediated by these areas (e.g., Albert, 2000; McNamara & Albert, 2004; Raymer et al., 2001). Such facilitation was presumed to reflect in part augmented attentional systems associated with activation of different language output systems (Alexander, 2006; Crosson et al., 2005). Beversdorf et al. (2007), for example, proposed that medication targeting the noradrenergic system can help suppress background neural activation, thus improving the efficiency with which persons with aphasia perform lexical-semantic searches. However, such proposals remain speculative, as most aphasia pharmacotherapy studies do not include behavioral measures of attention, leaving open the question of whether the language gains observed are necessarily modulated by the resolution of patients' attention deficits (Murray, 2002, 2004).

More recently, as a result of aphasia language treatment, efforts have been made to identify neural changes in attention networks induced by language therapy (Marcotte et al., 2013). Specifically, persons with aphasia who were administered intensive language treatment demonstrated improved connectivity of the default mode network (DMN) following treatment. The authors compared DMN connectivity between persons with aphasia and age-matched peers without aphasia, using a global measure of connectivity termed *functional integration* (Marrelec et al., 2008). For all participants, measures were taken during a naming task as well as before and after intensive lexical training (semantic feature training). Treatment was expected to result in increased integration values, with improved connectivity between anterior and posterior cortices. Results indicated that among aphasic participants, in whom evidence of DMN connectivity was observed pretreatment, increased connectivity in posterior regions posttreatment was found. This neural reorganization was coupled with language performance gains, but the correlation between the two failed to reach significance, probably due to sample size limitations. Whether the therapy-induced neural plasticity actually reflects changes in attention systems is difficult to determine in the absence of an analysis of the participants' cognitive profiles. Also, as the authors themselves point out, the extent to which the findings are interpretable is limited by the fact that they compared DMN connectivity pre- and posttreatment without reference to resting state value, which is the standard practice in neuroimaging DMN connectivity studies (e.g., Binder et al., 1999; Zhang & Raichle, 2010). Nonetheless, the results of the study highlight the potential value of analyzing DMN connectivity as a tool to be incorporated into the assessment and possibly treatment of aphasia.

Cumulative evidence from studies of attention and language performance among persons with and without aphasia suggests that attention and linguistic functions are intertwined in the brain and that these interdependencies account, at least in part, for some of the variability in language performance observed under suboptimal conditions. Although models elucidating the specific mechanisms underlying these attention-language links remain to be further developed, an initial understanding of how different attention components contribute to language performance in aphasia is emerging, along with a more detailed understanding of their neural underpinnings. These insights are increasingly used for the development of novel neurally based assessments and treatment programs of attention in aphasia by capitalizing on preserved right hemisphere networks or by targeting the neurochemistry of attention-related neurotransmission systems to alleviate the detrimental effects of impaired attention on language performance. In the context of this book, we are suggesting that these neurocognitive systems are engaged in reshaping poststroke language-dedicated neural networks, the activation of which is guided by principles of neural multifunctionality.

Such a multifunctional approach could help explain, for example, why posttreatment language activation patterns observed following anomia treatment implicate "nontraditional" language areas (e.g., Fridriksson et al., 2006, 2007). In addition, they could account in part for the dynamic nature of such treatment-induced changes, as short-term treatment effects have been found to be mediated by domain-general brain regions that support cognitive skills such as attention, compared with longer-term effects, which have been associated with activation of more traditional language areas (e.g., Menke et al., 2009). We revisit this idea in more detail in the concluding chapter of the book.

References

Albert, M. L. (2000). Toward a neurochemistry of naming and anomia. In Y. Grodzinsky, L. Shapiro, & D. Swinney (Eds.), *Language and the brain* (pp. 157–165). San Diego, CA: Academic Press.

Albert, M. L., & Bear, D. (1974). Time to understand. A case study of word deafness with reference to the role of time in auditory comprehension. *Brain, 97*(2): 373–384.

Alexander, M. P. (2006). Impairments of procedures for implementing complex language are due to disruption of frontal attention processes. *Journal of the International Neuropsychological Society, 12*, 236–247.

Alexander, M. P., Stuss, D. T., Shallice, T., Picton, T. W., & Gillingham, S.M.E. (2005). Impaired concentration in patients with frontal damage: deficits from two anatomically distinct lesion sites. *Neurology, 65*, 572–579.

Anderson, B. (1996). Semantic neglect? *Journal of Neurology, Neurosurgery & Psychiatry, 60*(3), 349–350.

Baars, B.J. (2007) Attention and consciousness. In B. J. Baars, & N. M. Gage (Eds.), *Cognition, brain, and consciousness: introduction to cognitive neuroscience* (pp. 225–253). Academic Press.

Badre, D., & Wagner, A. D. (2007). Left ventrolateral prefrontal cortex and the cognitive control of memory. *Neuropsychologia, 45*(13) 2883–2901.

Barker-Collo, S. L., Feigin, V. L., Lawes, C. M., Parag, V., Senior, H., & Rodgers, A. (2009). Reducing attention deficits after stroke using attention process training: a randomized controlled trial. *Stroke, 40*, 3293–3298.

Bartolomeo, P. de Schotten, M., & Chica, A. B. (2012). Brain networks of visuospatial attention and their disruption in visual neglect. *Frontiers in Human Neuroscience, 6*, 110.

Beversdorf, D. Q., Narayanan, A., Hillier, A., & Hughes, J. D. (2007). Network model of decreased context utilization in autism spectrum disorder. *Journal of Autism and Developmental Disorders, 37*(6), 1040–1048. doi:10.1007/s10803-006-0242-7

Binder, J. R., Frost, J. A., Hammeke, T. A., Bellgowan, P. S., Rao, S. M., & Cox, R.Z.W. (1999). Conceptual processing during the conscious resting state, a functional MRI study. *Journal of Cognitive Neuroscience, 11*, 80–95.

Blumstein, S. E., Katz, B., Goodglass, H., Shrier, R., & Dworetsky, B. (1985). The effects of slowed speech on auditory comprehension in aphasia. *Brain and Language, 24*(2), 246–265.

Borod, J. C., Carper, M., Goodglass, H., & Naeser, M. (1984). Aphasic performance on a battery of constructional, visuospatial, and quantitative tasks: factorial structure and CT scan localization. *Journal of Clinical Neuropsychology, 6*(2), 189–204.

Cahana-Amitay, D., Albert, M. L., & Oveis, A. (2014). Psycholoinguistics of aphasia pharmacotherapy: asking the right questions. *Aphasiology, 28*(2), 133–154.

Cahana-Amitay, D., Albert, M. L., Pyun, S.-B., Westwood, A., Jenkins, T., Wolford, S., & Finley, M. (2011). Language as a stressor in aphasia. *Aphasiology, 25*(5), 593–614. DOI:10.1080/02687038.2010.541469.

Cherry, E. C. (1953). Some experiments on the recognition of speech, with one and with two ears. *The Journal of the Acoustical Society of America, 25*(5), 975–979.

Coelho, C. A. (2005). Direct attention training as a treatment for reading impairment in mild aphasia. *Aphasiology, 19*(3–5), 3–5.

Connor, L. T., Albert, M. L., Helm-Estabrooks, N., & Obler, L. K. (2000). Attentional modulation of language performance. *Brain and Language, 71*, 52–55.

Connor, L. T., & Fucetola, R. P. (2011). Assessment of attention in people with aphasia: challenges and recommendations. *Perspectives on Neurophysiology and Neurogenic Speech and Language Disorders, 21*, 55–63.

Conroy, P. J., Snell, C., Sage, K. E., & Lambon Ralph, M. A. (2012). Using phonemic cueing of spontaneous naming to predict item responsiveness to therapy for anomia in aphasia. *Archives of Physical Medicine and Rehabilitation, 93*(Suppl 1), S53–S60.

Copland, D. A., Cherney, H. J., & Murdoch, B. E. (2002). Hemispheric contributions to lexical ambiguity resolution: evidence from individuals with complex language impairment following left-hemisphere lesions. *Brain and Language, 81*, 131–143.

Corbetta, M., Kincade, M. J., Lewis, C., Snyder, A. Z., & Sapir, A. (2005). Neural basis and recovery of spatial attention deficits in spatial neglect. *Nature Neuroscience, 8*(11), 1602–1610.

Corbetta, M., & Shulman, G. L. (2002). Control of goal-directed and stimulus-driven attention in the brain. *Nature Reviews Neuroscience, 3*(3), 201–215.

Coslett, H. B. (1999). Spatial influences on motor and language function. *Neuropsychologia, 37*(6), 695–706.

Craik, F.I.M., & Lockhart, R. S. (1972). Levels of processing: a framework for memory research. *Journal of Verbal Learning and Verbal Behavior, 11*, 671–684.

Crosson, B. (2000). Systems that support language processes: attention. In S. E. Nadeau, L. J. G. Rothi, & B. Crosson (Eds.), *Aphasia and language: theory to practice* (pp. 372–398). New York: Guilford Press.

Crosson, B., Fabrizio, K. S., Singletary, F., Cato, M., Wierenga, C. E., Parkinson, R. B., … Rothi, L. J. (2007). Treatment of naming in nonfluent aphasia through manipulation of intention and attention: a phase 1 comparison of two novel treatments. *Journal of the International Neuropsychological Society, 13*(4), 582–594.

Crosson, B., Moore, A. B., Gopinath, K., White, K. D., Wierenga, C. E., Gaiefsky, M. E., … Gonzalez Rothi, L. J. (2005). Role of the right and left hemispheres in recovery of function during treatment of intention in aphasia. *Journal of Cognitive Neuroscience, 17*(3), 392–406.

Desimone, R., & Duncan, D. (1995). Neural mechanisms of selective visual attention. *Annual Review of Neuroscience, 18*, 193–222.

Dotson, V. M., Singletary, F., Fuller, R., Koehler, S., Moore, A. B., Gonzalez Rothi, L. J., & Crosson, B. (2007). Treatment of word-finding deficits in fluent aphasia through the manipulation of spatial attention: preliminary findings. *Aphasiology, 22*(1), 103–113.

Driver, J., Eimer, M., Macaluso, E., & van Velzen, J. (2004). Neurobiology of human spatial attention: modulation, generation, and integration. In N. Kanwisher & J. Duncan (Eds.), *Attention and performance*. Oxford, UK: Oxford University Press.

Duncan, J. (2006). EPS mid-career award 2004: Brain mechanisms of attention. *The Quarterly Journal of Experimental Psychology, 59*(1), 2–27.

Erickson, R. J., Goldinger, S. D., & LaPointe, L. L. (1996). Auditory vigilance in aphasic individuals: detecting nonlinguistic stimuli with full or divided attention. *Brain and Cognition, 30*(2), 244–253.

Fan, J., Fossella, J., Sommer, T., Wu, Y., & Posner, M. I. (2003). Mapping the genetic variation of executive attention onto brain activity. *Proceedings of the National Academy of Sciences of the United States of America, 100*(12), 7406–7411.

Fan, J., McCandliss, B. D., Fossella, J., Flombaum, J. I., & Posner, M. I. (2005). The activation of attentional networks. *Neuroimage, 26*, 471–479.

Fan, J., McCandliss, B. D., Sommer, T., Raz, A., & Posner, M. I. (2002). Testing the efficiency and independence of attentional networks. *Journal of Cognitive Neuroscience, 14*(3), 340–347.

Fedorenko, E., Duncan, J., & Kanwisher, N. (2012). Language-selective and domain-general regions lie side by side within Broca's area. *Current Biology, 22*, 2059–2062.

Filley, C. M. (2002). The neuroanatomy of attention. *Seminars in Speech and Language, 23*, 89–98.

Fridriksson, J., Morrow-Odom, L., Moser, D., Fridriksson, A., & Baylis, G. (2006). Neural recruitment associated with anomia treatment in aphasia. *Neuroimage, 32*(3), 1403–1412.

Fridriksson, J., Moser, D., Bonilha, L., Morrow-Odom, K., Shaw, H., Fridriksson, A., … Rorden, C. (2007). Neural correlates of phonological and semantic-based anomia treatment in aphasia. *Neuropsychologia, 45*, 1812–1822.

Gitelman, D. R. (2003). Attention and its disorders. *British Medical Bulletin, 65*, 21–34.

Gold, B. T., & Buckner, R. L. (2002) Common prefrontal regions coactivate with dissociable posterior regions during controlled semantic and phonological tasks. *Neuron, 35*, 803–812.

Gonzalez-Rothi, L. J. (1995). Theory and clinical intervention: one clinician's view. In J. Cooper (Ed.), *Aphasia treatment: current approaches and research opportunities* (Vol. 2, pp. 91–98). Bethesda, MD: National Institute on Deafness and Other Communcation Disorders.

Hagoort, P. (1993). Impairments of lexical-semantic processing in aphasia: Evidence from the processing of lexical ambiguities. *Brain and Language, 45,* 189–232.

Hardin, K., & Ramsberger, G. (2004).Treatment of attention in aphasia. Poster presented at the 2004 Clinical Aphasiology Conference, Park City, Utah.

Hardin, K., & Ramsberger, G. (2011). Treatment of attention to improve conversational success in aphasia. *Perspectives on Neurophysiology and Neurogenic Speech and Language Disorders, 21*(2), 72–77.

Helm-Estabrooks, N. (1992). *Aphasia diagnostic profiles.* Chicago: Riverside.

Helm-Estabrooks, N. (2002). Cognition and aphasia: a discussion and a study. *Journal of Communication Disorders, 35,* 171–186.

Helm-Estabrooks, N. (2011), Treating attention to improve auditory comprehension deficits associated with aphasia. *Perspectives on Neurophysiology and Neurogenic Speech and Language Disorders, 21,* 64–71.

Helm-Estabrooks, N., & Albert, M. L. (1991). *Manual of aphasia therapy.* Austin, TX: Pro-Ed.

Helm-Estabrooks, N., Connor, L. T., & Albert, M. L. (2000). Training attention to improve auditory comprehension in aphasia. *Brain and Language, 74,* 469–472.

Hinckley, J., & Nash, C. (2007). Cognitive assessment and aphasia severity. *Brain and Language, 103,* 195–196.

Hoffman, P., Jefferies, E., Ehsan, S., Hopper, S., & Lambon Ralph, M. (2009). Selective short-term memory deficits arise from impaired domain-general semantic control mechanisms. *Journal of Experimental Psychology: Learning, Memory, and Cognition, 35,* 137–156.

Hula, W. D., & McNeil, M. R. (2008). Models of attention and dual-task performance as explanatory constructs in aphasia. *Seminars in Speech and Language, 29*(3), 169–187.

Hula, W. D., McNeil, M. R., & Sung, J. E. (2007). Is there an impairment of language-specific attention processing in aphasia? *Brain and Language, 103,* 240–241.

Hunting-Pompon, R., Kendall, D., & Bacon Moore, A. (2011). Examining attention and cognitive processing in participants with self-reported mild anomia. *Aphasiology, 25*(6–7), 800–812.

James, W. (1890). *The principles of psychology* (Vol. 1). New York: Henry Holt.

Kahneman, D. (1973). *Attention and effort.* Englewood Cliffs, NJ: Prentice-Hall.

Kalbe, E., Reinhold, N., Brand, M., Markowitsch, J., & Kessler, J. (2005). A new test battery to assess aphasic disturbances and associated cognitive dysfunctions: German normative data on the aphasia check list. *Journal of Clinical and Experimental Neuropsychology, 27,* 779–794.

Kastner, S., & Ungerleider, L.G. (2000) Mechanisms of visual attention in the human cortex. *Annual Review of Neuroscience, 23,* 315–341.

Kastner, S., & Ungerleider, L. G. (2001). The neural basis of biased competition in the human visual cortex. *Neuropsychologia, 39,* 1263–1276.

Kimura, D. (1967). Functional asymmetry of the brain in dichotic listening. *Cortex, 3*(2), 163–178.

King, J. M., & Hux, K. (1996). Attention allocation in adults with and without aphasia: performance on linguistic and nonlinguistic tasks. *Journal of Medical Speech-Language Pathology, 4*, 245–256.

Kinomura, S., Larson, J., Gulyas, B., & Roland, P. E. (1996). Activation by attention of the human reticular formation and thalamic intralaminar nuclei. *Science, 271*, 511–515.

Korda, R. J., & Douglas, J. M. (1997). Attention deficits in stroke patients with aphasia. *Journal of Clinical and Experimental Neuropsychology, 19*(4), 525–542.

Kreindler, A., & Fradis, A. (1968). *Performances in aphasia: a neurodynamical diagnostic and psychological study*. Paris: Gauthier-Villars.

Kurland, J. (2011). The role that attention plays in language processing. *Perspectives on Neurophysiology and Neurogenic Speech and Language Disorders, 21*(2), 44–77.

Lambon Ralph, M., Snell, C., Fillingham, J., Conroy, P., & Sage, K. (2010). Predicting the outcome of anomia therapy for people with aphasia post CVA: both language and cognitive status are key predictors. *Neuropsychological Rehabilitation, 20*(2), 289–305.

Langner, R., & Eickhoff, S. B. (2012). Sustaining attention to simple tasks: a meta-analytic review of the neural mechanisms of vigilant attention. *Psychological Bulletin, 139*(4), 870–900.

LaPointe, L. L., & Erickson, R. J. (1991). Auditory vigilance during divided task attention in aphasic individuals. *Aphasiology, 5*(6), 511–520.

Laures, J. S. (2005). Reaction time and accuracy in individuals with aphasia during auditory vigilance tasks. *Brain and Language, 95*(2), 353–357.

Laures-Gore, J., DuBay, M., Duff, M. C., & Buchanan, T. W. (2010). Identifying behavioral measures of stress in individuals with aphasia. *Journal of Speech, Language, and Hearing Research, 53*, 1394–1400.

Laures-Gore, J., Heim, C., & Hsu, Y. S. (2007). Assessing cortisol reactivity to a linguistic task as a marker of stress in individuals with left hemisphere stroke and aphasia. *Journal of Speech, Language, and Hearing Research, 50*(2), 493–507.

Laures, J. S., Odell, K., & Coe, C. (2003). Arousal and auditory vigilance in individuals with aphasia during a linguistic and nonlinguistic task. *Aphasiology, 17*(12), 1133–1152.

Lavie, N., Hirst, A., de Fockert, J., & Viding, E. (2004). Load theory of selective attention and cognitive control. *Journal of Experimental Psychology: General, 133*(3), 339–354.

Lupyan, G., & Mirman, D. (2013). Linking language and categorization: evidence from aphasia. *Cortex, 49*(5), 1187–1194.

Marcotte, K., Perlbarg, V., Marrelec, G., Benali, H., & Ansaldo, A. I. (2013). Default-mode network functional connectivity in aphasia: therapy-induced neuroplasticity. *Brain and Language, 124*, 45–55.

Marien, P., Baillieux, H., De Smet, H. J., Engelborghs, S., Wilssens, I., Paquier, P., & De Deyn, P. P. (2009). Cognitive, linguistic and affective disturbances following right superior cerebellar artery infarction: a case study. *Cortex, 45*, 527–536.

Marrelec, G., Bellec, P., Krainik, A., Duffau, H., Pelegrini-Issac, M., Lehericy, S., … Doyon, J. (2008). Regions, systems, and the brain: Hierarchical measures of functional integration in fMRI. *Medical Image Analysis, 12*(4), 52–63.

Martin, R. C., & Allen, C. (2008). A disorder of executive function and its role in language processing. *Seminars in Speech and Language, 29*, 201–210.

McNamara, P., & Albert, M. (2004). Neuropharmacology of verbal perseveration. *Seminars in Speech and Language, 25*(4), 309–321.

McNeil, M. R. (1983). Aphasia: neurological considerations. *Topics in Language Disorders, 1*, 1–19.

McNeil, M. R. (1997). Resource allocation theory: clinical applications. Paper presented at the annual meeting of the Academy of Neurologic Communication Disorders and Sciences, Boston.

McNeil, M. R., Odell, K., & Tseng, C. (1991). Toward the integration of resource allocation into a general theory of aphasia. *Clinical Aphasiology, 20*, 21–39.

McNeil, M. R., Doyle, P. J., Hula, W. D., Rubinsky, H. J., Fossett, T.R.D., & Matthews, C. T. (2004). Using resource allocation theory and dual-task methods to increase the sensitivity of assessment in aphasia. *Aphasiology, 18*(5–7), 521–542.

Menke, R., Meinzer, M., Kugel, H., Deppe, M., Baumgärtner, A., Schiffbauer, H., … Breitensten, C. (2009). Imaging short- and long-term training success in chronic aphasia. *BMC Neuroscience, 10*, 118.

Mirsky, A. F., Anthony, B., Duncan, C., Ahearn, M., & Kellam, S. (1991). Analysis of the elements of attention: a neuropsychological approach. *Neuropsychology Review, 2*(2), 109–145.

Miyake, A., Just, M.A., & Carpenter, P. A. (1994). Working memory constraints on the resolution of lexical ambiguity: maintaining multiple interpretations in neutral contexts. *Journal of Memory and Language, 33*, 175–202.

Mort, D. J., Malhotra, P, Mannan, S. K., Rorden, C.,Pambakian, A., Kennard, C., & Husain, M. (2003). The anatomy of visual neglect. *Brain, 126*, 1986–1997.

Murray, L. L. (1997). Auditory processing in individuals with mild aphasia: a study of resource allocation. *Journal of Speech, Language & Hearing Research, 40*(4), 792–809.

Murray, L. L. (1999). Attention and aphasia: theory, research and clinical implications. *Aphasiology, 13*, 91–112.

Murray, L. L. (2000). The effects of varying attentional demands on the word-retrieval skills of adults with aphasia, right hemisphere brain-damage or no brain-damage. *Brain and Language, 72*, 40–72.

Murray, L. L. (2002). Attention deficits in aphasia: presence, nature, assessment, and treatment. *Seminars in Speech and Language, 23*(2), 107–116.

Murray, L. L. (2004). Cognitive treatments for aphasia: should we and can we help attention and working memory problems? *Medical Journal of Speech-Language Pathology, 12*, xxi–xxxviii.

Murray, L. L. (2012). Attention and other cognitive deficits in aphasia: presence and relation to language and communication measures. *American Journal of Speech-Language Pathology, 21*(2), S51–S64A.

Murray, L. L., Holland, A. L., & Beeson, P. M. (1997). Grammaticality judgments of mildly aphasic individuals under dual task conditions. *Aphasiology, 11*, 993–1016.

Murray, L. L., Keeton, R. J., & Karcher, L. (2006). Treating attention in mild aphasia: evaluation of attention process training-II. *Journal of Communication Disorders, 39*, 37–61.

Myachykov, A.V., & Posner, M. I. (2005). Attention in language. In L. Itti, G. Rees, & J. Tsotsos (Eds.), *Neurobiology of attention* (pp. 324–329). New York: Academic Press/Elsevier.

Nicholas, M., Sinotte, M., & Helm-Estabrooks, N. (2005). Using a computer to communicate: effect of executive function impairments in people with severe aphasia. *Aphasiology, 19*(10–11), 1052–1065.

Nicholas, M., Sinotte, M., & Helm-Estabrooks, N. (2011). C-speak aphasia alternative communication program for people with severe aphasia: importance of executive functioning and semantic knowledge. *Neuropsychological Rehabilitation, 21*(3), 322–366.

O'Donnell, B. F. (2002). Forms of attention and attentional disorders. *Seminars in Speech and Language, 23*(2), 99–106.

Oksala, N. K., Jokinen, H., Melkas, S., Oksala, A., Pohjasvaara, T., Hietanen, M., & Erkinjuntti, T. (2009). Cognitive impairment predicts poststroke death in long-term follow-up. *Journal of Neurology, Neurosurgery, and Psychiatry, 80*, 1230–1235.

Pashler, H. (1984). Evidence against late selection: stimulus quality effects in previewed displays. *Journal of Experimental Psychology: Human Perception and Performance, 10*(3), 429–448.

Pashler, H. (1990). Do response modality effects support multiprocessor models of divided attention? *Journal of Experimental Psychology: Human Perception and Performance, 16*(4), 826–842.

Pashler, H. (1994). Overlapping mental operations in serial performance with preview. *Quarterly Journal of Experimental Psychology, 47*, 161–191.

Peach, R. K., Newhoff, M., & Rubin, S. S. (1992). Attention in aphasia as revealed by event-related potentials: a preliminary investigation. *Clinical Aphasiology, 21*, 323–333.

Peach, R., Rubin, S., & Newhoff, M. (1994). A topographic event-related potential analysis of the attention deficit for auditory processing in aphasia. *Clinical Aphasiology, 22*, 81–96.

Petersen, S. E., & Fiez, J. A. (1993). The processing of single words studied with positron emission tomography. *Annual Review of Neuroscience, 16*, 509–530.

Petry, M., Crosson, B., Gonzalez Rothi, L. J., Bauer, R., & Schauer, C. (1994). Selective attention and aphasia in adults: preliminary findings. *Neuropsychologia, 32*(11), 1397–1408.

Piazza, J. R., Almeida, D. M., Dmitrieva, N. O., & Klein, L. C. (2010). Frontiers in use of biomarkers of health in research on stress and aging. *The Journals of Gerontology Series B: Psychological Sciences and Social Sciences, 65*(5), 513–525.

Posner, M. I. (1992). Attention as a cognitive and neural system. *Current Directions in Psychological Science, 1*, 11–14.

Posner, M. I., & Peterson, S. E. (1990). The attention system of the human brain. *Annual Review of Neuroscience, 13*, 25–42.

Posner, J. B., Saper, C. B., Schiff, N. D., & Plum, F. (1982). *Plum and Posner's diagnosis of stupor and coma.* New York: Oxford University Press.

Ramsberger, G. (2005). Achieving conversational success in aphasia by focusing on nonlinguistic cognitive skills: a potentially promising new approach. *Aphasiology, 19*(10/11), 1066–1073.

Ramsberger, G., & Hardin, K. (2011). Treatment of attention to improve conversational success in aphasia. *Perspectives on Neurophysiology and Neurogenic Speech and Language Disorders, 21*, 72–77.

Raymer, A. M., Bandy, D., Adair, J. C., Schwartz, R. L., Williamson, D.J.G., Gonzalez-Rothi, L. J., & Heilman, K. M. (2001). Effects of bromocriptine in a patient with crossed nonfluent aphasia: A case report. *Archives of Physical Medicine and Rehabilitation, 82*(1), 139–144.

Robertson, I. H., Ward, T., Ridgeway, V., & Nimmo-Smith, I. (1994). *The test of everyday attention*. Edmunds, UK: Thames Valley Testing.

Rogalsky, C., & Hickok, G. (2009). Selective attention to semantic and syntactic features modulates sentence processing networks in anterior temporal cortex. *Cerebral Cortex, 19*, 786–796.

Sarter, M., Gehring, W., & Kozak, R. (2005). More attention must be paid: the neurobiology of attentional effort. *Brain Research Reviews, 51*, 145–160.

Shallice, T. (2006). Contrasting domains in the control of action: the routine and the non-routine. In M. Johnson, & Y. Munakata (Eds.), *Attention and performance XXI: processes of change in brain and cognitive development* (pp. 3–29). New York: Oxford University Press.

Shallice, T., Stuss, D. T., Alexander, M. P., Picton, T. W., & Derkzen, D. (2008). The multiple dimensions of sustained attention. *Cortex, 44*(7), 794–805.

Shiffrin, R. M., & Schneider, W. (1977). Controlled and automatic human information processing: II. Perceptual learning, automatic attending and a general theory. *Psychological Review, 84*(2), 127–190.

Silkes, J.P.T., McNeil, M. R., & Drton, M. (2004).Simulation of aphasic naming performance in normal adults. *Journal of Speech, Language and Hearing Research, 47*(3), 610–623.

Sinotte, M. P., & Coelho, C. A. (2007). Attention training for reading impairment in mild aphasia: a follow-up study. *NeuroRehabilitation, 22*(4), 303–310.

Snyder, H. R., Banich, M. T., & Munakata, Y. (2011). Choosing our words: retrieval and selection processes recruit shared neural substrates in left ventrolateral prefrontal cortex. *Journal of Cognitive Neuroscience, 23*(11), 3470–3482.

Sohlberg, M. M., McLaughlin, K. A., Pavese, A., Heidrich, A., & Posner, M. (2001). Evaluation of attention process training and brain injury education in persons with acquired brain injury. *Journal of Clinical and Experimental Neuropsychology, 22*, 656–676.

Sohlberg, M. M., & Mateer, C. A. (1986). *Attention process training* (APT). Puyallup, WA: Association for Neuropsychological Research and Development.

Sohlberg, M. M., & Mateer, C. A. (2001). *Cognitive rehabilitation: an integrative neuropsychological approach*. New York: Guilford Press.

Sohlberg, M. M., Avery, J., Kennedy, M., Ylvisaker, M., Coelho, C., Turkstra, L., & Yorkston, K. (2003). Practice guidelines for direct attention training. *Journal of Medical Speech-Language Pathology, 11*(3), xix–xxxix.

Stroop, J. R. (1935). Studies of interference in serial verbal reactions. *Journal of Experimental Psychology, 18*, 643–662.

Sturm, W., & Willmes, K. (1991). Efficacy of a reaction training on various attentional and cognitive functions in stroke patients. *Journal of Neuropsychological Rehabilitation, 1*(4), 259–280.

Sturm, W., Willmes, K., Orgass, B., & Hartje, W. (1997). Do specific attention deficits need specific training? *Neuropsychological Rehabilitation, 7*(2), 81–103.

Stuss D. T., Shallice T., Alexander M. P., & Picton, T. W. (1995). A multidisciplinary approach to anterior attentional functions. *Annals of the New York Academy of Sciences, 769*, 191–209.

Stuss, D. T., Alexander, M. P., Shallice, T., Picton, T. W., Binns, M. A., Macdonald, R., … Katz, D. I. (2005). Multiple frontal systems controlling response speed. *Neuropsychologia, 43*(3), 396–417.

Stuss, D. T., Binns, M. A., Murphy, K. J., & Alexander, M. P. (2002). Dissociations within the anterior attentional system: effects of task complexity and irrelevant information on reaction time speed and accuracy. *Neuropsychology, 16*, 500–513.

Styles, E. A. (1997). *The psychology of attention*. East Sussex, UK: Psychology Press.

Tatemichi, T. K., Desmond, D. W., Stern, Y., Paik, M., Sano, M., & Bagiella, E. (1994). Cognitive impairment after stroke: frequency, patterns, and relationship to functional abilities. *Journal of Neurology, Neurosurgery, and Psychiatry, 57*, 202–207.

Thompson-Schill, S. L., D'Esposito, M., Aguirre, G. K., & Farah, M. J. (1997). Role of left inferior prefrontal cortex in retrieval of semantic knowledge: a reevaluation. *Proceedings of the National Academy of Sciences, USA, 94*, 14792–14797.

Thompson-Schill, S. L., Swick, D., Farah, M. J., D'Esposito, M., Kan, I. P., & Knight, R. T. (1998).Verb generation in patients with focal frontal lesions: a neuropsychological test of neuroimaging findings. *Proceedings of the National Academy of Sciences of the United States of America, 26*, 14792–14797.

Treisman, A. (1993). The perception of features and objects. In A. D. Baddeley & L. Weiskrantz (Eds.), *Attention: selection, awareness, and control: a tribute to Donald Broadbent* (pp. 5–35). New York: Clarendon Press/Oxford University Press.

Tseng, C.-H., McNeil, M. R., & Milenkovic, P. (1993). An investigation of attention allocation deficits in aphasia. *Brain and Language, 45*(2), 276–296.

Van Zomeren, A. H., & Brouwer, W. H. (1994). *Clinical neuropsychology of attention*. New York: Oxford University Press.

Wagner, A. D., Paré-Blagoev, E. J., Clark, J., & Poldrack, R. A. (2001). Recovering meaning: left prefrontal cortex guides controlled semantic retrieval. *Neuron, 31*(2), 329–338.

Weintraub, S. (2000). Neuropsychological assessment of mental state. In M. M. Mesulam (Ed.), *Principles of behavioral and cognitive neurology* (2nd ed., pp. 121–173). New York: Oxford University Press.

Wickens, C. D. (1984). Processing resources in attention. In R. Parasuraman & R. Davies (Eds.), *Varieties of attention* (pp. 63–101). New York: Academic Press.

Wickens, C. D. (1989). Attention and skilled performance. In D. Holding (Ed.), *Human skills* (pp. 71–105). New York: Wiley.

Zhang, D., & Raichle, M. E. (2010). Disease and the brain's dark energy. *Nature Reviews Neurology. 6*(1), 15–28.

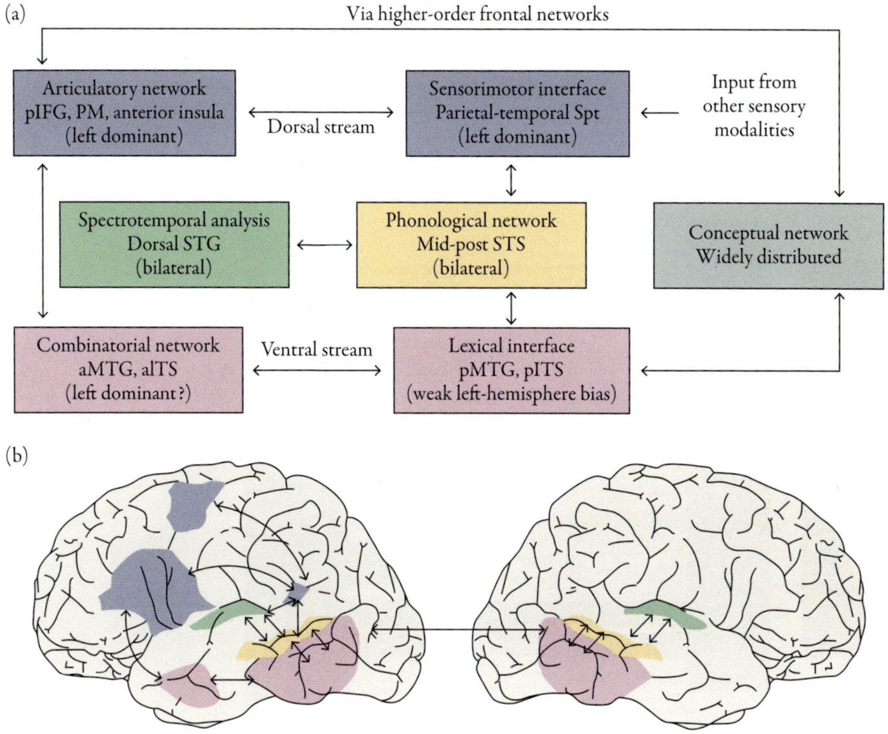

FIGURE 2.1 Dorsal-ventral streams.

Source: Adapted from Cahana-Amitay, D., & Albert, M. L. (2014). Brain and language: evidence for neural multifunctionality. *Behavioural Neurology*, Figure 1.

Reprinted under the Creative Commons Attribution License from Cahana-Amitay, D., and Albert, M. L. (2014). Brain and language: evidence for neural multifunctionality. *Behavioural Neurology*, http://dx.doi.org/10.1155/2014/260381. Hindawi, copyright 2014.

STS, superior temporal sulcus; STG, superior temporal gyrus; aITS, anterior inferior temporal sulcus; aMTG, anterior middle temporal gyrus; pIFG, posterior inferior frontal gyrus; PM, premotor cortex.

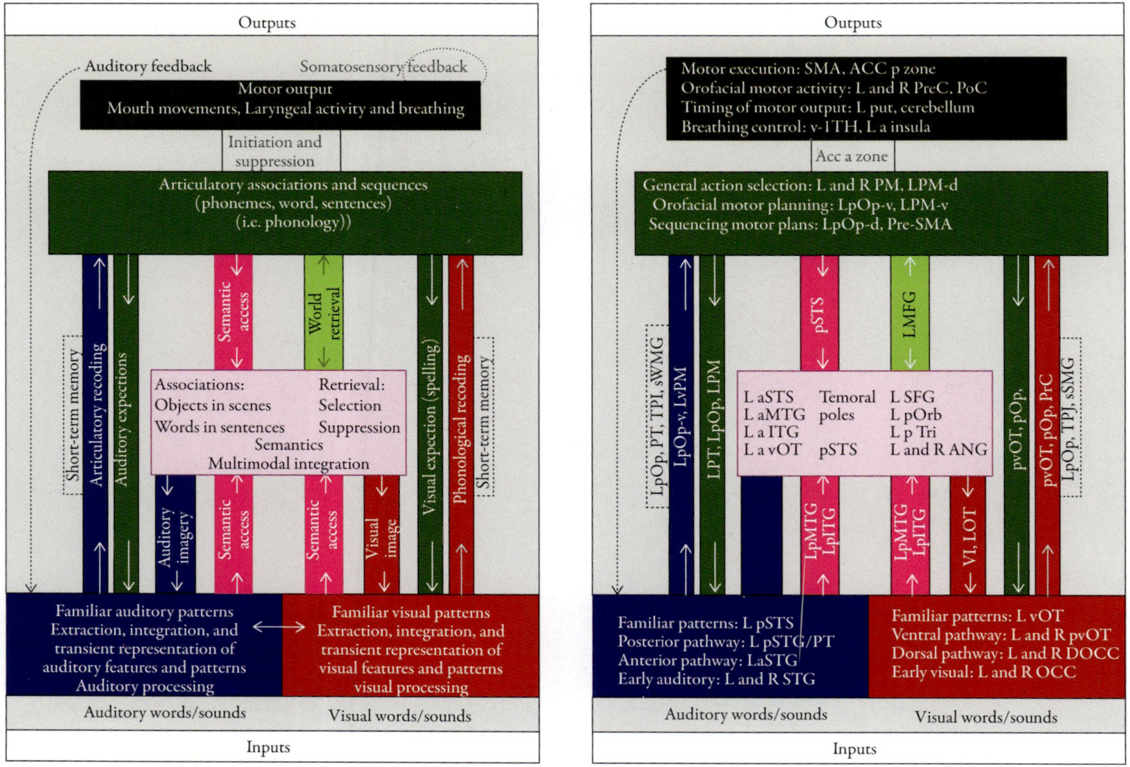

FIGURE 2.2 Brain-function mappings.

Source: Adapted from Cabana-Amitay, D., & Albert, M. L. (2014). Brain and language: evidence for neural multifunctionality. *Behavioural Neurology*, Figure 2. Reprinted under the Creative Commons Attribution License from Cabana-Amitay, D. and Albert, M.L. (2014). Brain and language: evidence for neural multifunctionality. *Behavioural Neurology*, http://dx.doi.org/10.1155/2014/260381. Hindawi, copyright 2014.

a, anterior; A, auditory cortex; ACC, anterior cingulate; AG, angular gyrus; c, caudate; CB, cerebellum; d, dorsal; GP, globus pallidus; IFS, inferior frontal sulcus; IOG, inferior occipital gyrus; ITG, inferior temporal gyrus; MFG, middle frontal gyrus; MTG, middle temporal gyrus; Occ, occipital; OT, occipitotemporal; p, posterior; PO, parietal operculum; pOp, pars opercularis; pOrb, pars orbitallis; pTri, pars triangularis; PT, planum temporale; poC, postcentral; preC, precentral; PM, premotor; PUT, putamen; SFG, superior frontal gyrus; SMA, supplementary motor cortex; STG, superior temporal gyrus; STS, superior temporal sulcus; SMG, supramarginal gyrus; TPJ, temporoparietal junction; Tb, thalamus; v, ventral; VI, lobule VI (medial anterior); VII, lobule VII (lateral posterior).

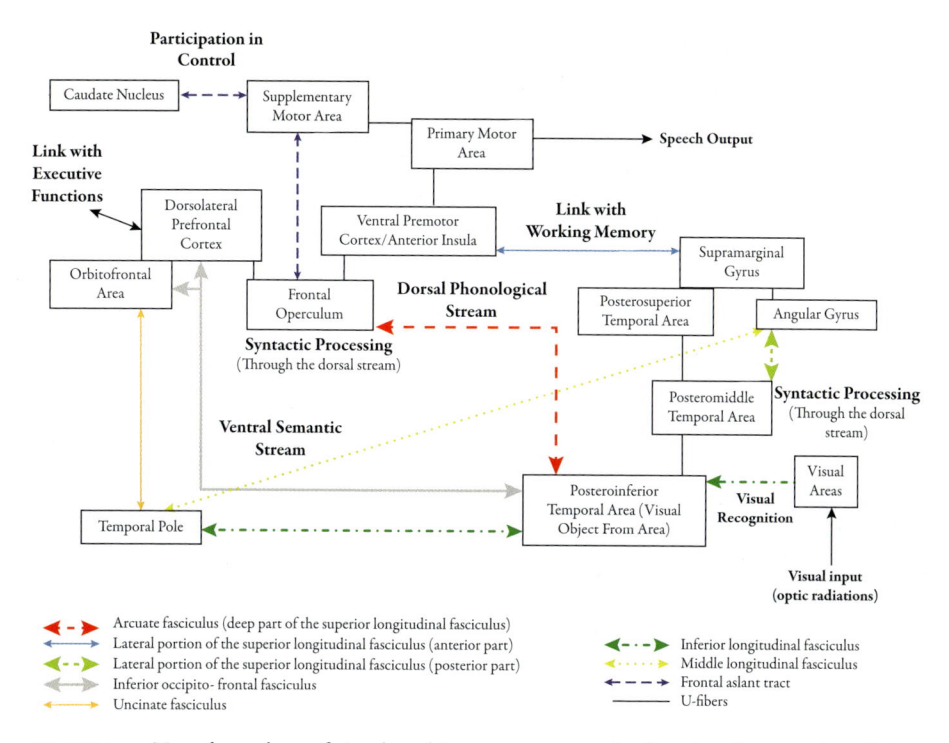

FIGURE 2.3 Neural correlates of visual-working memory-executive functions-language interlinks.

Source: Reprinted by permission from Elsevier Limited [Brain and Language] from Figure 2 in Duffau, H., Moritz-Gasser, S., & Mandonnet, E. (2014). A re-examination of neural basis of language processing: proposal of a dynamic hodotopical model from data provided by brain stimulation mapping during picture naming. *Brain and Language, 131,* 1-10, copyright 2014.

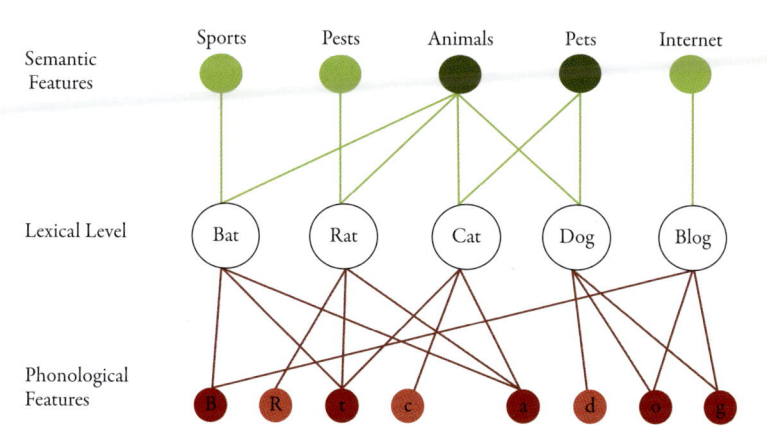

FIGURE 5.2 Levels of activation during lexical processing. Shaded circles reflect shared features; activation of connections in the model is bidirectional.

Source: Based on the lexical access framework developed by Dell, G. S., Schwartz, M. F., Martin, N., Saffran, E. M., & Gagnon, D. A. (1997). Lexical access in aphasic and nonaphasic speakers. *Psychological Review, 104*(4), 801–838.

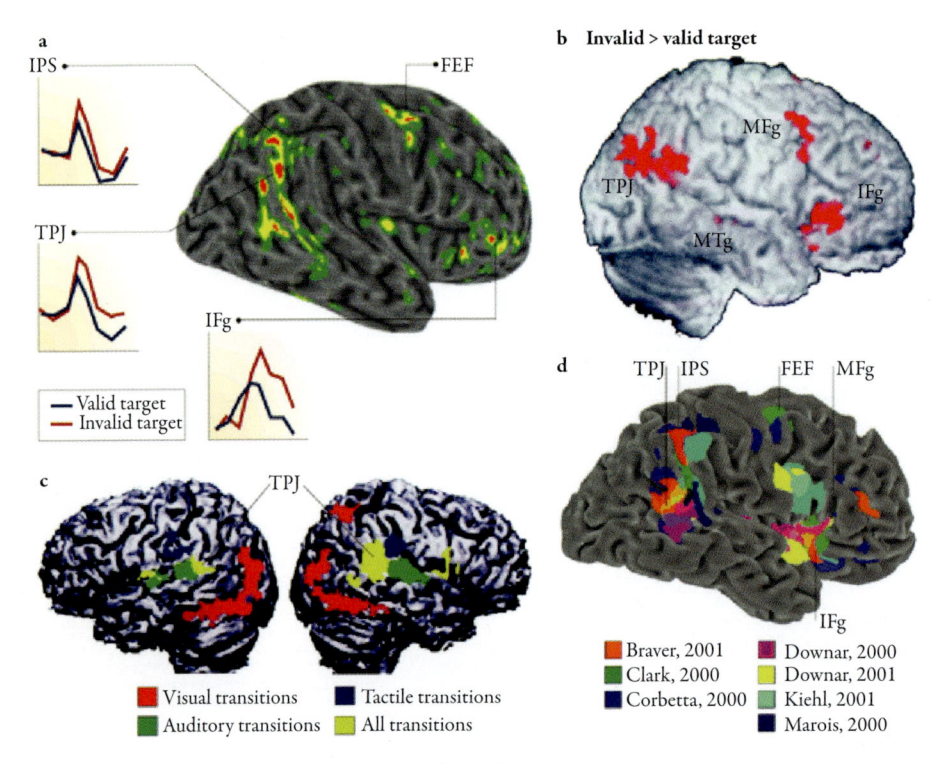

FIGURE 4.1 The functional neuroanatomy of attention systems.

Reprinted by permission from Macmillan Publishers Ltd [Nature Review Neuroscience], Corbetta, M. & Shulman, G.L. (2002). Control of goal-directed and stimulus-driven attention in the brain. Nature Review Neuroscience, 3(3), 1602-1610, copyright 2002.

(a) Human brain activity produced by attending to a location. Subjects see an arrow that cues one of two locations and covertly attend to the location indicated in preparation for a target at that location. The functional magnetic resonance imaging (fMRI) response is averaged over 13 subjects. The graphs show the time course of the fMRI signal after the cue. Signals are transient in occipital regions but sustained (gray arrow) in the parietal cortex and frontal eye field (FEF). (b) Human brain activity produced by attending to a direction of motion. Subjects see an arrow that cues a direction of motion and prepare for a subsequent target moving in that direction. The response is averaged over 14 subjects. The graphs contrast the response seen when the arrow cues a direction of motion with that observed when a cue instructs the subject to view the display passively. Directional cues produce sustained signals in frontal (FEF) and parietal (aIPs, pIPs) areas but transient signals in occipital areas (MT+). (c) *Left:* meta-analysis of studies of visual attention. Subjects expected a simple visual attribute, such as location or direction of motion, or a more complex array. Foci of activation from the expectation period are smoothed and projected onto the visible human brain. The area of maximal overlap between studies is in the pIPs. The figure shows regions that are activated by attending to and detecting visual stimuli (preparatory activity has been averaged with visual- and motor-detection activity). (d) Anticipatory activity in a macaque V3A neuron during a memory-guided task. (adapted with permission from Ref. 27 © 2000 The American Physiological Society). The graph shows the single-unit activity as the monkey performs two tasks while fixating the center of the screen. In the fixation task, a small stimulus is presented peripherally and the monkey is rewarded for maintaining fixation. In the memory-guided task, the monkey has to remember the location of the stimulus and after a variable delay make a saccade to that location. Activity is increased in the memory-guided task before stimulus onset, perhaps reflecting attention to the stimulus location.

aIPs, anterior intraparietal sulcus; Fus, fusiform cortex; MT+, middle temporal complex; pIPs, posterior IPs; vIPs, ventral IPs (junction of the vIPs and transverse occipital sulcus); PoCes, postcentral sulcus; PrCes, precentral sulcus; SFs, superior frontal sulcus; SPL, superior parietal lobule. Right: meta-analysis of imaging studies of visual attention and detection.

Source: Corbetta, M., & Shulman, G. L. (2002). Control of goal-directed and stimulus-driven attention in the brain. *Nature Reviews Neuroscience, 3*(3), 201–215, Figure 6. Reprinted by permission from Macmillan Publishers Ltd [Nature Review Neuroscience], copyright 2002.

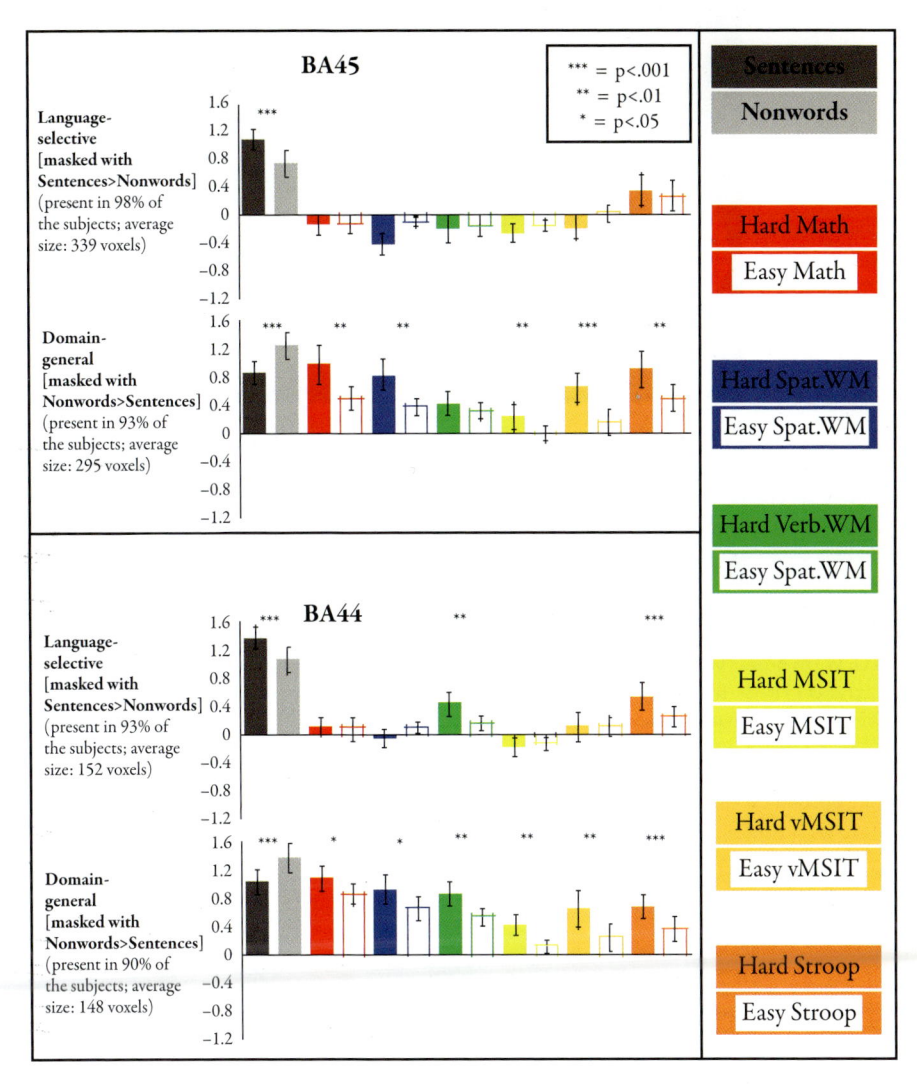

FIGURE 4.2 Representation of language and domain-general brain structures.
*Functional profiles of language-selective and domain-general functional ROIs. Magnitude of response (in percent signal change from the fixation baseline) of language-selective and domain-general regions within BA45 (top box) and BA44 (bottom box) to each of the two conditions in each of the seven tasks. Language-selective regions are defined by intersecting BA45/44 with sentences > nonwords activation, and domain-general regions are defined by intersecting BA45/44 with nonwords > sentences activation. All magnitudes shown are estimated from data independent of those used to define the regions; responses to the sentences and nonwords are estimated using a left-out run. Error bars represent SEM by participants. *P <.05; **P <.01; ***P <.001. In the math task, participants added smaller versus larger numbers; in the spatial and verbal working memory (WM) tasks, participants kept in memory fewer versus more locations or digits, respectively; and in the three cognitive control tasks (MSIT, vMSIT, Stroop), participants had to inhibit a prepotent but task-irrelevant response and choose instead the task-relevant response. Source:* Reprinted under the Creative Commons Attribution License from Fedorenko, E., Duncan, J., & Kanwisher, N. (2012). Language-selective and domain-general regions lie side by side within Broca's area. *Current Biology, 22,* 2059–2062, Figure 2.

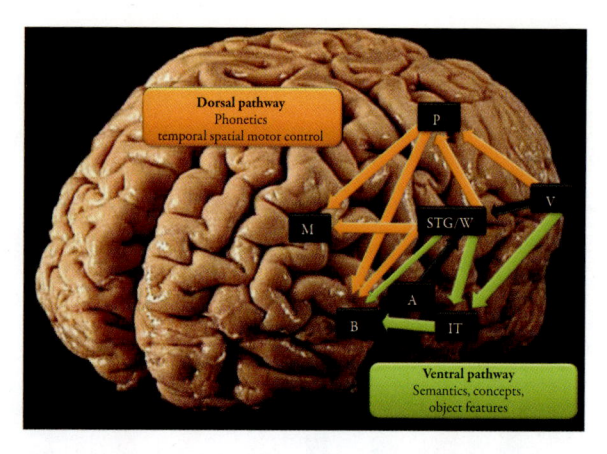

FIGURE 7.1 Neural parallels between apraxia and aphasia. The dorsal route (orange) comprises pathways from the parietal cortex (P) and posterior part of the superior temporal gyrus (STG/W) to the premotor area (M) and to Broca's area (B), connected via the arcuate/superior longitudinal fasciculus. The dorsal route may process phonetic information to produce verbal output without accessing word meaning. Word repetition may rely on this route, as evidenced by the phonemic paraphasia caused by damage to this pathway. The dorsal route may also be involved when guiding the hand to target objects via temporal spatial control combined with visual/tactile feedback. Damage to this route may impair gesture imitation. The ventral route (green) comprises pathways from the superior temporal gyrus (STG/W) to Broca's area (B) via the extreme capsule, and from the anterior part of the superior temporal gyrus (IT) to the frontal operculum via the uncinated fasciculus. Injury to the ventral pathway may result in sensory aphasia. It may also cause apraxia accompanied with difficulties with actual tool use.

A, auditory cortex; *M,* motor-related areas; *V,* visual cortex. *Source:* From Kobayashi, S., & Ugawa, Y. (2013). Relationships between aphasia and apraxia. *Journal of Neurology and Translational Neuroscience, 2*(1), 1028, Figure 2. Reprinted under the Creative Commons Attribution License.

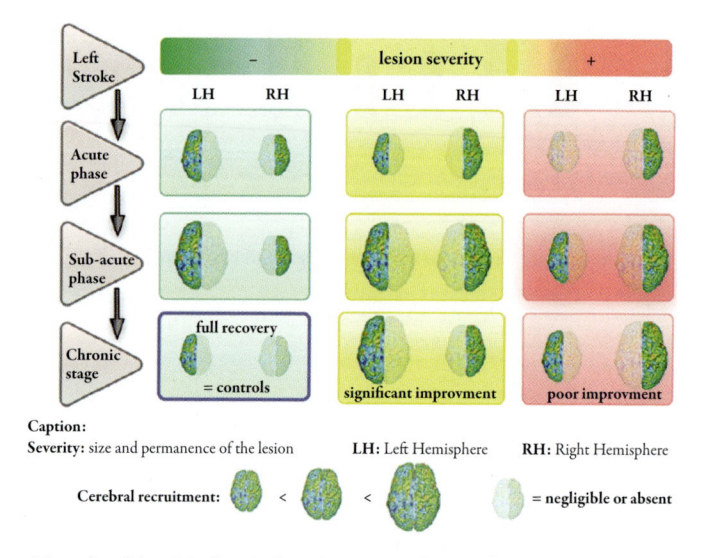

FIGURE 9.1 The role of the right hemisphere in recovery from aphasia. A possible interpretation of the controversial results about the role of the right hemisphere during recovery from aphasia: recruitment depending of lesion severity and time poststroke.

Source: From Anglade, C., Thiel, A., & Ansaldo, A. I. (2014). The complementary role of the cerebral hemispheres in recovery from aphasia after stroke: a critical review of the literature. *Brain Injury, 28(2),* 138-145. Reprinted by permission from Informa Healthcare [Brain Injury], copyright 2014.

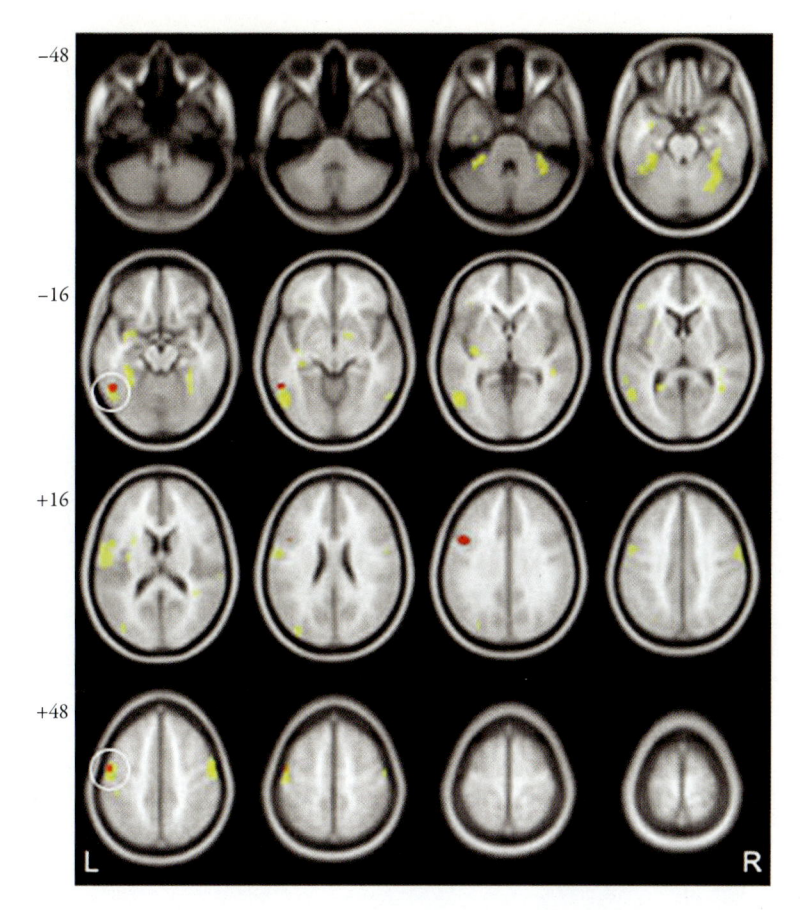

FIGURE 8.1 Neural correlates of visual and responsive naming in Hamberger's et al.'s (2013) study.
GLM results for visual and description naming. There was visual naming activation (yellow, VN > VC) in the bilateral parahippocampal gyrus and fusiform gyrus (row 1, fourth panel), temporooccipital cortex (row 2, bottom clusters), and bilateral pre/postcentral and inferior frontal gyrus (row 3 and 4). There was description naming activation (red, DN > DC) in left temporo-occipital cortex (row 2, left two panels), left inferior frontal gyrus (row 3, third panel), and left precentral gyrus (row 4, first panel). Regions of overlap for description and visual naming are indicated with circles (temporo-occipital cortex, second row, and pre/post central gyrus, fourth row). Source: **From Hamberger, M.J., Habeck, C.G., Pantazatos, S.P., Williams, A.C., & Hirsch, J. (2013). Shared space, separate processes: Neural activation patterns for auditory description and visual object naming in healthy adults.** *Human Brain Mapping 35*(6), 2507-2520, figure 1. Reprinted by permission from John Wiley and Sons [Human Brain Mapping], copyright 2013.

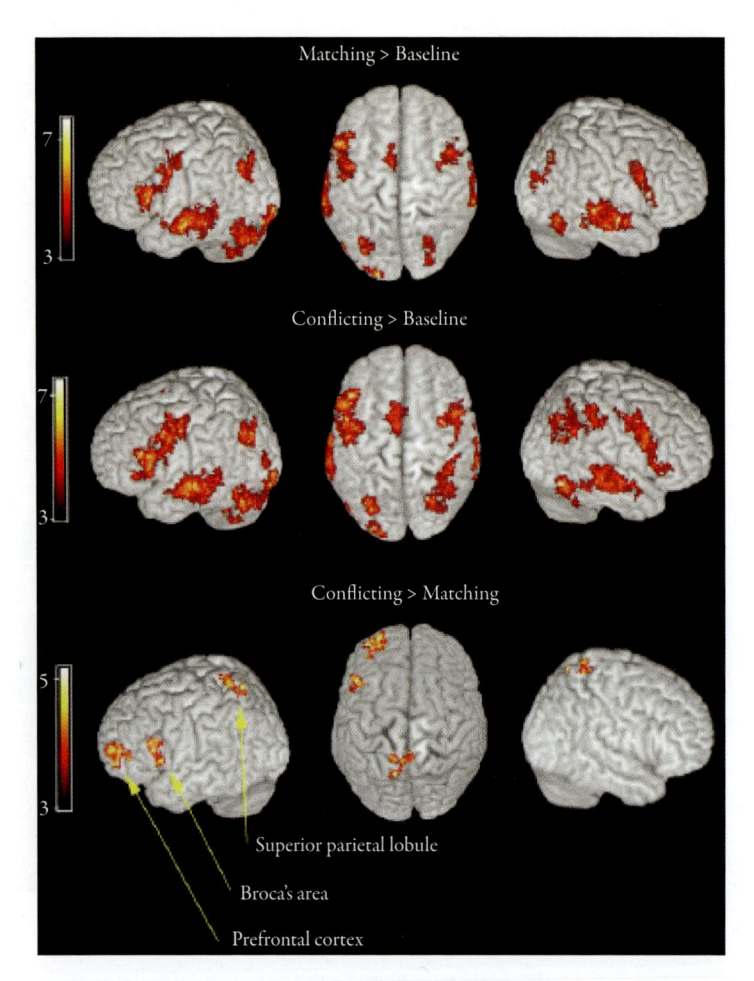

FIGURE 8.2 Brain activation in response to audiovisual processing.

Across-subjects (N = 10) z statistical maps overlaid on an anatomical template. Matching audiovisual speech activated the auditory and visual cortical areas as well as the inferior frontal, premotor, and the visual-parietal areas bilaterally (upper panel). Conflicting audiovisual speech caused a similar but more extensive pattern of brain activity (middle panel). The difference in the contrast conflicting N matching AV-stimulation reached significance in three left-hemisphere areas: Broca's area (BA44/45), the superior parietal lobule (BA7), and the prefrontal cortex (BA10) (lower panel). In the contrast matching N conflicting no statistically significant voxels were detected. Activation maps were thresholded using clusters determined by voxelwise Z N 3.0 and a cluster significance threshold of P b.05, corrected for multiple comparisons. *Source*: From Ojanen, V., Möttönen, R., Pekkola, J., Jääskeläinen, I.P., Joensuu, R., Autti, T., & Sams, M. (2005). Processing of audiovisual speech in Broca's area, *Neuroimage, 25*, 333-338, figure 2. Reprinted by permission from Elsevier Limited [NeuroImage], copyright, 2005.

5

The Role of Memory Functions in Recovery from Aphasia

Introduction

At this point in the book, the claim that some people with aphasia may also exhibit memory deficits alongside their language impairments should come as no surprise. Indeed, many studies have reported memory decrements in aphasia involving different memory types and severities (e.g., Allen, Martin, & Martin, 2012; Baldo, Katseff, & Dronkers, 2012; Beeson, Bayles, Rubens, & Kaszniak, 1993; Burgio & Basso, 1997; Butters et al., 1970; Caplan & Waters, 1994; Caspari et al., 1998; Coughlin, 1979; Dalla Barba et al., 1996; Gandha et al., 1983; Gordon, 1983; Gvion & Friedmann, 2012; Harris Wright & Fergadiotis, 2012; Kasselimis et al., 2013; Kinsbourne, 1972; Lang & Quitz, 2012; Laures-Gore, Marshall, & Verner, 2011; Leff et al., 2009; Martin & Ayala, 2004; Martin & Saffran, 1997; Mayer & Murray, 2012; Miyake, Carpenter, & Just, 1994; Murray, Ramage, & Hopper, 2001; Ostergaard & Meudell, 1984; Potagas et al., 2011; Turksta, 2001; Vallila-Rohter & Kiran, 2013). These studies once again point to the interconnectedness of language functions and nonverbal domains of cognition and underscore the essential role of these interconnections in shaping the long-term changes in language performance observed in aphasia recovery.

Early studies of the contributions of memory functions to language performance in aphasia were framed in a neuroanatomical context, which considered whether complex memory functions remain distinct from or interact with linguistic processes subserved by the left temporal lobe (e.g., Coughlin, 1979; Kinsbourne, 1972; Gordon,

1983). Researchers examined whether particular temporal regions support both verbal and nonverbal cognitive processes (Coughlin, 1979) or represent distinguishable components such as memory span and linguistic load (Kinsbourne, 1972; Gordon, 1983). Although the advent of neuroimaging and advances in methods of neuropsychological assessment have led to finer-grained analyses concerning the relationships between memory, language, aphasia, and the brain, the precise nature of these interdependencies still remains to be uncovered. Our goal in this chapter, then, is to expose the threads of evidence emerging from these different strands of research relating to the mutual influences of language and memory in health and disease.

To this end we will first introduce the central theoretical models put forth to explain behavioral and neural processes underlying memory-language interactions, drawing on theoretical distinctions among working memory, short-term memory, and long-term memory (e.g., Baddeley, 2003). These models can largely be grouped into three approaches that differ in the extent to which they assume that language and memory constitute distinct components (see, in this regard, N. Martin, 2000): (1) *independent* but *cooperative*, which argues that the language processor independently generates the phonological forms that enter the verbal short-term memory system (e.g., Shallice, 1988); (2) *interactive*, which implicates both systems in the temporary storage of multilevel linguistic representations (e.g., R. Martin & Lesch, 1996); and (3) *unified*, where both systems are assumed to share the same activation patterns when forming linguistic representations (N. Martin & Saffran, 1997). These models have propelled the development of new approaches to aphasia rehabilitation over the past three decades, harnessing memory-based notions to interventions that maximize retention, learning, and generalization (e.g., Friedman, 2000; N. Martin, 2000; Murray et al., 2001; Stout & Murray, 2001; Vallila-Rohter & Kiran, 2013).

We place particular emphasis on findings from recent neuroimaging studies that clearly point to a need to expand the neuroanatomical maps one typically considers in theories of aphasia recovery to include neural structures critically associated with memory functions, such as the hippocampus (Menke et al., 2009; Meinzer et al., 2010). These newly discovered patterns of brain activation are exactly what one would expect in a system with the fundamental characteristics of neural multifunctionality in which, as pointed out in Chapter 2, *constant* and *dynamic interaction* exists among neural networks subserving cognitive (and other nonlinguistic) functions with neural networks specialized for language functions.

Memory: Multiple Classifications

Memory is not a unitary construct (e.g., Cabeza & Moscovitch, 2013; Squire & Wixted, 2011). Over the years, researchers have sliced and spliced this concept along many axes in an attempt to capture its different facets, such as the *type* of information to be remembered (explicit/implicit; declarative/nondeclarative), the *duration* of the information to be retained and processed (short-/long-term/working memory), the *content* of the processed information (verbal/nonverbal; semantic/phonological), and even the *modality* in which it is presented (visual/auditory). As different frameworks evolved, questions about information decay and the consolidation of information have been considered, specifically with regard to the extent to which persons can encode incoming information, maintain it in storage, and retrieve it during task performance. We would do a great disservice to the thousands of books and research publications on memory if we tried to review the entire range of concepts that have been proposed over time. Instead, in what follows we narrow the discussion to those concepts that have been studied most extensively in relation to language performance, particularly among persons with aphasia.

EXPLICIT/IMPLICIT, DECLARATIVE/PROCEDURAL MEMORY
SYSTEMS AND THEIR NEURAL UNDERPINNINGS

A central distinction has been drawn between two memory systems: (1) *explicit memory*, the function of which is to remember factual information ("what"), and (2) *implicit memory*, whose role is to remember habitual aspects of memory performance ("how") (e.g., Curran & Schacter, 2013; Squire, 2004). This classification was designed to capture, for example, the difference between the type of information processing required for remembering that you bought a pair of shoes and the type of information processing necessary for remembering that when you purchase something you should pay with cash, check, or credit card.

The systems of explicit and implicit memory have also been termed *declarative* and *nondeclarative/procedural* systems (e.g., Eichenbaum & Cohen, 2001; Mishkin et al., 1984; Poldrack & Packard, 2003; Schacter & Tulving, 1994; Squire, 2007; Squire & Knowlton, 2000; Ullman, 2004). The declarative system has been assumed to consist of two subcomponents: (1) *semantic*, to support memories of facts, and (2) *episodic*, to mediate memories of particular events (recently reviewed in Roediger & Craik, 2014). It is argued that this system participates in rapid learning, interacts with multiple mental systems, and involves conscious recollection (e.g., Ullman, 2004). The procedural system, in contrast, has been assumed to be an unconscious process that contributes to the learning of context-based, rule-governed new and/or established skills (e.g., Knowlton, Mangels, & Squire, 1996; Packard & Knowlton, 2002; Poldrack, Prabhakaran, Seger, & Gabrieli, 1999; White, 1997; Wise, Murray, & Gerfen, 1996).

Brain structures subserving the declarative memory system are assumed to consist of hierarchically organized mediotemporal structures, including the hippocampus and the entorhinal, perirhinal, and parahippocampal cortices (Squire & Knowlton, 2000; Suzuki & Eichenbaum, 2000; Ullman, 2004). The hippocampus projects to the mammillary bodies and parts of the thalamus. These areas have been implicated in the encoding, consolidation, and retrieval of new and existing memories (e.g., Alvarez & Squire,

1994; Buckner & Wheeler, 2001; Eichenbaum & Cohen, 2001; Squire & Knowlton, 2000). The declarative system is tightly linked to a "ventral" stream of information flow (Goodale & Milner, 1992; Ungerleider & Mishkin, 1982), from which it receives perceptual representations of objects and their relations for long-term storage (Goodale, 2000).

Other brain structures implicated in the encoding, selection, and retrieval of declarative information involve prefrontal regions, especially the ventrolateral prefrontal cortex—the inferior frontal gyrus and Brodmann's areas 44, 45, and 47 (e.g., Buckner & Wheeler, 2001; Thompson-Schill et al., 1997; Wagner et al., 1998). These frontal structures have been shown to be further fractionated into neural structures dedicated to processing of specific types of linguistic information: BA 6/44 mediating processing of phonological information and BA 45/47 supporting processing of semantic information (e.g., Poldrack et al., 1999). We return to a more detailed description of these structures later in the chapter in discussing the neural correlates of working memory, focusing on the temporal features of memory processing (see also Chapter 3, where we review the role of these structures in relation to the framework of semantic control).

It is noteworthy that these cortical structures have also been implicated in the processing of procedural memory, especially in sequence learning (linear and hierarchical) (e.g., Conway & Christiansen, 2001; Dominey et al., 2003; Goschke et al., 2001). In fact, the processing of procedural memory system has been linked to a web of brain structures involving frontal/basal-ganglia connections, parietal and superior temporal cortices, and the cerebellum (e.g., De Renzi, 1989; Heilman, Watson, & Gonzalez-Rothi, 1997; Hikosaka et al., 2000; Mishkin et al., 1984; Schacter & Tulving, 1994; Squire & Zola, 1996). The basal ganglia are of particular importance in this regard as they have been found to be highly relevant to aspects of learning related to memory consolidation (e.g., Doya, 2000; Packard & Knowlton, 2002; White, 1997). The interconnections of the basal ganglia are organized into functionally distinct circuits, each receiving projections at the neostriatum (at the caudate or the putamen) from cortical or subcortical sources. These projections follow direct and indirect pathways ending at designated frontal destinations, inhibiting and disinhibiting different cortical functions (e.g., Alexander & Crutcher, 1990; Alexander, DeLong, & Strick, 1986; Middletown & Strick, 2000).

Unfortunately, for all their presumed clarity, the functional neuroanatomical maps of the memory systems just described have been found to be untenable (Cabeza & Moscovitch, 2013). For example, prefrontal cortical regions have been reported to mediate both declarative and nondeclarative information (e.g., Badre & Wagner, 2007). The same can be said for medial temporal structures (e.g., Dew & Cabeza, 2011; Henke, 2010). Rather than fractionating memory into isolable neural systems, Cabeza and Moscovitch (2013) have recently proposed to view the neural correlates of memory through a *component process framework*, in which region-specific neural configurations contribute to multiple cognitive tasks simultaneously. Under such a view, a model with a "prefrontal-specific subregion" component would predict activation of the left anterior ventrolateral prefrontal cortex in implicit memory tasks, semantic and episodic memory tasks, and conceptual priming tasks but not automatic conceptual processing, which may be associated with brain activation in left temporal cortical regions.

The component interactions in this framework are defined as "process-specific alliances" (Cabeza & Moscovitch, 2013). These alliances comprise small brain regions that are temporarily activated to meet task demands associated with the performance of a given cognitive task. Each component in the alliance has a particular function, and together they converge to yield a complex operation. These small neural bundles are dismantled once task demands are met, unlike larger-scale neural networks, whose connections continue to hold (evidenced, for example, in resting-state brain activation patterns) (Doucet et al., 2011; Wig, Schlagger, & Petersen, 2011; Yeo et al., 2011). The stable links among components in the larger networks can affect which transient alliances are created, but they do not directly govern them. We note with interest that our model of the neural multifunctionality of language is aligned in many respects with the component process framework of Cabeza and Moscovitch in that the operations within our neural multifunctionality model rest on the interaction of "neural cohorts" mediating multiple interactive functions in cognitive, emotional, motor, and perceptual domains.

Theoretical accounts linking the neural correlates of declarative and procedural memory systems to language functions from a multifunctional perspective are limited. A notable exception is Ullman's (2004) declarative/procedural model, which was mentioned in Chapter 2 and which we briefly repeat here. Within his framework, neuroanatomical structures share the burden of processing declarative and procedural memory and language functions by drawing on functional similarities between these systems. Thus temporal networks that mediate the encoding, consolidation, and retrieval of new memories in declarative memory are also assumed to subsume noncompositional, irregular, unpredictable forms in the mental lexicon. Similarly, frontal, basal ganglia, parietal, and cerebellar structures supporting nondeclarative rule-based operations are assumed to play a role in the sequencing and hierarchical organization of grammatical structures. These processes are assumed to be accomplished via dynamically interactive neural networks, which, in the course of information processing, operate cooperatively, complimentarily, and competitively.

Long-Term, Short-Term, and Working Memory: A Window into Memory-Language Dependencies

Theoretical models that elucidate the nature of the relationship between memory and language functions have been more concerned with the *temporal* aspects of memory processing (i.e., the duration associated with information retention and its manipulation). This emphasis is likely linked to the general observation that persons with aphasia typically have preserved semantic knowledge, the "what" but show impaired *access* to their semantic system, the "how" (Antonucci & Reilly, 2008; Reilly, 2008; see also the discussions of semantic control in Chapter 3 and mechanisms of attention allocation in Chapter 4). Moreover, deficits in verbal short-term memory have been identified as one of the most central and lingering characteristics of aphasic language impairment (Attout, Van der Kaa, George, & Majerus, 2012; Martin, Saffran, & Dell, 1996; Majerus, Van der Linden, Poncelet, & Metz-Lutz, 2004).

Historically, time-focused models of memory were developed in the context of Hebb's (1949) seminal work, which identified two types of memory: *long-term memory* (LTM), leading to long-lasting changes in the brain, and *short-term memory* (STM), implicating transient electrical brain activation. This distinction inspired much of the early work on memory in cognitive psychology, which proposed that information processing in the human brain involved a mechanism for temporarily storing small amounts of information (e.g., Adams & Dijksstra, 1966; Brown 1958; Peterson & Peterson, 1959; Pilsbury & Sylvester, 1940).

A breakthrough proposal was Atkinson & Shiffrin's (1968) well-known two-component sequential model of memory, according to which information from the environment was assumed to be briefly stored in STM, which controlled the flow of information to prevent its decay en route to the more permanent LTM. In this model, STM was assumed to subsume a wide array of complex cognitive functions, including long-term learning, reasoning, and language comprehension.

In early research on this topic, evidence of double dissociations between the STM and LTM systems among persons with brain damage served to confirm this two-component model. A case in point was that of H.M., who, following surgery to his hippocampi to relieve symptoms of epilepsy, lost his ability to create ongoing memories (LTM) but retained his capacity to perform short-term tasks (STM), such as repetition (Milner, 1966). In addition, persons with mediotemporal damage were shown to have impaired LTM but preserved STM (Baddeley & Warrington, 1970), whereas persons with conduction aphasia were found to demonstrate the exact opposite pattern (Shallice & Warrington, 1970).

Unfortunately this model fell short by failing to account for the preservation of complex cognitive abilities typically observed among persons with conduction aphasia but not predicted by a model with a unitary STM component. Moreover, studies of retention of verbal information in STM revealed differential effects of speech sounds and word meaning on immediate recall, emphasizing the need to develop a finer-grained theoretical model of memory. For example, phonological similarity among words (e.g., "cat," "cap"), rather than their semantic relatedness (e.g., "cat," "dog"), was found to impede immediate recall of short word lists (Baddeley, 1966), with the opposite being true when participants were presented with longer lists (greater than 10 items) involving a number of practice trials (Baddeley & Hitch, 1974). Relatedly, effective long-term learning of new words was shown only when word meaning rather than phonological information was encoded (Craik & Lockhart, 1972).

In the face of these empirical problems, Baddeley and Hitch (1974) proposed a three-component parallel processing working memory (WM) system, which shifted the exploration of the nature of *memory-language* dependencies in a new direction (e.g., Baddeley, Gathercole, Papagno, 1998; Collete, Van der Linden, & Poncelet, 2000). This newer model was conceived as a limited-capacity system designed to temporarily store and manipulate information, just as complex cognitive processes are concurrently performed (Baddeley, 2003, 2007; Baddeley, Chincotta, & Adlam, 2001). In this context, it is important to note the distinction between the concepts of STM and WM. Although the two overlap, STM is associated with temporary storage of information, whereas WM is associated with the manipulation of the stored information, and is therefore more strongly tied to executive function systems (N. Martin et al., 2012).

The components of the Baddeley and Hitch model included domain-specific buffers, "slave" systems, governed by a domain-general cognitive control mechanism: (1) a verbal-acoustic storage component, termed *the phonological loop*, engaged in the processing of verbal information; (2) a visuospatial component, called the *visuospatial sketchpad*, involved in the processing of visuospatial material; and (3) a limited-capacity *central executive system*, which controls behavior (Baddeley, 1986, 2001). This executive system is assumed to operate in much the same way as the *supervisory attention system* (Norman & Shallice, 1980, 1986) mentioned in Chapter 3 (i.e., suppression of unwanted responses through the inhibition of irrelevant information, incompatible with task goals). Efficient operation of the central executive was found to be highly dependent on resource demands placed on working memory capacity. For example, the simultaneous performance of two tasks did not present a challenge to task performers unless WM load exceeded three items (Baddeley & Hitch, 1974).

The phonological loop, the component most directly linked to the processing of linguistic information, was assumed to have two roles. First, to store dissolvable traces of verbal memory (decay of which is estimated at approximately 2 seconds) in a *phonological input store*; second, to refresh these traces through online subvocal rehearsal, termed *articulatory rehearsal process*. The proposed phonological store readily explained Baddeley's (1966) observation that phonologically similar words are more difficult to recall ("cap," "cat," "can") compared with phonologically dissimilar items ("cat," "cow," "jam"). Empirical support for the rehearsal process has been found in studies of word-length effects on immediate serial recall, which showed decline in recall as word length within the list increased—a pattern that disappeared with the insertion of irrelevant sound sequences (Baddeley, Thomson, & Buchanan, 1975). The argument is that the irrelevant sounds block rehearsal and, consequently, the retention of the memory trace; also, when stimuli are presented visually, they stop registration of phonological information through subvocalization. Overt articulation does not appear to be necessary for rehearsal, as persons with dysarthria have been shown to demonstrate the word-length effect (Baddeley & Wilson, 1985). Additionally, persons with dyspraxia impairing their speech-motor plan for articulation fail to show any signs of rehearsal (Caplan & Waters,

1995), suggesting that motor planning and not articulation as such is at the heart of rehearsal.

To increase the empirical validity of his original model, Baddeley added a fourth component to his WM mechanism—an *episodic buffer* (Baddeley, 2000, 2007, 2010). This buffer was assumed to be a consciously accessible temporary store of up to four "episodes" that interface with perceptual information and long-term memory, allowing for the storage of a multimodal code combing different types of information (e.g., visual with phonological). With such a mechanism in place, the new model was able to account for effects on word recall that extend well beyond word lists, as in our increased ability to retain words when they are presented in sentential context (Baddeley, 2007). Figure 5.1 illustrates the components of this revised model.

Some have challenged the Baddeley view of WM as being too domain-specific. Cowan (1988), for example, suggested an *embedded processes* model, in which the activation of generic representational formats, organized hierarchically in memory, was assumed. Roughly speaking, a cluster of traces in LTM is activated in response to external stimulation, which gives rise to the content of STM. Within this cluster an event within a smaller subset constitutes the focus of attention, where they are maximally activated in service of cognitive processing. Memory traces that enter the center of attention are selected by an *attention orienting system*, which responds to stimulus novelty. Over time, if unchanged, stimulus novelty may wear off, resulting in habituation and trace "deactivation." In addition, traces may migrate outside the scope of attention in the presence of interference from previously presented stimuli. Traces that remain outside the focus on attention are minimally activated, primarily at the perceptual level.

Despite differences between Baddeley's and Cowan's models, both emphasize the contribution of central-attention limited-capacity systems to individual differences in sustaining working memory representations. In doing so, they highlight the tight links between higher-order cognitive processes associated with working memory and goal-directed behaviors related to executive abilities (Just & Carpenter, 1992). A useful way to distinguish the two is to consider working memory as a work space in which information is stored and manipulated and executive functions, as abilities that organize

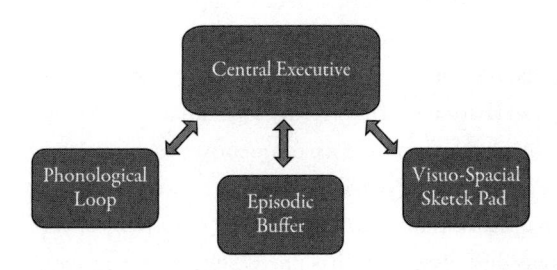

FIGURE 5.1 Multicomponent model of working memory
Source: Based on the model proposed by Baddeley, A. D. (2010). Working memory. *Current Biology, 20*(4), R136–R140.

working memory representations to enhance efficiency of information processing (e.g., Carpenter, Just, & Reichle, 2000; Connor, MacKay, & White, 2000).

Hasher and Zacks's (1988) well-known framework of *attention control* is a good example of a proposal linking WM and executive functions via *inhibitory mechanisms*. Briefly, within this framework, information in WM is automatically activated in response to internal/external stimuli engaging three interrelated inhibitory processes: (1) *access*, which is concerned with directing attention to goal-relevant information by suppressing intervening irrelevant information; (2) *deletion*, which is responsible for clearing information from conscious awareness as it becomes irrelevant to prevent "cluttering" of the WM system; and (3) *restraint*, which governs strong responses. Evidence for these components can be found in literature on aging, which reliably demonstrates (1) reductions in older persons, compared with younger adults, in processing efficiency in the presence of distraction, including an increase in response times to targets that are conceptually related to one another (Connelly, Hasher, & Zacks, 1991); (2) a decrease in the ability to rule out alternative interpretations of structurally ambiguous sentences (Hamm & Hasher, 1992); and (3) impaired ability to inhibit overlearned responses (May, Hasher, & Bhatt, 1994). Although this model has been used to account for changes in language performance, especially in the aging population, it was not proposed to deal specifically with linguistic processes.

With the emergence of Baddeley's model of WM, there was a surge of psycholinguistic proposals meant to relate WM and language functions, with a particular focus on sentence comprehension (e.g., Caplan & Waters, 1999; 2013; Caramazza et al., 1981; Fedorenko, Gibson, & Rhode, 2006; Friedrich et al., 1984; Gordon et al., 2002; King & Just, 1991; Lauro et al., 2010; Papagno et al., 2007; McDonald & Christiansen, 2002). These were backed by behavioral observations obtained from a variety of studies, including (1) interference effects meant to distinguish the operation of the phonological loop and central executive (e.g., King & Just, 1991), (2) tongue twisters (Acheson & Madonald, 2011; Keller, Carpenter & Just, 2003; Perfetti & McCutchen, 1982; Zhang & Perfetti, 1993), and (3) correlations of performance on memory span tasks and reading comprehension (e.g., Just & Carpenter, 1992; Miyake, Carpenter, & Just, 1994; Waters & Caplan, 1996). In a meta-analysis, Daneman & Merikle (1996) observed that performance of complex rather than storage memory span tasks reliably accounted for variability in sentence comprehension among adults. They also noted that tasks comprised of numerical stimuli predicted comprehension performance, indicating effects of WM that go beyond those associated with verbal WM (Engle et al., 1992; Kane et al., 2004).

One of the most influential models proposed in this context is that of Just and Carpenter (1992). They set out to capture the role of WM in sentence comprehension, proposing a memory limited-capacity mechanism that can support the storage and manipulation of linguistic elements provided that the activation of these elements is kept above a minimal threshold. If the activation threshold falls below the minimum required, linguistic processing is scaled back, as activation is reallocated to other elements being stored and processed in WM. This reallocation results in reduced speed and reduced efficiency of information processing. Thus, impaired sentence comprehension, measured by speed and accuracy, is expected when total activation demands on WM exceed available activation capacity. It is noteworthy that decreased processing speed has been considered by some to be the primary source of reductions in working memory and other cognitive functions (e.g., Salthouse, 1996). Others, however, have argued for some level of dissociability between the two as they relate to language comprehension in aging (e.g., Waters & Caplan, 2005).

Confirmatory findings for the Just and Carpenter (1992) model have been reported in studies exploring the effects of WM capacity as measured, for example, by reading spans, on comprehension of syntactically complex sentences, and sentences with ambiguities (e.g., King & Just, 1992; Just & Carpenter, 1992). The argument was that increased WM capacity enhances integration of syntactic and nonsyntactic information, evidenced, for instance, in faster reading times for sentences with disambiguating nonsytactic information among persons with greater WM capacity of sentences as compared with sentences with no such information.

This account had been extended by Miyake and colleagues (1994) to patterns of sentence comprehension among persons with aphasia whose deficits were attributed to a quantitative drop in WM capacity compared with adults with no aphasia. A comparable reduction in WM capacity was demonstrated among neurologically intact adults whose WM capacity was taxed by increased speech rate, who then became very much aphasic-like. Clearly, as Waters and Caplan (1996) have pointed out, general WM problems do not always result in decrements in sentence comprehension (Waters et al., 1991). Instead, they proposed an additional WM resource pool specifically dedicated to the online, obligatory, tacit processing of linguistic information underlying sentence structure and meaning (e.g., Caplan & Waters, 1999).

The extent to which WM can be divided into two separate resource pools in service of sentence comprehension, one dedicated to linguistic processing and the other more generally to verbally mediated cognitive processes (as in Caplan & Waters, 1999), remains a topic of debate. Fedorenko, Gibson, and Rhode (2006), for example, used a dual-task paradigm to examine whether participants' reading times of sentences of varying levels of syntactic complexity were affected by the concurrent demand to remember up to three nouns of differing semantic relatedness to the nouns in the target sentences. They reasoned that under Caplan and Waters's approach, the words in the recall lists and the words in the target sentences would be stored separately and not interact with one another. However, they found that reading times increased for the most syntactically complex sentences (those containing object- rather than subject-relative clauses) with the presentation of semantically similar memory nouns (for a counterargument, see Caplan & Waters, 2013).

MacDonald & Christiansen (2002) also challenged the Caplan and Waters (1999) view of WM-language interlinks, arguing for a connectionist approach in which capacity and processing are inseparable and where performance is constrained through interactions between biological factors and language experience. In adopting this approach they claim to have avoided the "proliferation of little domains of working memory" (MacDonald & Christiansen, 2002, p. 50). Our discussion here is not intended to settle this controversy, but we will note that proposing a proliferation of components, in and of itself, is no basis for ruling out a theoretical account. A prime example is Cabeza and Moscovitch's (2013) components approach, just discussed, which entails neural activation of multiple "process-specific alliances" in the course of task performance.

Even within the Caplan and Waters (1999) approach, further refinements of the WM in sentence comprehension have been proposed. These included differentiation of the respective contributions of WM to the *online* and *offline* properties of sentence processing (Caplan & Waters, 1999; Newman et al., 2013). The assumption is that online sentence comprehension, in which interpretive processes involving integration of syntactic, thematic, prosodic, propositional, and discursive features, engage episodic memory by utilizing event knowledge to form an event representation. At the offline stage, postinterpretive processes occur and derive, through executive-based processes, the appropriate meaning from the WM representation generated during sentence processing. Neuroimaging data have been used to support this suggestion, as discussed below.

Relatedly, Caplan and Waters (2013) have proposed to depart from conceptualizing mechanisms of short-term/WM as support systems to sentence processing toward a knowledge/schema-based mechanism they term *long-term working memory*. This shift is anchored in part in their empirically based observation that short-term memory recall tasks do not necessarily reflect memory processes activated during sentence parsing and interpretation: "retrieval in sentence comprehension is not easily related to retrieval in any laboratory STM task" (Caplan & Waters, 2013, p. 259). This long-term WM component supports skilled memory (e.g., memorizing the digits of *pi* beyond 3.14) and has been shown to be immune to performance interruptions (Ericsson & Kintsch, 1995). By and large, under this newer approach linguistic input is assumed to activate long-term memory items—which are related in long-term WM by associations, patterns, and schemas to form a memory representation—leaving short-term memory to handle maintenance of the retrieval cues of these items. The engagement of the short-term WM mechanism is triggered by incremental comprehension failure, which is directly determined by task demands. In the face of such failure, participants invoke controlled comprehension mechanisms correlated with short-term/WM measures, which improve performance. Support for this claim come from Caplan et al.'s (2011) reading comprehension study, in which they found positive correlations between short-term/WM measures and self-paced reading times as well as between short-term/WM measures and task performance.

The appeal to long-term memory mechanisms in this context ties us back to the declarative/procedural literature reviewed above (e.g., Ullman, 2004), highlighting once again the multifunctional nature of the systems discussed here. Caplan and Waters (2013) correctly state that more detailed elucidation of the mechanisms of encoding, storage, and retrieval in procedural memory will be required before their role in sentence processing can be fully evaluated.

A somewhat different view of memory and language interlinks has been proposed by several scholars of aphasia, who have argued that verbal short-term memory (STM) is not a specialized system but rather consists of temporary activations of memory-language representations integral to the language processing system (Acheson & MacDonald, 2009; Berndt & Mitchum, 1990; N. Martin, 2000; N. Martin & Saffran, 1992; 1997; R. Martin & He; 2004; R. Martin & Romani, 1994; Ruchkin, Grafman, Cameron, & Berndt, 2003). The underlying assumption in this framework is that because language tasks span over time, they necessarily implicate a mechanism that supports ongoing activation of a word's representation, which enables its comprehension, production, and repetition. Based on the work of Dell and colleagues (Dell & O'Seaghdha, 1991; 1992; Gagnon et al., 1997; Martin, Dell, Saffran, & Schwartz, 1994; Schwartz et al., 1994), it has been assumed that the spreading activation of linguistic information spans three levels—semantic, lexical, and phonological—schematically represented in the "lexical network" in Figure 5.2.

The dependency between STM and language is thus manifested through the ability to maintain the phonological and semantic representation of a word as it is being processed individually or as part of a larger sequence. Much of the evidence supporting this model comes from the aphasia literature, to which we return later in the chapter.

SHORT-TERM/WORKING MEMORY-LANGUAGE INTERLINKS:
EVIDENCE FOR NEURAL CORRELATES

Claims about the neural correlates of short-term and working memory systems related to language functions (mostly sentence processing) have been based on studies of

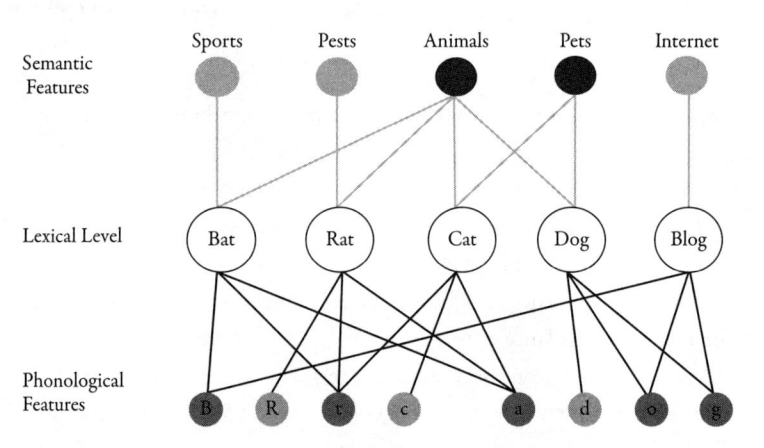

FIGURE 5.2 Levels of activation during lexical processing. Shaded circles reflect shared features; activation of connections in the model is bidirectional (See color insert.)

Source: Based on the lexical access framework developed by Dell, G. S., Schwartz, M. F., Martin, N., Saffran, E. M., & Gagnon, D. A. (1997). Lexical access in aphasic and nonaphasic speakers. *Psychological Review, 104*(4), 801–838.

associations and dissociations of phonological loop and central executive operations among persons with focal brain damage (e.g., Caplan & Waters, 1996; Grossman et al., 1991; R. Martin, 1990; Rochon & Saffran, 1995), as well as on neuroimaging studies of brain activation patterns contrasting persons with high and low memory spans performing central executive versus parsing and interpretive tasks (e.g., Fiebach, Schleswsky, & Friederici, 2001; Fiebach, Vos, & Friederici, 2004).

By and large, short-term/WM systems have been argued to involve frontal regions, which mediate articulatory, vocal, and/or subvocal processes, and parietal structures, which engage phonological processing and storage (Buchsbaum, Padmanabhan, & Berman, 2011; Paulesu, Frith, & Frackowiak, 1993; Schweickert & Boruff, 1986). Evidence for distinct storage and rehearsal mechanisms of working memory has been found in studies of persons with phonological loop deficits (e.g., Vallar & Papagno, 2002), in whom damage to Brodmann's area 44 has been associated with storage problems and injury to Brodmann's areas 6 and 40 to impaired rehearsal (Baddeley, 2003). Additional support comes from findings in brain studies of healthy adults, among whom better WM capacity not only predicted faster reading times and more accurate comprehension but was also associated with increased functional connectivity and decreased, higher-efficiency neural activation of brain structures in language networks elicited in response to task performance (e.g., Prat et al., 2007).

In addition, there has been much interest in the role that Broca's area plays in subserving WM-language interlinks (e.g., Fiebach et al., 2005; Newman & Just, 2005). We have already called attention to the apparent overlap between brain structures mediating WM and language functions in Chapter 2, in relation to the works of Friederici and colleagues (e.g., Friederici, 2012; Friederici & Gierhan, 2013; Makuuchi & Friederici, 2013). In this respect, of particular interest are the brain structures assumed to support the processing of syntactically complex sentences, where linguistic information is transferred from BA44 to the posterior temporal cortex in a top-down fashion (e.g., when examination of sentential context is called for). Friederici and colleagues proposed that because activation of both BA44 and the temporal cortex has been associated with syntactic processing and because the dorsal portion of BA44 and the inferior frontal sulcus have been related to syntactic working memory, working memory is likely involved in the processing of syntactically complex sentences (see also Caplan & Waters, 1999; Makuuchi, Bahlmann, Anwander, & Friederici, 2009). Specifically, Makuuchi and Friederici (2013) proposed hierarchical processing of linguistic information from visual word-form regions (fusiform gyrus) through working memory areas (inferior frontal sulcus and intraparietal sulcus) to language regions (pars opercularis and the middle temporal gyrus), demonstrating increased connectivity with a greater processing load.

In a recent neuroimaging study exploring the effects of WM capacity on sentence comprehension, Newman et al. (2013) found differential brain activation patterns for online reading of syntactically complex sentences (object relatives) and offline probe recognition. Specifically, they demonstrated that online sentence processing was mediated by WM capacity (greater memory capacity leading to better language performance) via the posterior cingulate/precuneus region, a nontraditional language structure; effects of WM on offline probe recognition, however, activated BA 45 in the left inferior frontal gyrus. Additionally, their connectivity analyses implicated two distinct neural networks in service of sentence processing: (1) a network comprising the middle temporal and the anterior portion of the inferior frontal gyrus to support semantic processing (see discussion of Friederici above and in Chapter 2) and (2) a network involving the posterior cingulate and BA 45 to mediate generation of *event* representations via memory-based processes. Evidence for their proposal comes from the observation that the cingulate region has been implicated in semantic, episodic, and visuospatial memory processing (e.g., Binder et al., 2009) as well as in narrative comprehension (e.g., Yarkoni et al., 2008).

Neuroimaging studies have also revealed the involvement of subcortical circuitry, especially that of the basal ganglia, in mediating verbal working memory (e.g., Crosson, Benjamin, & Levy, 2007; Moore et al., 2013). The contribution of these structures has been attributed to effects of WM-related cognitive mechanisms, such as suppression/inhibition, on the efficiency and accuracy of semantic processing, as in Crosson and colleagues' works (e.g., Crosson et al., 2003), which we reviewed in Chapter 3 and 4. Moore et al. (2013) explored brain activation during the encoding, maintenance, and retrieval of words in a semantic relatedness task in order to focus more directly WM effects. Participants were first shown a target word and asked to remember it. Their task was to determine the semantic relatedness of that word (encoding) to a decision word presented later in the experiment (retrieval). In between, the participants were shown distractor pairs of words and were also asked assess their semantic relatedness to the target (maintenance). This procedure was designed to prevent rehearsal of the target word. Findings indicated that encoding activated left inferior frontal structures as well as the caudate and thalamus bilaterally; maintenance activated the medial thalamus and posterior cingulate regions; and retrieval activated the left inferior frontal sulcus and posterior parietooccipital cortices. Because the authors did not report performance on independent measures of WM, it is difficult to assess whether the neural patterns associated with "maintenance" performance reflect WM capacity, as opposed, for example, to inhibitory control. It may very well be impossible to isolate these functions completely, but a distinction at some level would be expected if indeed executive processes, such as inhibition, manipulate the content of working memory representations, as is commonly assumed (e.g., Carpenter, Just, & Reichle, 2000).

Memory Deficits and Aphasia

Much of the work on memory impairments in stroke-based aphasia has focused on effects associated with short-term and/or working memory (STM/WM) system(s) (Mayer & Murray, 2012). STM, for example, has been shown to negatively affect the processing of sounds, meanings, phrases, and sentences (e.g., Allport, 1984; Heilman, Scholes, & Watson, 1976; Martin & Ayala, 2004; Martin & He, 2004). Few studies have examined the effects of long-term memory (LTM) on language performance in aphasia (e.g., Beeson et al., 1993; Burgio & Basso, 1997; Dalla Barba et al., 1997; Risse, Rubens, & Jordan, 1984). Studies have used mixed methodologies and do not converge on a clear picture regarding LTM abilities in this population (Murray et al., 2001).

In what follows, we thus focus our review on studies that explore STM/WM effects on language performance in aphasia, including the methods used to assess these memory impairments, the behavioral observations that have emerged from different studies, and the neural correlates associated with these patterns.

SHORT-TERM MEMORY/WORKING MEMORY ASSESSMENT IN APHASIA

The assessment of STM/WM problems among persons with aphasia has largely relied on performance on subsets of standardized memory tests, such as the Wechsler Memory Scale-Revised (Wechsler, 1987). In these tests, participants are asked to recall items that are serially presented to them either in order of presentation (forward span) or in reverse (backward span). Backward span is more difficult for persons both with and without aphasia (e.g., Laures-Gore et al., 2010; Wechsler, 2003), as it implicates the storage, retention, and manipulation of verbal information, presumably via the phonological loop (e.g., Baddeley, 2007). Because these tests usually involve a linguistic component, they necessarily conflate memory and language functions, making it difficult to determine whether they are actually tests of "memory" (Mayer & Murray, 2012; Stout & Murray, 2001). However, isolating the assessment of language from components of STM/WM system(s) in aphasia may be untenable (e.g., Lang & Quitz, 2012). Even temporary maintenance of nonlinguistic shapes in memory has been found to be affected by verbal distraction (Postle, D'Esposito, & Corkin et al., 2005).

To make up for this inherent "task impurity," researchers have also opted to characterize STM/WM problems in aphasia by varying stimulus types during memory testing. Gutbrod et al. (1989), for example, compared WM capacity in aphasic participants as well as others with damage to the right hemisphere using a self-ordered pointing task to pictures of faces and line drawings of real objects, which required participants to successively point to pictures in a stack without repeating the same picture twice. The persons with aphasia, but not those with right hemisphere damage had greater difficulties pointing to most stimuli, even though they were able to use semantic information to sort them correctly on a separate sorting task. The authors interpreted this pattern as a deficit in strategizing memorization for category clustering. This interpretation implies, however, the involvement of other cognitive abilities, such as planning, which extend beyond the scope of WM. (Evidence that categorization abilities among persons with aphasia rely on cognitive control mechanisms can be found in Lupyan & Mirman, 2013.)

Indeed, some of the most commonly used tests of STM/WM tap overlapping cognitive constructs (for related comments, see also Chapter 3). Consider, for example, the *n-back test*, the use of which has increased in popularity in aphasia studies over the past 10 years (e.g., Christensen & Harris Wright, 2010; Friedmann & Gvion, 2003; Harris Wright & Fergadiotus, 2012; Wright et al., 2007). This task requires a person to determine if an item presented in a sequence matches an item shown *n* steps prior, with the number of steps usually ranging from one to three. This complex process involves, encoding and interpretation of the letters or digits to be recalled, maintenance of the number of steps that matches *n*, and suppression of elements presented further back in the list. This process thus implicates all the important components of working memory—temporary storage and manipulation of information. But it also involves additional executive functions, such as updating (e.g., Miyake et al., 2000), or speeded recognition (Kane et al., 2007), which once again points to the blurry boundaries among the specific cognitive constructs underlying performance on such a task. The face validity of this task has also proven mixed, and its reliability with clinical population remains underdetermined (Harris Wright & Fergadiotus, 2012; Mayer & Murray, 2012).

However, as Mayer and Murray (2012) point out, the *n*-back test does offer several methodological advantages, which renders it useful for evaluating WM in aphasia. These include (1) simple verbal instructions, which enable its administration to persons with comprehension deficits, (2) a focus on recognition rather than retrieval, which facilitates performance for persons with impaired language production, (3) measurement of reaction time, which allows the detection of general cognitive impairment, and (4) stimulus flexibility, as it can be used successfully with both verbal and nonverbal materials.

A good example of the dynamic nature of the *n*-back test can be found in a study by Christensen and Harris Wright (2010), who compared aphasic and nonaphasic participants on an n-back test in order to differentiate activation of verbal from nonverbal WM in aphasia during confrontation naming. They asked the participants to recall, at levels of one and two back, three types of pictorial stimuli that varied in terms of their linguistic load—high load (namable fruits), semilinguistic (namable monochromatic shapes, or "fribbles"), and nonlinguistic (nonnamable blocks). They found that both groups had difficulty at the two-back level, but the aphasic participants showed greater memory decrements and also demonstrated poorer performance on both the seminamable and nonnamable items. This finding was taken to reflect the role of linguistic knowledge in supporting WM memory performance.

BEHAVIORAL OBSERVATIONS

Although impaired STM performance need not be associated with language impairment in aphasia (e.g., Basso, Spinnler, Vallar, & Zanobio, 1982; Beeson et al., 1993; Majerus et al., 2004; R. Martin et al., 1994; Saffran & Marin, 1975; Vallar & Baddeley, 1984; Warrington et al. 1971), the consensus is that STM/WM tasks pose a challenge for many persons with aphasia, reflecting memory limitations that are negatively associated with their language performance (e.g., Baldo & Dronkers, 2006; Beeson et al., 1993; Caplan & Waters, 1999; Caspari et al., 1998; Christensen & Wright, 2010; Friedmann & Gvion, 2003; Gvion & Friedmann, 2012; Harris Wright et al., 2007; Laures-Gore et al., 2010; Rönnberg et al., 1996; Sung et al., 2009; Ween et al., 1996).

A prime example is the deficit patterns of phonological STM and repetition abilities reported for persons with conduction aphasia (e.g., Baldo & Dronkers, 2006; Baldo, Klostermann, & Dronkers, 2008; Kohn, 1992; Lang & Quitz, 2012). These patients have been shown to have limited STM (with a typical span of one to three items), impaired verbatim repetition of sentences they understand perfectly well (Hanten & Martin, 2000; Martin, 1993; Martin et al., 1994; Willis & Gathercole, 2001) and poor comprehension of sentences with multiple and/or arbitrary lexical elements (Caplan & Waters, 1999; Martin et al., 1994; Vallar & Baddeley, 1984; Waters et al., 1991). Another example is the relationship between STM impairment and word production in deep dysphasia. Such patients may show severely reduced STM spans (even less than one), along with word repetition or naming errors comprising semantic paraphasias, phonemic paraphasias, and nonword substitutions (Martin et al., 1996; Martin & Saffran, 1992).

These and similar findings have served as the foundation for the development of a memory-language model, mentioned earlier in the chapter, in which activation of verbal short-term memory (STM) is subsumed by the processing of phonological and semantic information (Acheson & MacDonald, 2009; Berndt & Mitchum, 1990; N. Martin, 2000; N. Martin & Saffran, 1992, 1997; R. Martin & He; 2004; R. Martin & Romani, 1994; Ruchkin, Grafman, Cameron, & Berndt, 2003). In this model, the retention of verbal material relies on the type of linguistic information to be processed—phonological or semantic (e.g., Martin & Romani, 1994; N. Martin & Saffran, 1997; R. Martin & He; 2004; R. Martin & Lesch, 1996). Recall that according to Dell and colleagues, the processing of this information occurs at three levels—semantic, semantic-lexical, and phonological—which interact with one another as words are processed over time (Dell & O'Seaghdha, 1991; 1992; Gagnon et al., 1997; Martin et al., 1994; Schwartz et al., 1994).

With such a mechanism in place, findings of double dissociations between processing of phonological and semantic information in persons with aphasia can be readily explained. For example, this mechanism could explain why persons with phonological deficits show better recall of list-initial items (primacy effects), based on preserved semantic knowledge, compared with persons who have semantic deficits. The latter demonstrate better recall of list-final items (recency effects) based on their unimpaired phonological system (N. Martin & Saffran, 1997).

In this model, then, persons with phonological deficits have problems retaining phonological information, and those with lexicosemantic impairments have difficulties maintaining semantic information—problems that can extend to sentence-level processing (e.g., Leff et al., 2009; Martin & Feher, 1990; Papagno et al., 2012; Vallar et al., 1992; Vallar & Papagno, 2002). The assumption is that activation of damaged language networks changes the *rate* of decay of phonological and semantic representations (e.g., N. Martin & Saffran, 1992, 1997). Within this framework, phonological information is assumed to be activated earlier than semantic information in the process of lexical selection and is presumably more severely affected by increases in decay rate. Thus, in repetition tasks, overly rapid decay may cause deficient language performance in which phonological processing is adversely affected, shifting lexical selection to more semantically based information. In mild cases, activation of the phonological representations may be retained sufficiently long to perform single-word tasks.

The notion that phonological and/or semantic deficits in aphasia represent a processing problem of access to linguistic information has prompted a surge of studies exploring the relationship between STM and *executive functions*. For example, problems manipulating semantic information, previously attributed to a breakdown in the activation of semantic information, have been reinterpreted as deficits of executive control (e.g., Allen et al., 2012; Hoffman et al., 2012; N. Martin et al., 2012), which lead to interference effects of previously presented task-relevant information (Hamilton & R. Martin, 2007) or to an inability to adhere to task-appropriate demands (e.g., Hoffman et al., 2009; see also studies cited in Chapters 3 and 4).

N. Martin and colleagues (2012) specifically demonstrated effects of WM load on accuracy of judgments of rhymes and synonyms, which respectively tap phonological and semantic knowledge. They found that, for persons with aphasia, increased working memory load (i.e., an increase in number of items retained in WM) reduced judgment accuracy in both task types. Abstract but not concrete words posed a particular challenge in the semantic task. As it happens, these semantic effects were also found among neurologically intact controls and were associated with reduced inhibition and semantic short-term memory. Poor inhibition predicted less accurate performance on the rhyming task. Based on these findings, the authors argue that the WM load built into task demands drives the extent to which verbal STM and executive functions engage in language processing.

Of course not all research converges on the nature of the relationship between semantic STM and executive functions, since some researchers have found no links between measures of executive functions and the performance of semantic STM tasks (e.g., Badre et al., 2010) while others have reported more generalized effects of executive impairment on semantic STM and semantic processing (e.g., Hoffman et al., 2009). For a recent study exploring these contrasting views, see Allen and Martin (2012).

Other studies have been more focused on exploring the effects of WM on sentence comprehension (e.g., Caspari et al., 1998; Sung et al., 2009; Tompkins et al., 1994). For example, Caspari et al. (1998) used a complex reading span task, modeled on Daneman and Carpenter's (1980) reading span test, which evaluates sentence-final-word recall abilities. Participants were asked to remember the last word of sentences in increasingly longer sets presented to them. The highest number of sentence-final words recalled was taken as that individual's reading span. The authors found that listening span, Western

Aphasia Battery (WAB) aphasia quotients, and reading span scores were significantly and positively correlated among persons with aphasia. Based on these findings, they argued that WM predicts sentence comprehension. This interpretation is aligned with Just and colleagues' conceptualization of WM-language interlinks (e.g., Just & Carpenter, 1992; King & Just, 1991; MacDonald et al., 1992; Miyake et al., 1994), according to which reduced WM capacity interferes with sentence comprehension in the face of concurrent increased memory load.

As we pointed out earlier in this chapter, such a unified approach to the relationship between WM and language has encountered several empirical problems, most notably with the observation that in aphasia, poor reading span is not necessarily associated with failed sentence comprehension (Waters et al., 1991). The alternative suggested by Caplan and colleagues—"the separate language resource theory"—has received support in several subsequent studies (e.g., Friedmann & Gvion, 2003; Gvion & Friedmann, 2012; Wright et al., 2007).

For example, Friedmann & Gvion (2003) demonstrated that while participants with conduction and agrammatic aphasia both show reduced WM abilities (indicated by poor performance on a one-level *n*-back task and several span tests), they each demonstrate distinct patterns of sentence comprehension, reflecting distinct WM-language dependencies: phonological versus semantic-syntactic. A subsequent study (Gvion & Friedmann, 2012) further teased apart the role of phonological WM among persons with conduction aphasia. These persons showed preserved comprehension of sentences containing relative clauses, which require semantic-syntactic reactivation of an antecedent. In contrast, they demonstrated poor paraphrasing of sentences with ambiguous words and judgment of sentences containing rhymes, which implicate long-distance phonological reactivation of words presented earlier in the sentence. These results clearly emphasize the need to consider the type of linguistic information assessed in characterizing the nature of the relationship between WM and language functions. Findings by Wright et al. (2007) lend further support to this argument. Although the WM of their aphasic participants declined as *n*-back level increased (from one to two), they found that participants performed better on semantic-back tasks versus phonological- and syntactic-back tasks. In addition, among aphasic participants with impaired comprehension of syntactically complex sentences, they found the most severe syntactic-back WM problems.

NEURAL CORRELATES OF SHORT-TERM MEMORY/WORKING MEMORY IN APHASIA

Early lesion studies of STM problems among persons with aphasia have pointed to brain damage affecting multiple cortical structures comprising the inferior parietal lobule, the posterior portion of the superior temporal gyrus, the middle temporal gyrus, and anterior perisylvian structures including Broca's area (Gordon, 1983; Smith & Jonides, 1998; Warrington et al., 1971). However, some have argued that neural structures supporting

STM do not always map onto the classical "language" regions, pointing to the independence of STM and language representations in the brain (Koenings et al., 2011).

However, if language functions subsume STM, as has been assumed by many researchers whose work we reviewed in this chapter, we would not expect the processing of phonological and semantic to be mediated by traditional language areas. This idea is consistent with findings from several studies exploring the neural bases of phonological and semantic word substitutions in aphasia (e.g., Cloutman et al., 2009; Hillis et al., 2001, 2006; Schwartz et al., 2009, 2012; Walker et al., 2011). For example, in a voxel-based lesion symptom mapping study of 64 aphasic participants, Schwartz et al. (2009) found evidence for the involvement of the left anterior temporal cortex in semantic errors produced by aphasic persons, which clearly argues against the classical attribution of these errors to Wernicke's area.

In a subsequent voxel-based lesion symptom mapping study, Schwartz and colleagues (2012) examined the neural underpinnings of phonological errors in a sample of 106 aphasic participants. They found evidence for the involvement of brain structures in the dorsal stream, including the premotor cortex, pre- and postcentral gyri, supramarginal gyrus, and, minimally, the posterior temporal and temporoparietal cortices, indicating a far more anterior map for these types of errors than previously thought. Interestingly, the investigators compared these phonological maps with those obtained from semantic errors and found no overlap between them.

Indeed, converging evidence suggests that STM and language functions do in fact share some of the same neural substrates (Acheson, Hamidi, Binder, & Postle, 2011; Baldo & Dronkers, 2006; Baldo, Katseff, & Dronkers, 2012; Koenigs et al., 2011; Leff et al., 2009; Martin & Allen, 2008). For example, structural neuroimaging analyses from over 200 persons with focal brain damage indicated that damage to the left inferior frontal and posterior temporal cortices is associated with STM deficits as measured by digit span and impaired language functions as measured by naming and command comprehension (Koenigs et al., 2011). Similarly, in a voxel-based lesion symptom mapping study of persons with aphasia, evidence has been provided that auditory verbal short-term memory span and repetition are most critically mediated by cortical regions in left posterior temporoparietal cortex, the same regions of the brain considered to be crucial for comprehension of spoken language (Baldo, Katseff, & Dronkers, 2012).

Another study, also using voxel-based analysis, addressed similar questions regarding theories of short-term memory function that make specific predictions about the functional anatomy of auditory short-term memory and its role in language comprehension (Leff et al., 2009). The authors analyzed high-resolution structural magnetic resonance images from 210 stroke patients and employed a novel voxel-based analysis to test the relationship between auditory short-term memory and speech comprehension. Using digit span as an index of auditory short-term memory capacity, they found that the structural integrity of a posterior region of the superior temporal gyrus and sulcus predicted auditory short-term memory capacity; they demonstrated further that the integrity of this region also predicts the ability to comprehend spoken sentences.

Even finer-grained observations have been made by Buchsbaum et al. (2011), who identified the posterior portion of the *planum temporale*, area Spt (Sylvian-parietal-temporal), as a crucial structure damaged in conduction aphasia. They demonstrated maximal lesion overlap in 14 persons with conduction aphasia in area Spt, which they defined through an aggregate fMRI analysis of 105 participants performing a phonological WM task. Because of the involvement of this region in sensorimotor integration, they suggest reinterpreting conduction aphasia as a disorder of this system. We return to this idea in Chapters 7 and 8.

However, a question has arisen as to whether these deficits are the consequence of the left hemispheric lesions per se and not due to the presence of aphasia. To address this question, Kasselimis and colleagues (2013) tested groups of persons with left hemispheric lesions with and without aphasia on verbal and visuospatial span tasks. The group with aphasia was found to have impaired performance on the memory tasks, regardless of lesion localization, while the group without aphasia did not. The authors offered the tentative conclusion that memory deficits in patients with left hemisphere lesions might thus perhaps be dependent on the presence of aphasia.

Memory Systems, Aphasia Recovery, and Treatment

N. Martin and colleagues have explored the relationship between lexical-semantic and/or phonological deficits and STM impairments in the course of aphasia recovery (e.g., N. Martin, 2008, 2009; N. Martin & Ayala, 2004; N. Martin et al., 1996; N. Martin & Gupta, 2004). Several major findings emerged from their studies: first, that improved memory span is significantly associated with increased repetition abilities in the course of aphasia recovery (N. Martin et al., 1996); second, that error patterns can evolve from one type to another in the course of aphasia recovery within a single case; and third, that size of memory span, measured by repetition and pointing responses, is positively correlated with severity of phonological and semantic impairment, with greater memory deficits related to more severe cases of aphasia (N. Martin & Ayala, 2004).

These findings have had considerable impact on the design of aphasia assessment and treatment studies (e.g., Abel et al., 2009). The choice of therapy targets in anomia treatment studies, for example, has been driven by the particular linguistic deficit patients exhibit—semantic or phonological (e.g., Abel et al., 2014; Dell et al., 1997; Fridriksson et al., 2005, 2007; Maher & Raymer, 2004; Martin & Laine, 2000; Nickles, 2002; Renvall et al., 2003; Wambaugh et al., 2004; Wisenburn & Mahoney, 2009; Wisenburn, 2010). Thus phonologically based treatments would be administered to those with phonological impairments and semantic-based treatments to those with semantic impairments (e.g., Fridriksson et al., 2005; Wambaugh et al., 2004). Unfortunately a meta-analysis by Wisenburn and Mahoney (2009) revealed no conclusive evidence for which types of linguistic- or memory-based therapy are optimal for which types of aphasic patients.

Moreover, it is unclear whether such therapy outcomes are in fact related to measures of STM/WM. In one study, for example, nonverbal visuospatial WM was associated with posttherapy improvements in naming and comprehension (Seniów, Litwin, & Leśniak, 2009). In another study, measures of nonverbal recall from episodic or semantic memory were correlated with language therapy outcomes but not with patterns of language performance during spontaneous recovery (Goldenberg et al., 1994). In yet another study, STM training was not shown to affect language-therapy outcomes at all (e.g., Murray, Keeton, & Karcher, 2006).

Other studies have directly explored the relationship between changes in verbal STM/WM and language treatment outcomes. For example, in a study targeting sentence repetition in a person with mild aphasia, Francis, Clark, and Humphreys (2003) were able to demonstrate a concomitant increase in sentence recall as measured by sentence length and forward and backward span measures. Similar findings were reported by Koenig-Bruhin and Studer-Eichenberger (2007), who examined immediate and delayed recall of noun compounds and sentences in a person with conduction aphasia.

The extent to which the effects of memory training on specific aspects of aphasia generalize to untreated items also remains unclear, as shown in an intervention study of sentence repetition using filled and unfilled delays between stimuli and responses to improve phonological and semantic STM; this study failed to find generalization to untrained items (Kalinyak-Fliszar, Kohen, & Martin, 2011). Mixed findings have also emerged from a recent aphasia study of STM treatment, in which effects of STM training through listening span and serial word recognition were examined in relation to word- and sentence-level comprehension (Salis, 2012). Posttreatment STM abilities improved, with some evidence of generalization to untrained sentence comprehension items but no effects on single-word comprehension. The author interpreted these findings in terms of positive changes in the rate of decay of linguistic information at the sentence level.

More compelling evidence for effects of STM training on language treatment outcomes among persons with aphasia was found in a case study by Kalinyak et al. (2012), which targeted activation and maintenance of phonological and semantic information in a person with conduction aphasia. The investigators reasoned that treatment targeting the ability to maintain linguistic activation over time will enhance generalization effects to untrained items. The participant showed improvements on standardized language measures, STM-based measures, and generalization to untrained items but only when the items trained first were phonologically more complex.

The phonological and semantic components of STM have been shown to have distinct effects on aphasic patients' abilities to learn new linguistic information. Freedman and R. Martin (2001) examined five aphasic participants with differential patterns of STM deficits whereby patients with more phonological than semantic STM problems had trouble learning new phonological material but were able to acquire semantically based forms while patients with more semantic than phonological STM problems showed the reverse. One patient with semantic STM was not able to engage in any long-term learning at all. The authors interpreted these findings as evidence for the relevance of phonological and semantic STM to the establishment of representation in long-term memory (LTM). However, the long-term effects of such interventions are not always as straightforward. For example, in a recent case study, Winans et al. (2012) found modest positive effects of WM treatment on sentence span and sentence comprehension that did not carry over at follow-up assessment.

LEARNING IN APHASIA TREATMENT

Few memory-related aphasia treatment studies have focused on the role of *learning* in shaping therapy outcomes (e.g., Fillingham et al., 2003). Some interventions have specifically explored whether or *implicit learning* leads to treatment gains (e.g., Friedman, 2000). Implicit learning refers to a process in which the relationship between two items is established through incidental learning, with no awareness of existing regularities and no use of explicit strategies. Such learning has been found to be extremely efficacious for persons with agrammatic aphasia with WM problems who, unlike healthy controls, were able to master auditory word sequencing only under implicit conditions (controls learned under both implicit and explicit conditions) (Schuchard & Thompson, 2012, 2014).

Relatedy, several studies have examined the method of *errorless learning*, which is designed to minimize the participant's errors by providing him or her with the correct answer to begin with, preventing incorrect response-stimulus pairings (Friedman, 2000). This method has been found to be extremely useful for persons with memory impairments (Baddeley & Wilson, 1994; Clare et al., 1999, 2000; Evans et al., 2000) and has triggered interest in its impact on persons with aphasia in whom, as noted throughout this chapter, memory problems are frequently observed (Fillingham et al., 2003, 2006; McKissok & Ward, 2007).

Most anomia treatment protocols rely to some degree on aspects of errorless learning, with emphasis primarily on error reduction through cueing (e.g., Best et al., 2002; Fillingham et al., 2003; Greenwald et al., 1995; Howard et al., 1985; Miceli et al., 1996). The theoretical motivation underlying this approach is that the processing of feedback relies on explicit memory, whose deliberate nature makes it more immune to interference effects from incorrect responses (e.g., Baddeley & Wilson, 1994). Because explicit memory appears to remain intact among persons with anomia, these patients stand to benefit from such input (McKissock & Ward, 2007).

Miceli et al. (1996), for example, demonstrated training benefits at 17 months, when aphasia treatment involved error reduction through the introduction of cues with increasingly reduced specificity. This approach represents a "staircase" method, in which a participant is presented with incrementally more difficult stimuli/cues (e.g., Morris et al., 1996). This very approach, however, may fail to maximize treatment benefits, as it is often the presentation of "complex" material first that leads to better treatment outcomes (e.g., Kiran, 2007; Thompson et al., 2003). In other studies using error elimination (e.g., instructing a participant to talk about a picture but to refrain from naming it), partial benefits have been observed for untrained items (Frattali & Kang, 2004). Such studies often include "semantic" treatment, in which word-picture pairings are used to create semantic associations (Marshall, Pound, White-Thomson, & Pring, 1990; Pring, Hamilton, Harwood, & Macbride, 1993; Pring, White-Thomson, Pound, Marshall, & Davis, 1990).

In a meta-analysis by Fillingham et al. (2003), however, errorless learning failed to show particular benefits over other techniques and reportedly offered only very limited long-term gains. Specifically, presence or type of feedback to participants appears to make no difference in treatment outcome (e.g., Fillingham et al., 2005a,b; 2006; McCandliss et al., 2002). In the work of Fillingham et al. (2006), the strongest predictor of treatment outcome was the number of naming attempts the participant made. McKissok and Ward (2007), however, found that treatment in which a correct response was provided by the experimenter was efficacious whether or not participants were allowed to err. That is, comparable benefits were observed in the errorless condition, where the correct name was supplied before the participant's response, and in the errorful with feedback condition, where the participant first attempted to name and was then supplied with the correct label.

Interestingly, Fillingham et al. (2006) have shown that the better responders to both leaning methods (errorless and nonerrorless) were those with better recall, better working memory, and better executive function abilities but not those with better language scores. The authors suggest that such persons can learn effectively even in a nonerrorless environment in which they are required to filter out errorful trials (see also McCandliss et al., 2002). However, in a recent study exploring nonlinguistic learning in aphasia using a paired associate and feedback task, Vallila-Rohter and Kiran (2013) found that the ability of persons with aphasia to correctly categorize novel animals (as measured by the percentage of features shared with one of two prototypes) was not related to standardized cognitive measures.

Some have argued that most aphasia treatment studies targeting learning mechanisms are in fact studies of "relearning," since they rely on training of familiar exemplars (Tuomiranta et al., 2012). Studies exploring novel word learning among persons with aphasia have shown benefits resulting from implicit incidental learning (e.g., Grossman & Carey, 1987; Tuomiranta et al., 2011), although the long-term benefits from these interventions have not been assessed systematically (Breitenstein et al., 2004; Gupta et al., 2006; Kelly & Armstrong, 2009). In a recent aphasia treatment study, however, phonemic cueing was shown to enhance long-term maintenance of newly acquired novel items measured at 6 months postintervention (Tuomiranta et al., 2012). The two participants differed in terms of their lexical-semantic processing abilities at baseline and showed slightly different learning patterns. While both benefitted from phonemic cues, the person with greater semantic difficulty showed poorer learning during treatment, decreased recognition of the trained items, and reduced recall of semantic definitions postintervention. Interestingly, this participant's lesion included the hippocampus, suggesting that this region may play a critical role in effective word learning, as discussed below.

NEURAL STRUCTURES IN STUDIES OF MEMORY-RELATED APHASIA TREATMENT

There is a growing literature describing the neural underpinnings of phonological and semantic-based treatments of anomia, although these studies do not typically include direct assessments of STM/WM abilities (e.g., Abel et al., 2014; Fridriksson et al., 2007; Meizner et al., 2008; Rochon et al., 2010; Schwartz et al., 2009, 2012). Findings from these studies reinforce the notion that neural substrates involved in therapy-induced aphasia recovery involve either bilateral or left perilesional brain structures (e.g., Cornelissen et al., 2003; Fridriksson et al., 2006, 2007, 2012; Leger et al., 2002; Meizner et al., 2007, 2008; Menke et al., 2009; Naeser et al., 2005; Vitali et al., 2007).

Rochon et al. (2010), for example, compared the neural correlates associated with phonological and semantic tasks following a phonologically based intervention in two persons with aphasia. In both patients, post treatment scans demonstrated changes in the activation of left-frontal and temporal brain structures. Fridriksson et al. (2007) contrasted semantic and phonological cueing in the treatment of two nonfluent and one fluent aphasic patient. The nonfluent participants improved in naming and showed neural activity bilaterally in the precuneus; the participant with fluent aphasia demonstrated a reduction in naming errors with increased activity in the right entorhinal cortex and posterior thalamus—brain structures not typically associated with language functions.

In a recent model-based group study of anomia treatment, Abel et al. (2014) detected differential neural patterns among their participants, who had phonological or semantic naming deficits ($n = 14$). The study involved a 4-week treatment of naming in which increasing hierarchies of semantic and phonological cues were administered. The participants with phonological impairment showed distinct therapy-induced effects. Their naming gains were positively predicted by brain activation in the left inferior frontal gyrus and pars opercularis but negatively predicted by the right caudate nucleus. Following therapy, they showed a reduction in activation decreases of left temporoparietal cortices; naming of trained items resulted in less activation decreases in the left superior temporal gyrus, precuneus, bilateral thalamus, and right caudate.

Participants with semantic impairments showed a slightly different pattern. They relied on activation of the right inferior frontal gyrus and pars triangularis; following therapy, they demonstrated a reduction in activation decreases in the left superior temporal gyrus, caudate, paracentral lobule, and right rolandic operculum.

A comparison of the intervention types—phonological or semantic—also revealed differential brain activation patterns. Employment of semantic cues implicated the right superior parietal lobule while the use of phonological cues involved bilateral anterior and midcingulate, right precuneus, and left mid/superior frontal gyrus.

The authors concluded that the two patient groups used distinct brain regions to support their naming abilities: the phonologic group utilized preserved left hemisphere structures while the semantic group showed more compensatory right-sided brain activation. Benefits of training were associated with the activation of brain areas typically linked to nonlinguistic cognitive functions, such as strategizing and monitoring, although the authors do not specifically mention memory functions.

Very few studies have explored the neural bases of *learning* in aphasia treatment (Vallila-Rohter & Kiran, 2013). This gap is especially surprising, since the development of the errorless learning approach was anchored in Hebb's (1961) conceptualization of neural plasticity, whereby neurons that fire together strengthen the connection established between them and enhance their potential concurrent reactivation in subsequent occasions. Advances in computational neuroscience have led to further suggestions about the role of feedback in altering the strength of connections among "neuron-like" processing nodes (e.g., McClleland et al., 1999). Specifically, the connection among nodes has been shown to remain unchanged when the system is reinforced by self-errors but not under errorless learning conditions. Based on this observation, it has been argued that errorless learning might, in fact, facilitate treatment-based reshaping of neural networks in the aphasic brain (Fillingham et al., 2003).

The few neuroimaging studies exploring the neural underpinnings of learning in aphasia treatment have pointed to the importance of the hippocampal formation for therapy gains. For example, in an early computed tomography study, Goldenberg and Spatt (1994) found that persons with temporobasal lesions were less successful at aphasia therapy than patients in whom these structures were spared. They proposed that such damage disconnects the hippocampal formation and perisylvian language areas and so hinders explicit learning of linguistic information.

Additional support for this proposal comes from more recent neuroimaging studies of aphasia treatment. For example, in a diffusion tensor imaging study by Meinzer et al. (2010), the structural integrity of fiber tracts surrounding the hippocampus was related to positive aphasia therapy outcomes. Comparable neural structures have also been implicated in studies of healthy adult learners engaged in novel lexical or syntactic learning tasks (Breinstein et al., 2005; Maguire & Firth, 2004; Opitz & Friederici, 2003).

An important contribution to our understanding of the role of learning in aphasia treatment comes from Menke et al. (2009), who contrasted the short- and long-term effects of naming training, showing differential brain activation patterns. Short-term therapy gains were mediated by increased bilateral activation of the hippocampus, the right precuneus, and the cingulate gyrus and bilaterally in the fusiform gyrus; long-term effects implicated well-established language regions. These findings suggest that aphasia therapy involves a *dynamic* process of treatment-induced neural changes, much in line with our view of neural multifunctionality espoused throughout the book.

Thus, little by little, chapter by chapter, the overall thrust of this book embraces a unifying theory of the neural mulitfunctionality of language in the context of aphasia recovery, much in the spirit of Hickok's (2014) attempts to lay out an integrative neural model of language and motor-sensory processing. We will return to this topic in Chapter 7.

References

Abel, S., Huber, W., & Dell, G. S. (2009). Connectionist diagnosis of lexical disorders in aphasia. *Aphasiology, 23*(11), 1353–1378.

Abel, S., Weiller, C., Huber, W., & Willmes, K. (2014). Neural underpinnings for model-oriented therapy of aphasic word production. *Neuropsychologia, 57,* 154–165.

Acheson, D. J., Hamidi, M., Binder, J. R., & Postle, B. R. (2011). A common neural substrate for language production and verbal working memory. *Journal of Cognitive Neuroscience, 23*(6), 1358–1367. doi:10.1162/jocn.2010.21519

Acheson, D. J., & MacDonald, M. C. (2009). Verbal working memory and language production: common approaches to the serial ordering of verbal information. *Psychological Bulletin, 135,* 50–68.

Acheson, D. J., & MacDonald, M.C. (2011).The rhymes that the reader perused confused the meaning: phonological effects during on-line sentence comprehension. *Journal of Memory and Language, 65,* 193–207.

Adams, J. A., & Dijkstra, S. (1966). Short-term memory for motor responses. *Journal of Experimental Psychology, 71,* 314–318.

Alexander, G. E., & Crutcher, M. D. (1990). Functional architecture of basal ganglia circuits: neural substrates of parallel processing. *Trends in Neurosciences, 13*(7), 266–271.

Alexander, G. E., DeLong, M. R., & Strick, P. L. (1986). Parallel organization of functionally segregated circuits linking basal ganglia and cortex. *Annual Review of Neuroscience, 9*(1), 357–381.

Allen, C. M., Martin, R. C., & Martin, N. (2012). Relations between short-term memory deficits, semantic processing, and executive function. *Aphasiology, 26*(3–4), 428–461.

Allport, D. A. (1984). Speech production and comprehension: one lexicon or two? In W. Prinz & A. F. Sanders (Eds.), *Cognition and motor processes* (pp. 209–228). Berlin: Springer Verlag.

Alvarez, P., & Squire, L. R. (1994). Memory consolidation and the medial temporal lobe: a simple network model. *Proceedings of the National Academy of Sciences of the United States of America, 91*(15), 7041–7045.

Antonucci, S. M., & Reilly, J. (2008). Semantic memory and language processing: a primer. *Seminars in Speech and Language, 29*(1), 5–17.

Atkinson, R. C., & Shiffrin, R. M. (1968). Human memory: a proposed system and its control processes. In K. W. Spence & J. T. Spence (Eds.), *The psychology of learning and motivation* (Vol. 2, pp. 89–195). New York: Academic Press.

Attout, L., Van der Kaa, M. A., George, M., & Majerus, S. (2012). Dissociating short-term memory and language impairment: the importance of item and serial order information. *Aphasiology, 26*(3–4), 355–382.

Baddeley, A. D. (1966). Short-term memory for word sequences as a function of acoustic, semantic and formal similarity. *The Quarterly Journal of Experimental Psychology, 18*, 362–365.

Baddeley, A. D. (1986). *Working memory*. New York: Clarendon/Oxford University Press.

Baddeley, A. D. (2000). The episodic buffer: A new component of working memory? *Trends in Cognitive Sciences, 4*(11), 417–423.

Baddeley, A. D. (2001). Is working memory still working? *American Psychologist, 56*(11), 851.

Baddeley, A. D. (2003). Working memory and language: an overview. *Journal of Communication Disorders, 36*, 189–208.

Baddeley, A. D. (2007). Working memory: multiple models, multiple mechanisms. In H. L. Roediger, Y. Dudai, & S. M. Fitzpatrick (Eds.), *Science of memory: concepts* (pp. 151–153). Oxford, UK: Oxford University Press.

Baddeley, A. D. (2010). Working memory. *Current Biology, 20*(4), R136–R140.

Baddeley, A., Chincotta, D., & Adlam, A. (2001). Working memory and the control of action: evidence from task switching. *Journal of Experimental Psychology: General, 130*(4), 641–657.

Baddeley, A., Gathercole, S., & Papagno, C. (1998). The phonological loop as a language learning device. *Psychological Review, 105*(1), 158–173.

Baddeley, A. D., & Hitch, G. (1974). Working memory. In G. H. Bower (Ed.), *The psychology of learning and motivation: advances in research and theory* (Vol. 8, pp. 47–89). New York: Academic Press.

Baddeley, A., Thomson, N., & Buchanan, M. (1975). Word length and the structure of short-term memory. *Journal of Verbal Learning and Verbal Behavior, 14*, 575–589.

Baddeley, A. D., & Warrington, E. K. (1970). Amnesia and the distinction between long- and short-term memory. *Journal of Verbal Learning and Verbal Behavior, 9*, 176–189.

Baddeley, A., & Wilson, B. (1985). Phonological coding and short-term memory in patients without speech. *Journal of Memory and Language, 24*(4), 490–502.

Baddeley, A., & Wilson, B. A. (1994). When implicit learning fails: amnesia and the problem of error elimination. *Neuropsychologia, 32*, 53–68.

Badre, D., & Wagner, A. D. (2007). Left ventrolateral prefrontal cortex and the cognitive control of memory. *Neuropsychologia, 45*(13), 2883–2901.

Baldo, J. V., Klostermann, E. C., & Dronkers, N. F. (2008). It's either a cook or a baker: patients with conduction aphasia get the gist but lose the trace. *Brain and Language, 105*(2), 134–140.

Baldo, J., & Dronkers, N. (2006). The role of inferior parietal and inferior frontal cortex in working memory. *Neuropsychology, 20*, 529–538.

Baldo, J. V., Katseff, S., & Dronkers, N. F. (2012). Brain regions underlying repetition and auditory-verbal short-term memory deficits in aphasia: evidence from voxel-based lesion symptom mapping. *Aphasiology, 26*(3–4), 338–354.

Barde, L. H., Schwartz, M. F., Chrysikou, E. G., & Thompson-Schill, S. L. (2010). Reduced short-term memory span in aphasia and susceptibility to interference: contribution of material-specific maintenance deficits. *Neuropsychologia, 48*(4), 909–920.

Basso, A., Spinnler, H., Vallar, G., & Zanobio, M. (1982). Left hemisphere damage and selective impairment of auditory verbal short-term memory. A case study. *Neuropsychologia, 20*(3), 263–274.

Beeson, P. M., Bayles, K. A., Rubens, A. B., & Kaszniak, A. W. (1993). Memory impairment and executive control in individuals with stroke-induced aphasia. *Brain and Language*, *45*(2), 253–275.

Berndt, R. S., & Mitchum, C. C. (1990). Auditory and lexical information sources in immediate recall: evidence from a patient with deficit to the phonological short-term store. In G. Vallar & T. Shallice (Eds.), *Neuropsychological impairments of short-term memory*. New York: Cambridge University Press.

Best, W., Herbert, R., Hickin, J., Osborne, F., & Howard, D. (2002). Phonological and orthographic facilitation of word-retrieval in aphasia: immediate and delayed effects. *Aphasiology*, *16*(1–2), 151–168.

Binder J. R., Desai, R. H., Graves, W. W., & Conant, L. L. (2009). Where is the semantic system? A critical review and meta-analysis of 120 functional neuroimaging studies. *Cerebral Cortex*, *19*(12), 2767–2796.

Breinstein, C., Jansen, A., Deppe, M., Foerster, A., Sommer, J., Wolbers, T., & Knecht, S. (2005). Hippocampus activity differentiates good from poor learners of a novel lexicon. *Neuroimage*, *25*, 958–968.

Breitenstein, C., Kamping, S., Jansen, A., Schomacher, M., & Knecht, S. (2004). Word learning can be achieved without feedback: implications to aphasia therapy. *Restorative Neurology and Neuroscience*, *22*, 445–458.

Brown, J. (1958). Some tests of the decay theory of immediate memory. *Quarterly Journal of Experimental Psychology*, *10*(1), 12–21.

Buchsbaum, B. R., Baldo, J., Okadad, K., Berman, K. F., Dronkers, N., D'Esposito, M., & Hickok, G. (2011). Conduction aphasia, sensory-motor integration, and phonological short-term memory—an aggregate analysis of lesion and fMRI data. *Brain and Language*, *119*(3), 119–128.

Buchsbaum, B. R., Padmanabhan, A., & Berman, K. F. (2011). The neural substrates of recognition memory for verbal information: spanning the divide between short- and long-term memory. *Journal of Cognitive Neuroscience*, *23*(4), 978–991.

Buckner, R. L., & Wheeler, M. E. (2001). The cognitive neuroscience of remembering. *Nature Reviews Neuroscience*, *2*, 624–634.

Burgio, F., & Basso, A. (1997). Memory and aphasia. *Neuropsychologia*, *35*(6), 759–766.

Butters, N. Samuels, I., Goodglass, H., & Brody, B. (1970). Short-term visual and auditory memory disorders after parietal and frontal lobe damage. *Cortex*, *6*, 440–459.

Cabeza, R., & Moscovitch, M. (2013). Memory systems, processing modes, and components: functional neuroimaging evidence. *Perspectives on Psychological Science*, *8*(1), 49–55.

Caplan, D., & Waters, G. (1994). Articulatory length and phonological similarity in span tasks: a reply to Baddeley and Andrade. *Quarterly Journal of Experimental Psychology*, *47A*, 1055–1062.

Caplan, D., & Waters, G. (1996). Syntactic processing in sentence comprehension under dual-task conditions in aphasic patients. *Language and Cognitive Processes*, *11*, 525–551.

Caplan, D., & Waters, G. (2013). Memory mechanisms supporting syntactic comprehension. *Psychonomic Bulletin & Review*, *20*(2), 243–268.

Caplan, D., & Waters, G. S. (1995). Aphasic disorders of syntactic comprehension and working memory capacity. *Cognitive Neuropsychology*, *12*(6), 637–649.

Caplan, D., & Waters, G. S. (1999). Verbal working memory and sentence comprehension. *Journal of Behavioral and Brain Science, 22*(1), 77–94; discussion 95–126.

Caplan, D., Dede, G., Waters, G., Michaud, J., & Tripodis, Y. (2011). Effects of age, speed of processing, and working memory on comprehension of sentences with relative clauses. *Psychology and Aging, 26*(2), 439–450.

Caramazza, A., Basili, A., Keller, J. & Berndt, R. S. (1981). An investigation of repetition and language processing in a case of conduction aphasia. *Brain and Language, 14*, 235–271.

Carpenter, P. A., Just, M. A., & Reichle, E. D. (2000). Working memory and executive function: evidence from neuroimaging. *Current Opinion in Neurobiology, 10*, 195–199.

Caspari, I., Parkinson, S. R., LaPointe, L. L., & Katz, R. C. (1998). Working memory and aphasia. *Brain and Cognition, 37*, 205–223.

Christensen, S. C., & Harris Wright, H. (2010). Verbal and non-verbal working memory in aphasia: what three n-back tasks reveal. *Aphasiology, 24*(6), 752–762.

Clare, L., Wilson, B. A., Breen, K., & Hodges, J. R. (1999). Errorless learning of face–name associations in early Alzheimer's disease. *Neurocase, 5*, 37–46.

Clare, L., Wilson, B. A., Carter, G., Gosses, A., Breen, K., & Hodges, J. R. (2000). Intervening with everyday memory problems in early Alzheimer's disease: an errorless learning approach. *Journal of Clinical and Experimental Neuropsychology, 22*, 132–146.

Cloutman, L., Gottesman, R., Chaudhry, P., Davis, C., Kleinman, J. T., Pawlak, M., ... Hillis, A. E. (2009). Where (in the brain) do semantic errors come from? *Cortex, 45*(5), 641–649.

Collete, F., Van der Linden, M., & Poncelet, M. (2000). Working memory, long-term memory, and language processing: issues and future directions. *Brain and Language, 71*, 46–51.

Connelly, S. L., Hasher, L., & Zacks, R. T. (1991). Age and reading: the impact of distraction. *Psychology and Aging, 6*, 533–541.

Connor, L. T., MacKay, A. J., & White, D. A. (2000). Working memory: a foundation for executive abilities and higher-order cognitive skills. *Seminars in Speech and Language, 21*, 109–119.

Conway, C. M., & Christiansen, M. H. (2001). Sequential learning in non-human primates. *Trends in Cognitive Sciences, 5*(12), 539–546.

Cornelissen, K., Laine, M., Tarkiainen, A., Jarvensivu, T., Martin, N., & Salmelin, R. (2003). Adult brain plasticity elicited by anomia treatment. *Journal of Cognitive Neuroscience, 15*, 444–461.

Coughlin, A. K. (1979). Effects of localized cerebral lesions and dysphasia on verbal memory. *Journal of Neurology, Neurosurgery, and Psychiatry, 42*, 914–923.

Cowan, N. (1988). Evolving conceptions of memory storage, selective attention, and their mutual constraints within the human information processing system. *Psychological Bulletin, 104*, 163–191.

Craik, F.I.M., & Lockhart, R. S. (1972). Levels of processing: a framework for memory research. *Journal of Verbal Learning and Verbal Behavior, 11*(6), 671–684.

Crosson, B., Benefield, H., Cato, M. A., Sadek, J. R., Moore, A. B., Wierenga, C. E., ... Briggs, R. W. (2003). Left and right basal ganglia and frontal activity during language generation: contributions to lexical, semantic, and phonological processes. *Journal of the International Neuropsychological Society, 9*(7), 1061–1077.

Crosson, B., Benjamin, M., & Levy, I. (2007). Role of the basal ganglia in language and semantics: Supporting cast. In J. Hart Jr, & M. Kraut (Eds.), *Neural basis of semantic memory* (pp. 219–243). New York: Cambridge University Press.

Curran, T., & Schacter, D. L. (2013). Implicit memory and perceptual brain mechanisms. *Basic and Applied Memory Research: Theory in Context, 1*, 221–240.

Dalla Barba, G., Frasson, E., Mantovan, M.C., Gallo, A., & Denes, G. (1996). Semantic and episodic memory in aphasia. *Neuropsychologia, 34*(5), 361–367.

Dalla Barba, G., Mantovan, M. C., Ferruzza, E., & Denes, G. (1997). Remembering and knowing the past: a case study of isolated retrograde amnesia. *Cortex, 33*(1), 143–154.

Daneman, M., & Carpenter, P. A. (1980). Individual differences in working memory and reading. *Journal of Verbal Learning and Verbal Behavior, 19*, 450–466.

Daneman, M., & Merikle, P. M. (1996). Working memory and language comprehension: a meta-analysis. *Psychonomic Bulletin & Review, 3*(4), 422–433.

De Renzi, E. (1989). Apraxia. In F. Boller & J. Grafman (Eds.), *Handbook of neuropsychology* (pp. 245–263). New York: Elsevier Science.

Dell, G. S., & O'Seaghdha, P. G. (1991). Mediated and convergent lexical priming in language production: a comment on Levelt et al. (1991). *Psychological Review, 98*(4), 604–614.

Dell, G. S., & O'Seaghdha, P. G. (1992). Stages of lexical access in language production. *Cognition, 42*(1–3), 287–314.

Dell, G. S., Schwartz, M. F., Martin, N., Saffran, E. M., & Gagnon, D. A. (1997). Lexical access in aphasic and nonaphasic speakers. *Psychological Review, 104*(4), 801–838.

Dew, I. T., & Cabeza, R. (2011). The porous boundaries between explicit and implicit memory: behavioral and neural evidence. *Annals of the New York Academy of Sciences, 1224*, 174–190.

Dominey, P. F., Hoen, M., Blanc, J. M., & Lelekov-Boissard, T. (2003). Neurological basis of language and sequential cognition: evidence from simulation, aphasia, and ERP studies. *Brain and Language, 86*(2), 207–225.

Doucet, G., Naveau, M., Petit, L., Delcroix, N., Zago, L., Crivello, F., ... Joliot, M. (2011). Brain activity at rest: a multiscale hierarchical functional organization. *Journal of Neurophysiology, 105*(6), 2753–2763.

Doya, K. (2000). Complementary roles of basal ganglia and cerebellum in learning and motor control. *Current Opinion in Neurobiology, 10*(6), 732–739.

Eichenbaum, H., & Cohen, N. J. (2001). *From conditioning to conscious recollection: memory systems of the brain*. New York: Oxford University Press

Eichenbaum, H., & Cohen, N. J. (2001). *From conditioning to conscious recollection: memory systems of the brain*. New York: Oxford University Press.

Engle, R. W., Cantor, J., & Carullo, J. J. (1992). Individual differences in working memory and comprehension: a test of four hypotheses. *Journal of Experimental Psychology: Learning, Memory, and Cognition, 18*, 972–992.

Ericsson, K. A., & Kintsch, W. (1995). Long-term working memory. *Psychological Review, 102*(2), 211–245.

Evans, J. J., Wilson, B. A., Schuri, U., Andrade, J., Baddeley, A., Bruna, O., ... Taussik, I. (2000). A comparison of "errorless" and "trial and error" learning methods for teaching individuals with acquired memory deficits. *Neuropsychological Rehabilitation, 10*(1), 67–101.

Fedorenko, E., Gibson, E., & Rohde, D. (2006). The nature of working memory capacity in sentence comprehension: evidence against domain-specific resources. *Journal of Memory and Language, 54*(4), 541–553.

Fiebach, C. J., Schlesewsky, M., & Friederici, A. D. (2001). Syntactic working memory and the establishment of filler-gap dependencies: insights from ERPs and fMRI. *Journal of Psycholinguistic Research, 30*(3), 321–338.

Fiebach, C. J., Schlesewsky, M., Lohmann, G., von Cramon, D. Y., & Friederici, A. (2005). Revisiting the role of Broca's area in sentence processing: syntactic integration versus syntactic working memory. *Human Brain Mapping, 24*, 79–91.

Fiebach, C. J., Vos, S. H., & Friederici, A. D. (2004). Neural correlates of syntactic ambiguity in sentence comprehension for low and high span readers. *Journal of Cognitive Neuroscience, 16*(9), 1562–1575.

Fillingham, J. K., Hodgson, C., Sage, K., & Lambon Ralph, M. A. (2003). The application of errorless learning to aphasic disorders: a review of theory and practice. *Neuropsychological Rehabilitation, 13*(3), 337–363.

Fillingham, J. K., Sage, K., & Lambon Ralph, M. A. (2005a). Treatment of anomia using errorless versus errorful learning: are frontal executive skills and feedback important? *International Journal of Language and Communication Disorders, 40*(4), 505–523.

Fillingham, J. K., Sage, K., & Lambon Ralph, M. A. (2005b). Further explorations and an overview of errorless and errorful therapy for aphasic word-finding difficulties: the number of naming attempts during therapy affects outcome. *Aphasiology, 19*(7), 597–614.

Fillingham, J. K., Sage, K., & Lambon Ralph, M. A. (2006). The treatment of anomia using errorless learning. *Neuropsychological Rehabilitation, 16*(2), 129–154.

Francis, D. R., Clark, N., & Humphreys, G. W. (2003). The treatment of an auditory working memory deficit and the implications for sentence comprehension abilities in mild "receptive" aphasia. *Aphasiology, 17*, 723–750.

Frattali, C., & Kang, Y. K. (2004). An errorless learning approach to treating dysnomia. *Brain and Language, 91*(1), 177–178.

Freedman, M. L., & Martin, R. C. (2001). Dissociable components of short-term memory and their relation to long-term learning. *Cognitive Neuropsychology, 18*(3), 193–226.

Fridriksson, J., Holland, A., Beeson, P., & Morrow, K. L. (2005). Spaced retrieval treatment of anomia. *Aphasiology, 19*, 99–109.

Fridriksson, J., Morrow, K. L., Moser, D., Fridriksson, A., & Baylis, G. C. (2006). Neural recruitment associated with anomia treatment in aphasia. *NeuroImage, 32*, 1403–1412.

Fridriksson, J., Moser, D., Bonilha, L., Morrow-Odom, K. L., Shaw, H., Fridriksson, A., … Rorden, C. (2007). Neural correlates of phonological and semantic-based anomia treatment in aphasia. *Neuropsychologia, 45*(8), 1812–1822.

Fridriksson, J., Richardson, J. D., Fillmore, P., & Cai, B. (2012). Left hemisphere plasticity and aphasia recovery. *Neuroimage, 60*(2), 854–863.

Friederici, A. D. (2012). The cortical language circuit: from auditory perception to sentence comprehension. *Trends in Cognitive Science, 16*(5), 262–268.

Friederici, A. D., & Gierhan, S. M. (2013). The language network. *Current Opinion in Neurobiology, 23*(2), 250–254. doi: 10.1016/j.conb.2012.10.002

Friedman, R. B. (2000). The role of learning and memory paradigms in the remediation of aphasic disorders. *Brain and Language, 71*, 69–71.

Friedmann, N., & Gvion, A. (2003). Sentence comprehension and working memory limitation: a dissociation between semantic and phonological encoding. *Brain and Language, 86*, 23–39.

Friedrich, F. J., Glenn, C. G., & Marin, O. S. (1984). Interruption of phonological coding in conduction aphasia. *Brain and Language, 22*(2), 266–291.

Gagnon, D. A., Schwartz, M. F., Martin, N., Dell, G. S., & Saffran, E. M. (1997). The origins of formal paraphasias in aphasics' picture naming. *Brain and Language, 59*(3), 450–472.

Gandha, I., Dahmen, W., Hartje, W., Willmes, K., & Weniger, D. (1983). To what extent are the cognitive performances of Wernicke's aphasics disturbed by their own vocalizations? *Brain and Cognition, 2*(1), 12–24.

Goldenberg, G., & Spatt, J. (1994). Influence of size and site of cerebral lesions on spontaneous recovery of aphasia and on success of language therapy. *Brain and Language, 47*(4), 684–698.

Goodale, M. A. (2000). Perception and action in the human visual system. In Gazzaniga, M. S. (Ed.), *The new cognitive neurosciences* (pp. 365–378). Cambridge, MA: MIT Press.

Goodale, M. A., & Milner, A. D. (1992). Separate visual pathways for perception and actions. *Trends in Neurosciences, 15*(1), 20–25.

Gordon, P. C., Hendrick, R., & Levine, W. H. (2002). Memory-load interference in syntactic processing. *Psychological Science, 13,* 425–430.

Gordon, W. P. (1983). Memory disorders in aphasia—I. Auditory immediate recall. *Neuropsychologia, 21*(4), 325–339.

Goschke, T., Friederici, A. D., Kotz, S. A., & Van Kampen, A. (2001). Procedural learning in Broca's aphasia: dissociation between the implicit acquisition of spatio-motor and phoneme sequences. *Journal of Cognitive Neuroscience, 13*(3), 370–388.

Greenwald, M. L., Raymer, A. M., Richardson, M. E., & Rothi, L.J.G. (1995). Contrasting treatments for severe impairments of picture naming. *Neuropsychological Rehabilitation, 5,* 17–49.

Grossman, M., & Carey, S. (1987). Selective word-learning deficits in aphasia. *Brain and Language, 32,* 306–324.

Grossman, M., Carvell, S., Gollomp, S., Stern, M. B., Vernon, G., & Hurtig, H. I. (1991). Sentence comprehension and praxis deficits in Parkinson's disease. *Neurology, 41,* 1620–1628

Gupta, P., Martin, N., Abbs, B., Schwartz, M., & Lipinski, J. (2006). New word learning in aphasic patients: Dissociating phonological and semantic components. *Brain and Language, 99,* 8–9.

Gutbrod, K., Cohen, R., Mager, B., & Meier, E. (1989). Coding and recall of categorized material in aphasics. *Journal of Clinical and Experimental Neuropsychology, 11*(6), 821–841.

Gvion, A., & Friedmann, N. (2012). Does phonological working memory impairment affect sentence comprehension? A study of conduction aphasia. *Aphasiology, 26*(3–4), 494–535.

Hamilton, A. C., & Martin, R. C. (2007). Proactive interference in a semantic short-term memory deficit: role of semantic and phonological relatedness. *Cortex, 43*(1), 112–123.

Hamm, V. P., & Hasher, L. (1992). Age and the availability of inferences. *Psychology and Aging, 7,* 56–64.

Hanten, G., & Martin, R. C. (2000). Contributions of phonological and semantic short-term memory to sentence processing: evidence from two cases of closed head injury in children. *Journal of Memory and Language, 43,* 335–361.

Hasher, L., & Zacks, R. T. (1988). Working memory, comprehension, and aging: A review and a new view. In G.H. Bower (Ed.), *The psychology of learning and motivation* (Vol. 22, pp. 193–226). New York: Academic Press.

Hebb, D. O. (1949). *The organization of behavior.* New York: Wiley.

Hebb, D. O. (1961). *The organization of behavior: a neuropsychological theory.* New York: Science Editions.

Heilman, K. M., Watson, R. T., & Gonzalez-Rothi, L. J. (1997). Commentary on: The basal ganglia & apraxia by P. O. Pramstaller & C. David Marsden. *Neurology Network Commentary, 1*, 52–56.

Heilman, K. M., Scholes, R., & Watson, R. T. (1976). Defects of immediate memory in Broca's and conduction aphasia. *Brain and Language, 3*(2), 201–208.

Henke, K. (2010). A model for memory systems based on processing modes rather than consciousness. *Nature Reviews Neuroscience, 11*(7), 523–532.

Hickok, G. (2014). *The myth of mirror neurons: the real neuroscience of communication and cognition.* New York: Norton.

Hillis, A. E., Kleinman, J. T., Newhart, M., Heidler-Gary, J., Gottesman, R., Barker, P. B., ... Chaudhry, P. (2006). Restoring cerebral blood flow reveals neural regions critical for naming. *Journal of Neuroscience, 26*, 8069–8073.

Hillis, A. E., Wityk, R. J., Tuffiash, E., Beauchamp, N. J., Jacobs, M. A., Barker, P. B., & Selnes, O. A. (2001). Hypoperfusion of Wernicke's area predicts severity of semantic deficit in acute stroke. *Annals of Neurology, 50*(5), 561–566.

Hoffman, P., Jefferies, E., Ehsan, S., Hopper, S., & Lambon Ralph, M.A.L. (2009). Selective short-term memory deficits arise from impaired domain-general semantic control mechanisms. *Journal of Experimental Psychology: Learning, Memory, and Cognition, 35*(1), 137.

Hoffman, P., Jefferies, E., Ehsan, S., Jones, R. W., & Lambon Ralph, M. A. (2012). How does linguistic knowledge contribute to short-term memory? Contrasting effects of impaired semantic knowledge and executive control. *Aphasiology, 26*(3–4), 383–403.

Howard, D., Patterson, K., Franklin, S., Orchard Lisle, V., & Morton, J. (1985). Treatment of word retrieval deficits in aphasia: a comparison of 2 therapy methods. *Brain, 108*, 817–829.

Just, M. A., & Carpenter, P. A. (1992). A capacity theory of comprehension: individual differences in working memory. *Psychological Review, 99*(1), 122–149.

Kalinyak-Fliszar, M., Kohen, F., & Martin, N. (2011). Remediation of language processing in aphasia: Improving activation and maintenance of linguistic representations in (verbal) short-term memory. *Aphasiology, 25*(10), 1095–1131.

Kalinyak-Fliszar, M., Martin, N., & Kohen, F. (2012). Improving the maintenance of word representations in short-term memory to improve language function: acquisition and generalization effects. Presented at the 42nd Clinical Aphasiology Conference; Lake Tahoe, CA.

Kane, M. J., Conway, A. R., Hambrick, D. Z., & Engle, R. W. (2007). Variation in working memory capacity as variation in executive attention and control. In A. R. Conway, C. Jarrold, M. J. Kane, A. Miyake & J. N. Towse (Eds.), *Variation in working memory* (pp. 21–48). Oxford, UK: Oxford University Press.

Kane, M. J., Hambrick, D. Z., Tuholski, S. W., Wilhelm, O., Payne, T. W., & Engle, R. W. (2004). The generality of working memory capacity: a latent-variable approach to verbal and visuospatial memory span and reasoning. *Journal of Experimental Psychology: General, 133*, 189–217.

Kasselimis, D. S., Simos, P. G., Economou, A., Peppas, C., Evdokimidis, I., & Potagas, C. (2013). Are memory deficits dependent on the presence of aphasia in left brain damaged patients? *Neuropsychologia, 51*(9), 1773–1776.

Keller, T. A., Carpenter, P. A., & Just, M. A. (2003). Brain imaging of tongue-twister sentence comprehension: twisting the tongue and the brain. *Brain and Language, 84*(2), 189–203.
Kelly, H., & Armstrong, L. (2009). New word learning in people with aphasia. *Aphasiology, 23*(12), 1398–1417.
King, J., & Just, M. A. (1991). Individual differences in syntactic processing: the role of working memory. *Journal of Memory and Language, 30*(5), 580–602.
King, J., & Just, M. A. (1991). Individual differences in syntactic processing: the role of working memory. *Journal of Memory and Language, 30*, 580–602.
Kinsbourne, M. (1972). Contrasting patterns of memory span decrement in aging and aphasia. *Journal of Neurology, Neurosurgery and Psychiatry, 35*, 192–195.
Kiran, S. (2007). Semantic complexity in the treatment of naming deficits. *American Journal of Speech Language Pathology, 16*, 18–29.
Knowlton, B. J., Mangels, J. A., & Squire, L. R. (1996). A neostriatal habit learning system in humans. *Science, 273*(5280), 1399–1402.
Koenig-Bruhin, M., & Studer-Eichenberger, F. (2007). Therapy of short-term memory disorders in fluent aphasia: a single case study. *Aphasiology, 21*(5), 448–458.
Koenigs, M., Acheson, D. J., Barbey, A. K., Solomon, J., Postle, B. R., & Grafman, J. (2011). Areas of left perisylvian cortex mediate auditory–verbal short-term memory. *Neuropsychologia, 49*(13), 3612–3619.
Kohn, S. E. (1992). Conclusions: toward a working definition of conduction aphasia. In S. E. Kohn (Ed.), *Conduction aphasia* (pp. 151–156). Hillsdale, NJ: Erlbaum.
Lang, C.J.G., & Quitz, A. (2012). Verbal and nonverbal memory impairment in aphasia. *Journal of Neurology, 259*(8), 1655–1661.
Laures-Gore, J. S., DuBay, M., Duff, M. C., & Buchanan, T. W. (2010). Identifying behavioral measures of stress in individuals with aphasia. *Journal of Speech-Language Hearing Research, 53*, 1394–1400.
Laures-Gore, J. S., Marshall, R. M., & Verner, E. (2011). Digit span differences in aphasia and right brain damage. *Aphasiology, 25*(1), 43–56.
Lauro, L.J.R., Reis, J., Cohen, L. G., Cecchetto, C., & Papagno, C. (2010). A case for the involvement of phonological loop in sentence comprehension. *Neuropsychologia, 48*(14), 4003–4011.
Leff, A. P., Schofield, T. M., Crinion, J. T., Seghier, M. L., Grogan, A., Green, D. W., & Price, C. J. (2009). The left superior temporal gyrus is a shared substrate for auditory short-term memory and speech comprehension: evidence from 210 patients with stroke. *Brain, 132* (Pt. 12), 3401–3410.
Leger, A., Demonet, J. F., Ruff, S., Aithamon, B., Touyeras, B., Puel, M., … Cardebat, D. (2002). Neural substrates of spoken language rehabilitation in an aphasic patient: an fMRI study. *Neuroimage, 17*(1), 174–183.
Lupyan, G., & Mirman, D. (2013). Linking language and categorization: evidence from aphasia. *Cortex, 49*(5), 1187–1194.
MacDonald, M. C., & Christiansen, M. H. (2002). Reassessing working memory: a comment on Just & Carpenter (1992) and Waters & Caplan (1996). *Psychological Review, 109*, 35–54.
Maguire, E. A., & Firth, C. D. (2004). The brain network associated with acquiring semantic knowledge. *NeuroImage, 22*(1), 171–178.

Maher, L. M., & Raymer, A. M. (2004). Management of anomia. *Topics in Stroke Rehabilitation*, *11*(1), 10–21.

Majerus, S., Van der Linden, M., Poncelet, M., & Metz-Lutz, M. N. (2004). Can phonological and semantic short-term memory be dissociated? Further evidence from landau-kleffner syndrome. *Cognitive Neuropsychology*, *21*(5), 491–512.

Makuuchi, M., & Friederici, A. D. (2013). Hierarchical functional connectivity between the core language system and the working memory system. *Cortex*, *49*(9), 2416–2423. doi: 10.1016/j.cortex.2013.01.007

Makuuchi, M., Bahlmann, J., Anwander, A., & Friederici, A. D. (2009). Segregating the core computational faculty of human language from working memory. *Proceedings of the National Academy of Sciences of the United States of America*, *106*(20), 8362–8367.

Marshall, J., Pound, C., White-Thomson, M., & Pring, T. (1990). The use of picture/word matching tasks to assist word retrieval in aphasic patients. *Aphasiology*, *4*(2), 167–184.

Martin, N. (2000). Word processing and verbal short-term memory: how are they connected and why do we want to know? *Brain and Language*, *71*, 149–153.

Martin, N. (2008). The role of semantic processing in short-term memory and learning: evidence from aphasia. In A.Thorn & M. Page (Eds.), *interactions between short-term and long-term memory in the verbal domain* (p. 220–243). New York, NY: Psychology Press.

Martin, N., & Ayala, J. (2004). Measurement of auditory-verbal STM span in aphasia: effects of item, task, and lexical impairment. *Brain and Language*, *89*(3), 464–483.

Martin, N., Dell, G. S., Saffran, E. M., & Schwartz, M. F. (1994). Origins of paraphasias in deep dysphasia: testing the consequences of a decay impairment to an interactive spreading activation model of lexical retrieval. *Brain and Language*, *47*(4), 609–660.

Martin, N., & Gupta, P. (2004). Exploring the relationship between word processing and verbal short-term memory: evidence from associations and dissociations. *Cognitive Neuropsychology*, *21*(2–4), 213–228.

Martin, N., Kohen, F., Kalinyak-Fliszar, M., Soveri, A., & Laine, M. (2012). Effects of working memory load on processing of sounds and meanings of words in aphasia. *Aphasiology*, *26*(3–4), 462–493.

Martin, N., & Saffran, E.M. (1992). A computational account of deep dysphasia: evidence from a single case study. *Brain and Language*, *43*, 240–274.

Martin, N., & Saffran, E.M. (1997). Language and auditory-verbal short-term memory impairments: evidence for common underlying processes. *Cognitive Neuropsychology*, *14* (5), 641–682.

Martin, N., Saffran, E. M., & Dell, G. S. (1996). Recovery in deep dysphasia: evidence for a relation between auditory-verbal STM and lexical errors in repetition. *Brain and Language*, *52*, 83–113.

Martin, P. I., & Laine, M. (2000). Effects of contextual priming on word retrieval in anomia. *Aphasiology*, *14*(1), 53–70.

Martin, R.C. (1990). Neuropsychological evidence on the role of short-term memory in sentence processing. In G. Vallar & T. Shallice (Eds.), *Neuropsychological impairments of short-term memory* (pp. 390–427). Cambridge, UK: Cambridge University Press.

Martin, R. C. (1993). Short-term memory and sentence processing: evidence from neuropsychology. *Memory & Cognition*, *21*(2), 176–183.

Martin, R. C., & Allen, C. M. (2008). A disorder of executive function and its role in language processing. *Seminars in speech and language 29*(3), 201–210.

Martin, R. C., & Feher, E. (1990). The consequences of reduced memory span for the comprehension of semantic versus syntactic information. *Brain and Language, 38*(1), 1–20.

Martin, R. C., & He, T. (2004). Semantic short-term memory and its role in sentence processing: a replication. *Brain and Language, 89*(1), 76–82.

Martin, R. C., & Lesch, M. (1996). Associations and disassociations between language processing and list recall: implications for models of short-term memory. In S. Gathercole (Ed.), *Models of short-term memory* (pp. 149–178). Hove, UK: Erlbaum.

Martin, R. C., & Romani, C. (1994). Verbal working memory and sentence comprehension: a multiple-components view. *Neuropsychology, 8*, 506–523.

Martin, R. C., Shelton, J. R., & Yaffe, L. S. (1994). Language processing and working memory: neuropsychological evidence for separate phonological and semantic capacities. *Journal of Memory and Language, 33*, 83–111.

May, C. P., Hasher, L., & Bhatt, A. (1994). Time of day affects susceptibility to misinformation in younger and older adults. Presented at the Cognitive Aging Conference, Atlanta, GA.

Mayer, J. F., & Murray, L. L. (2012). Measuring working memory deficits in aphasia. *Journal of Communication Disorders, 45*(5), 325–339.

McCandliss, B. D., Fiez, J. A., Protopapas, A., Conway, M., & McClelland, J. L. (2002). Success and failure in teaching the [r]-[l] contrast to Japanese adults: tests of a Hebbian model of plasticity and stabilization in spoken language perception. *Cognitive, Affective, and Behavioral Neuroscience, 2*(2), 89–108.

McClelland, J., Thomas, A., McCandliss, B., & Fiez, J. (1999). Understanding failures of learning: Hebbian learning, competition for representational space, and some preliminary experimental data. *Progress in Brain Research, 121*, 75–80

MacDonald, M. C., Just, M. A., & Carpenter, P. A. (1992). Working memory constraints on the processing of syntactic ambiguity. *Cognitive Psychology, 24*, 56–98.

McKissok, S., & Ward, J. (2007). Do errors matter? Errorless and errorful learning in anomic picture naming. *Neuropsychological Rehabilitation, 17*(3), 355–373.

Meizner, M., Elbert, T., Djundja, D., Taub, E., & Rockstroh, B. (2007). Extending the constraint -induced movement therapy (CIMT) approach to cognitive functions: constraint-induced aphasia therapy (CIAT) of chronic aphasia. *NeuroRehabilitation, 22*(4), 311–318.

Meizner, M., Flaisch, T., Breitenstein, C., Wienbruch, C., Elbert, T., & Rockstroh, B. (2008). Functional re-recruitment of dysfunctional brain areas predicts language recovery in chronic aphasia. *Neuroimage, 39*(4), 2038–2046.

Meinzer, M., Mohammadi, S., Kugel, H., Schiffbauer, H., Floel, A., Albers, J., ... Deppe, M. (2010). Integrity of the hippocampus and surrounding white matter is correlated with language training success in aphasia. *Neuroimage, 53*(1), 283–290.

Menke, R., Meinzer, M., Kugel, H., Deppe, M., Baumgärtner, A., Schiffbauer, H., ... Breitenstein, C. (2009). Imaging short-and long-term training success in chronic aphasia. *BMC Neuroscience, 10*(1), 118.

Miceli, G., Amitrano, A., Capasso, R., & Caramazza, A. (1996). The treatment of anomia resulting from output lexical damage: analysis of two cases. *Brain and Language, 52*, 150–174.

Middletown, F. A., & Strick, P. L. (2000). Basal ganglia output and cognition: evidence from anatomical, behavior, and clinical studies. *Brain and Cognition, 42,* 183–200.

Milner, B. (1966). Amnesia following operation on the temporal lobes. In C.W.M. Whitty & O. L. Zangwill (Eds.), *Amnesia* (pp. 109–133). London: Butterworths.

Mishkin, M., Malamut, B., & Bachevalier, J. (1984). Memories and habits: two neural systems. In G. Lynch, J. L. McGaugh, & N. M. Weinberger (Eds.), *Neurobiology of learning and memory* (pp. 65–77). New York: Guilford.

Miyake, A., Carpenter, P., & Just, M. (1994). A capacity approach to syntactic comprehension disorders: making normal adults perform like aphasic patients. *Cognitive Neuropsychology, 11,* 671–717.

Miyake, A., Carpenter, P. A., & Just, M. A. (1994). A capacity approach to syntactic comprehension disorder: making normal adults perform like aphasic patients. *Cognitive Neuropsychology, 12,* 651–679.

Miyake, A., Friedman, N. P., Emerson, M.J., Witzki, A. H., Howerter, A., & Wager, T. D. (2000). The unity and diversity of executive functions and their contributions to complex "frontal lobe" tasks: a latent variable analysis. *Cognitive Psychology, 41,* 49–100.

Moore, A. B., Li, Z., Tyner, C. E., Hu, X., & Crosson, B. (2013). Bilateral basal ganglia activity in verbal working memory. *Brain and Language, 125,* 316–323.

Morris, J., Franklin, S., Ellis, A. W., Turner, J. E., & Bailey, P. J. (1996). Remediating a speech perception deficit in an aphasic patient. *Aphasiology, 10,* 137–158.

Murray, L. L., Keeton, R. J., & Karcher, L. (2006). Treating attention in mild aphasia: evaluation of attention process training-II. *Journal of Communication Disorders, 39*(1), 37–61.

Murray, L. L., Ramage, A. E., & Hopper, T. (2001). Memory impairments in adults with neurogenic communication disorders. *Seminars in Speech and Language, 22*(2), 127–136.

Murray. L. L., Ramage, M. S., & Hopper, T. (2001). Memory impairments in adults with neurogenic communication disorders. *Seminars in Speech and Language, 22*(1), 127–136.

Naeser, M. A., Martin, P. I., Nicholas, M., Baker, E. H., Seekins, H., Helm-Estabrooks, N., … Pascual-Leone, A. (2005). Improved naming after TMS treatments in a chronic, global aphasia patient: case report. *Neurocase, 11*(3), 183–193.

Newman, S., & Just, M. A. (2005). The neural bases of intelligence: a perspective based on functional neuroimaging. In R. J. Sternberg & J. Pretz (Eds.), *Cognition and intelligence: identifying the mechanisms of the mind* (pp. 88–103). New York: Cambridge University Press.

Newman, S. D., Malaia, E., Seo, R., & Cheng, H. (2013). The effect of individual differences in working memory capacity on sentence comprehension: an fMRI study. *Brain Topography, 26*(3), 458–467.

Nickels, N. (2002). Therapy for naming disorders: revisiting, revising and reviewing. *Aphasiology, 16,* 935–979.

Norman, D., & Shallice, T. (1980). *Attention to action: willed and automatic control of behaviour* (CHIP report 99). San Diego: University of California.

Norman, D. A., & Shallice, T. (1986). Attention to action: willed and automatic control of behaviour. In R. J. Davidson, G. E. Schwartz & D. Shapiro (Eds.), *Consciousness and self regulation: advances in research* (Vol. IV, pp. 1–18). New York: Plenum.

Opitz, B., & Friederici, A. D. (2003). Interactions of the hippocampal system and the prefrontal cortex in learning language-like rules. *NeuroImage, 19*(4), 1730–1737.

Ostergaard, A. L., & Meudell, P. R. (1984). Immediate memory span, recognition memory for subspan series of words, and serial position effects in recognition memory for supraspan series of verbal and nonverbal items in Broca's and Wernicke's aphasia. *Brain and Language, 22*(1), 1–13.

Packard, M. G., & Knowlton, B. J. (2002). Learning and memory functions of the basal ganglia. *Annual Review of Neuroscience, 25*(1), 563–593.

Papagno, C., Bricolo, E., Mussi, D., Daini, R., & Cecchetto, C. (2012). (Eye) tracking short-term memory over time. *Aphasiology, 26*(3–4), 536–555.

Papagno, C., Cecchetto, C., Reati, F., & Bello, L. (2007). Processing of syntactically complex sentences relies on verbal short-term memory: evidence from a short term memory patient. *Cognitive Neuropsychology, 24*(3), 292–311.

Paulesu, E., Frith, C. D., & Frackowiak, R. S. (1993). The neural correlates of the verbal component of working memory. *Nature, 362*(6418), 342–345.

Perfetti, C. A., & McCutchen, D. (1982). Speech processes in reading. In N. Lass (Ed.), *Speech and language: advances in basic research and practice* (pp. 237–269). New York: Academic Press.

Peterson, L. R. & Peterson, M. J. (1959). Short-term retention of individual items. *Journal of Experimental Psychology, 58*, 193–198.

Pilsbury, R. C., & Sylvester, A. (1940). Retroactive and proactive inhibition in immediate memory. *Journal of Experimental Psychology, 27*, 532–545.

Poldrack, R. A., & Packard, M. G. (2003). Competition between memory systems: converging evidence from animal and human studies. *Neuropsychologia, 41*, 245–251.

Poldrack, R. A., Prabakharan, V., Seger, C., & Gabrieli, J.D.E. (1999). Striatal activation during cognitive skill learning. *Neuropsychology, 13*, 564–574.

Poldrack, R. A., Wagner, A. D., Prull, M. W., Desmond, J. E., Glover, G. H., & Gabrieli, J. D. (1999). Functional specialization for semantic and phonological processing in the left inferior prefrontal cortex. *Neuroimage, 10*(1), 15–35.

Postle, B. R., D'Esposito, M., & Corkin, S. (2005). Effects of verbal and nonverbal interference on spatial and object visual working memory. *Memory & Cognition, 33*(2), 203–212.

Potagas, C., Kasselimis, D., & Evdokimidis, I. (2011). Short-term and working memory impairments in aphasia. *Neuropsychologia, 49*(10), 2874–2878.

Prat, C. S., Keller, T. A., & Just, M. A. (2007). Individual differences in sentence comprehension: a functional magnetic resonance imaging investigation of syntactic and lexical processing demands. *Journal of Cognitive Neuroscience, 19*(12), 1950–1963.

Pring, T., Hamilton, A., Harwood, A., & Macbride, L. (1993). Generalization of naming after picture/word matching tasks: only items appearing in therapy benefit. *Aphasiology, 7*(4), 383–394.

Pring, T., White-Thomson, M., Pound, C., Marshall, J., & Davis, A. (1990). Picture/word matching tasks and word retrieval: some follow-up data and second thoughts. *Aphasiology, 4*(5), 479–483.

Reilly, J. (2008). Semantic memory and language processing in aphasia and dementia. *Seminars in Speech and Language, 29*, 3–4.

Renvall, K., Laine, M., Laakso, M., & Martin, N. (2003). Anomia treatment with contextual priming: a case study. *Aphasiology, 17*(3), 305–328.

Risse, G. L., Rubens, A. B., & Jordan, L. S. (1984). Disturbances of long-term memory in aphasic patients a comparison of anterior and posterior lesions. *Brain, 107*(2), 605–617.

Rochon, E., & Saffran, E. M. (1995). A semantic contribution to sentence comprehension impairments in Alzheimer's disease. Poster presented at the Academy of Aphasia, San Diego.

Rochon, E., Leonard, C., Burianova, H., Laird, L., Soros, P., Graham, S., & Grady, C. (2010). Neural changes after phonological treatment for anomia: an fMRI study. *Brain and rLanguage, 114*(2), 164–179.

Roediger, H. L. III, & Craik, F. (Eds.). (2014). *Varieties of memory and consciousness: essays in honour of Endel Tulving.* Psychology Press.

Rönnberg, J., Larsson, C., Fogelsjöö, A., Nilsson, L. G., Lindberg, M., & Ängquist, K. A. (1996). Memory dysfunction in mild aphasics. *Scandinavian Journal of Psychology, 37*(1), 46–61.

Ruchkin, D. S., Grafman, J., Cameron, K., & Berndt, R. S. (2003). Working memory retention systems: a state of activated long-term memory. *The Behavioral and Brain Sciences, 26*(6), 709–728.

Saffran, E. M., & Marin, O. S. (1975). Immediate memory for word lists and sentences in a patient with deficient auditory short-term memory. *Brain and Language, 2*, 420–433.

Salis, C. (2012). Short-term memory treatment: patterns of learning and generalisation to sentence comprehension in a person with aphasia. *Neuropsychological Rehabilitation, 22*(3), 428–448.

Salthouse, T. A. (1996). The processing-speed theory of adult age differences in cognition. *Psychological Review, 103*(3), 403–428.

Schacter, D. L., & Tulving, E. (1994). *Memory systems.* Cambridge, MA: MIT Press.

Schuchard, J., & Thompson, C. (2014). Implicit and explicit learning in individuals with agrammatic aphasia. *Journal of Psycholinguistic Research, 43*(3), 209–224.

Schuchard, J., & Thompson, C. K. (2012). Implicit and explicit learning in aphasia. Presented at the 42nd Clinical Aphasiology Conference; Lake Tahoe, CA.

Schwartz, M. F., Saffran, E. M., Bloch, D. E., & Dell, G. S. (1994). Disordered speech production in aphasic and normal speakers. *Brain and Language, 47*(1), 52–88.

Schwartz, M. F., Faseyitan, O., Kim, J., & Coslett, H. B. (2012). The dorsal stream contribution to phonological retrieval in object naming. *Brain, 135*(Pt 12), 3799–3814.

Schwartz, M. F., Kimberg, D. Y., Walker G. M., Faseyitan, O., Brecher, A., Dell, G. S., & Coslett, H. B. (2009). Anterior temporal involvement in semantic word retrieval: voxel-based lesion-symptom mapping evidence from aphasia. *Brain, 132*(Pt 12), 3411–3427.

Schweickert, R., & Boruff, B. (1986). Short-term capacity: magic number or magic spell? *Journal of Experimental Psychology: Learning, Memory, and Cognition, 12*(3), 419–425.

Seniów, J., Litwin, M., & Leśniak, M. (2009). The relationship between non-linguistic cognitive deficits and language recovery in patients with aphasia. *Journal of the Neurological Sciences, 283*(1–2), 91–94.

Shallice, T. (1988). *From neuropsychology to mental structure.* Cambridge, UK: Cambridge University Press.

Shallice, T., & Warrington, E. K. (1970). Independent functioning of verbal memory stores: a neuropsychological study. *Quarterly Journal of Experimental Psychology, 22*, 261–273.

Smith, E. E., & Jonides, J. (1998). Neuroimaging analyses of human working memory. *Proceedings of the National Academy of Sciences, 95*(20), 12061–12068.

Squire, L. R. (2004). Memory systems of the brain: a brief history and current perspective. *Neurobiology of Learning and Memory, 82*, 171–177.

Squire, L. R. (2007). Rapid consolidation. *Science, 316*(5821), 57.

Squire, L.R., & Knowlton, B. J. (2000). The medial and temporal lobe, the hippocampus, and the memory systems of the brain. In M. S. Gazzaniga (Ed.), *The new cognitive neurosciences* (2nd ed., pp. 765–779). Cambridge, MA: MIT Press.

Squire, L. R., & Wixted, J. T. (2011). The cognitive neuroscience of human memory since H. M. *Annual Review of Neuroscience, 34*, 259–288.

Squire, L. R., & Zola, S. M. (1996). Structure and function of declarative and nondeclarative memory systems. *Proceedings of the National Academy of Sciences of the Unites States of America, 93*, 13515–13522.

Stout, J. C., & Murray, L. L. (2001). Assessment of memory in neurogenic communication disorders. *Seminars in Speech and Language, 22*(2), 139–148.

Sung, J. E., McNeil, M. R., Pratt, S. R., Dickey, M. W., Hula, W. D., Szuminsky, N. J., & Doyle, P. J. (2009). Verbal working memory and its relationship to sentence-level reading and listening comprehension in persons with aphasia. *Aphasiology, 23*(7–8), 1040–1052.

Suzuki, W. A., & Eichenbaum, H. (2000). The neurophysiology of memory. *Annals of the New York Academy of Sciences, 911*, 175–191.

Thompson, C., Shapiro, L., Kiran, S., & Sobecks, J. (2003). The role of syntactic complexity in treatment of sentence deficits in agrammatic aphasia: the complexity account of treatment efficacy (CATE). *Journal of Speech, Language and Hearing Research, 46*, 591–607.

Thompson-Schill, S. L., D'Esposito, M., Aguirre, G. K., & Farah, M. J. (1997). Role of left inferior prefrontal cortex in retrieval of semantic knowledge: a reevaluation. *Proceedings of the National Academy of Sciences of the United States of America, 94*(26), 14792–14797.

Tompkins, C. A., Bloise, C. G., Timko, M. L., & Baumgaertner, A. (1994). Working memory and inference revision in braindamaged and normally aging adults. *Journal of Speech, Language, and Hearing Research, 37*(4), 896–912.

Tuomiranta, L., Grönholm-Nyman, P., Kohen, F., Rautakoski, P., Laine, M., & Martin, N. (2011). Learning and maintaining new vocabulary in persons with aphasia: two controlled case studies. *Aphasiology, 25*(9), 1030–1052.

Tuomiranta, L., Rautakoski, P., Rinne, J. O., Martin, N., & Laine, M. (2012). Long-term maintenance of novel vocabulary in persons with chronic aphasia. *Aphasiology, 26*(8), 1053–1073.

Turksta, L. S. (2001). Treating memory problems in adults with neurogenic communication disorders. *Seminars in Speech and Language, 22(2),* 147–155.

Ullman, M. T. (2004). Contributions of memory circuits to language: the declarative/procedural model. *Cognition, 92*(1–2), 231–270.

Ungerleider, L. G. & Mishkin, M. (1982). Two cortical visual systems. In D. J. Ingle, M. A. Goodale, & R.J.W. Mansfield (Eds.), *Analysis of visual behavior* (pp. 549–86).Cambridge, MA: MIT Press.

Vallar, G., & Baddeley, A. D. (1984). Fractionation of working memory: neuropsychological evidence for a phonological short-term store. *Journal of Verbal Learning and Verbal Behavior, 23*(2), 151–161.

Vallar, G., & Papagno, C. (2002). Neuropsychological impairments of verbal short-term memory. In A. D. Baddeley, M. D. Kopelman, & B. A. Wilson (Eds.), *The handbook of memory disorders* (2nd ed; pp. 249–270). Chinchester, UK: Wiley.

Vallar, G., Corno, M., & Basso, A. (1992). Auditory and visual verbal short-term memory in aphasia. *Cortex, 28*(3), 383–389.

Vallila-Rohter, S. M., & Kiran, S. (2013). Non-linguistic learning and aphasia: evidence from a paired associate and feedback-based task. *Neuropsychologia, 51*(1), 79–90.

Vitali, P., Abutalebi, J., Tettamanti, M., Danna, M., Ansaldo, A., Perani, D., … Cappa, S. F. (2007). Training-induced brain remapping in chronic aphasia: a pilot study. *Neurorehabilitation and Neural Repair, 21*(2), 152–160.

Wagner, A. D., Schacter, D. L., Rotte, M., Koutstaal, W., Maril, A., Dale, A. M., … Buckner, R. L. (1998). Building memories: remembering and forgetting of verbal experiences as predicted by brain activity. *Science, 281*(5380), 1188–1191.

Walker, G. M., Schwartz, M. F., Kimberg, D. Y., Faseyitan, O., Brecher, A., Dell, G. S., & Coslett, H. (2011). Support for anterior temporal involvement in semantic error production in aphasia: new evidence from VLSM. *Brain and Language, 117*(3), 110–122.

Wambaugh, J., Cameron, R., Kalinyak-Fliszar, M., Nessler, C., & Wright, S. (2004). Retrieval of action names in aphasia: effects of two cueing treatments. *Aphasiology, 18*(11), 979–1004.

Warrington, E. K., Logue, V., & Pratt, R.T.C. (1971). The anatomical localisation of selective impairment of auditory short-term memory. *Neuropsychologia, 9*, 377–387.

Waters, G., & Caplan, D., (1996). Processing resource capacity and the comprehension of garden path sentences. *Memory & Cognition, 24*, 342–355.

Waters, G., & Caplan, D. (2005). The relationship between age, processing speed, working memory capacity, and language comprehension. *Memory, 13*(3–4), 403–413.

Waters, G. S., Caplan, D., & Hildebrandt, N. (1991). On the structure of verbal short-term memory and its functional role in sentence comprehension: evidence from neuropsychology. *Cognitive Neuropsychology, 8*(2), 81–126.

Wechsler, D. (1987). *WMS-R: Wechsler memory scale-revised: manual*. San Antonio, TX: Psychological Corporation.

Wechsler, D. (2003). *WISC-IV: administration and scoring manual*. San Antonio, TX: Psychological Corporation.

Ween, J. E., Verfaellie, M., & Alexander, M. P. (1996). Verbal memory function in mild aphasia. *Neurology, 47*(3), 795–801.

White, N. M. (1997). Mnemonic functions of the basal ganglia. *Current Opinion in Neurobiology, 7*, 164–169.

Wig, G. S., Schlaggar, B. L., & Petersen, S. E. (2011). Concepts and principles in the analysis of brain networks. *Annals of the New York Academy of the Sciences, 1224*, 126–146.

Willis, C. S., & Gathercole, S. E. (2001). Phonological short-term memory contributions to sentence processing in young children. *Memory, 9*, 349–363.

Winans, R., Hula, W., Friedman, B., Sperl, A., Swoyer, B., & Doyle, P. (2012). Treatment of working memory in a patient with moderate aphasia. Presented at the 42nd Clinical Aphasiology Conference; Lake Tahoe, CA.

Wise, S. P., Murray, E. A., & Gerfen, C. R. (1996). The frontal cortex-basal ganglia system in primates. *Critical Reviews in Neurobiology, 10*(3–4), 317–356.

Wisenburn, B, & Mahoney, K. (2009). A meta-analysis of word-finding treatments for aphasia. *Aphasiology, 23,* 1338–1352.

Wisenburn, B. (2010). An objective review of word finding treatments for aphasia. *Pennsylvania Speech-Language Hearing Association Journal, 1,* 4–18.

Wright, H. H., & Fergadiotis, G. (2012). Conceptualising and measuring working memory and its relationship to aphasia. *Aphasiology, 26*(3–4), 258–278.

Wright, H. H., Downey, R. A., Gravier, M., Love, T., & Shapiro, L. P. (2007). Processing distinct linguistic information types in working memory in aphasia. *Aphasiology, 21*(6–8), 802–813.

Yarkoni, T., Speer, N. K., & Jacks, J. M. (2008). Neural substrates of narrative comprehension and memory. *Neuroimage, 41*(4), 1408–1425.

Yeo, B. T., Krienen, F. M., Sepulere, J., Sabuneu, M. R., Lashkari, D., Hollinshead, M., ... Buckner, R. L. (2011). The organization of the human cerebral cortex estimated by intrinsic functional connectivity. *Journal of Neurophysiology, 106*(3), 1125–1165.

Zhang, S., & Perfetti, C. A. (1993). The tongue-twister effect in reading Chinese. *Journal of Experimental Psychology: Learning, Memory, and Cognition, 19*(5), 1082–1093.

6

The Role of Emotion in Recovery from Aphasia

Introduction

This chapter reviews our current understanding of the extent to which emotional changes in persons with aphasia following stroke participate in the molding of behavioral and neural changes associated with recovery of language functions. Although the emotional well-being of persons with aphasia has long been recognized as a central factor affecting their road to rehabilitative success (Code, 2003, 2010), the underlying mechanisms by which emotion interacts with language systems in the aphasic brain are still poorly understood (Cahana-Amitay et al., 2011). This gap persists despite early work clearly identifying stroke-induced negative changes in the emotional status of persons with aphasia. Goldstein (1942, 1948, 1959) and Luria (1970), for example, argued that aphasic persons "avoid the frustration, humiliation, anxiety, and catastrophic reaction that may be otherwise induced by the prospect of speaking defectively" (Sapir & Aronson, 1990, p. 504).

The studies we review here focus on two emotional states in aphasia: *depression* and *anxiety-induced stress dysregulation*. Our analysis is built upon three key findings. First, changes emotional states are common after stroke and frequently manifest as depression or anxiety (e.g., Chemerinski & Levine, 2006; Cohen, 1998; Robinson, 2006). Second, symptoms of depression and anxiety are commonly observed among persons with aphasia (e.g., Cahana-Amitay et al., 2011; Carota et al., 2001; Cohen, 1998; Gainotti, 1972, 1997; Laska et al., 2007; Sapir & Aronson, 1990; Small & Llano, 2009; Starkstein,

Fedoroff, Price, & Robinson, 1993). Third, nonpathological symptoms of depression and anxiety can negatively affect task performance even in healthy adults and hence likely play an important role in determining treatment outcomes among persons with emotional difficulties (Crocker et al., 2013).

Because there are many ways to interpret the term *emotion*, we first provide an operational definition for this concept (following Crocker et al., 2013) to clarify the sense in which we use this term throughout the chapter. We then briefly review ways in which depression and anxiety among nonaphasic persons can affect cognitive function (e.g., Bar Haim et al., 2007; Cisler et al., 2009; Gotlib & Joormann, 2010; McNally, 1998; Sass et al., 2010) and describe the neural bases of these effects (e.g., Levin et al., 2007; Miller, 2010). By way of example, we focus on emotion-based neural changes associated with executive functions (e.g., Levin et al., 2007; Snyder, 2013), as evidence relating such effects specifically to language performance is limited.

We then turn to a discussion of the occurrence of depression and anxiety-induced stress dysregulation in stroke-based aphasia (Cahana-Amitay et al., 2011; Carota et al., 2001; Cohen, 1998; Gainotti, 1972, 1997; Laska et al., 2007; Small & Llano, 2009; Sapir & Aronson, 1990; Starkstein, Fedoroff, Price, & Robinson, 1993). To the extent allowed by available evidence, we discuss their psychosocial aspects and neural mechanisms and their impact on aphasia recovery and rehabilitation outcome. We note findings from behavioral and biological interventions, especially aphasia pharmacotherapy studies (recently reviewed in Cahana-Amitay, Albert, & Oveis, 2014). Such studies offer a different window into the neural mechanisms associated with aphasia recovery from that provided by neuroimaging studies—a "neurochemical" view. Our focus on this "neurochemistry" prism derives in part from the relative lack of neuroimaging studies examining the effects of these emotional states on language functions in persons with aphasia. However, it also reflects the importance we attribute to systems of neurotransmission in the reshaping of the aphasic brain following stroke. Indeed, some have argued that neuropsychiatric problems following stroke implicate secondary neural damage (cell death, neural loss, and axonal degeneration) affecting brain structures beyond those associated with the initial locus of injury (e.g., Chen et al., 2014). As pointed out in Chapter 2, this perspective on language functions is a highly underdeveloped domain of inquiry, but it provides fertile ground for new ways of understanding of how language is created in the impaired and intact brain.

Emotion: Definition and Its Effects on Cognition

Before diving into how altered emotions in aphasia might affect recovery of language functions, we must first clarify the sense in which we use the term *emotion*. It can refer to one's general emotional state (e.g., feeling sad), to a situation-specific response (e.g., feeling anxious in response to a specific word), or to reactions to the content of the experimental stimuli (e.g., word lists of items with negative connotations). Some would argue, and rightly so, that the borders distinguishing these notions are somewhat blurry, especially if we consider the possibility that the neural systems dedicated for processing emotion (emotional state) and emotional language (content of the stimulus) may overlap and mutually affect one another (Niedenthal, 2007).

Indeed, the processing of words strongly connoting negative emotions has been shown to activate neural structures within networks subserving emotions (e.g., Citron, 2012) and to be affected by one's emotional state (e.g., Niedenthal, 2007). Healthy adults, for example, take longer to process sentences with unpleasant emotional content when frowning than they do to process pleasant sentences while smiling (Havas et al., 2007). The specific neural networks associated with such information processing have been argued to be primarily in the right hemisphere, although some findings indicate involvement of left-lateralized and/or bilateral neural structures (e.g., Atchley et al., 2003; Borod et al., 2002; Cato et al., 2004; Crosson et al., 1999; 2002; Demaree et al., 2005; Maddock & Buonocore, 1997; Maddock et al., 2003).

Such neural organization is consistent with reports concerning preserved abilities among persons with aphasia for processing emotional words (Kotz & Friederici, 2003; Landis, 2006; Landis et al., 1983; Ofek & Pratt, 2005; Ofek et al., 2013; Ortigue et al., 2004). For example, in an event-related potential study comparing cortical responses to emotional and neutral words, Ofek et al. (2013) demonstrated that while persons with aphasia showed some disrupted responses (smaller N1 and delayed P2 and P3 amplitudes), they were able to differentiate both word classes, just as their neurologically intact peers (as measured by larger P3 amplitudes for emotional words in both participant groups).

Cortical responses to negative words in both healthy and brain-damaged persons have been thought to reflect the activation of arousal and attention in response to threat (e.g., Kousta et al., 2009), which, according to some researchers, implicates greater processing resources (Holt et al., 2009). The neural basis of such activation encompasses structures in the limbic system, such as corticoamygdaloid circuits (Kissler et al., 2007; Ofek & Pratt, 2005) and rostral frontal and retrosplenial cortices (Cato & Crosson, 2006; Cato et al., 2004; Crosson et al., 1999, 2002). Note that Cato and Crosson (2006) found that rostral frontal and retrosplenial cortices were differentially activated in response to emotionally strong words depending on whether the words were incoming or outgoing; thus they proposed a finer-grained system for processing the emotional content of a word. According to this system, the emotional content of a word is considered a semantic feature that determines the word's emotional saliency. This saliency guides (1) the attention system in selection of task-relevant sensory input for further information processing, and (2) the intention system in the choice of action output for future execution.

In the remainder of the chapter, we will restrict our use of the term emotion to one's general emotional state rather than to the emotional content of the stimulus and focus on how altered emotional states in aphasia, manifested as depression and stress dysregulation, affect language performance. We adopt Crocker et al.'s (2013) definition, which views emotion as a multiprocess system that has specific physiological and behavioral manifestations (Kozak & Miller, 1982; Lang, 1968; Roseman, 2008) whose aim is to optimize adaptation to a person's successful/failed attempts to meet specific needs, goals, and concerns (Berenbaum et al., 2003). Specifically, we view emotion as a feeling state resulting from a comparison between expected and actual progress towards a given goal, where a mismatch leads to a change in emotion (a change in one's feeling state), which then affects future motivations *en route* to attaining that goal. These motivations then shape future expectations, which reinforce or alter subsequent emotions. This proposal indicates that emotion and motivation are interlinked but not completely overlapping (e.g., Chiew & Braver, 2011).

From a functional neuroanatomical perspective, the integration of emotional and cognitive information in the healthy brain has often been associated with brain structures in the left inferior frontal cortex and their interconnections with the limbic system (e.g., Denkova, Dolcos, & Dolcos, 2013; Dolcos et al., 2006; Ozawa, Matsuda, & Hiraki, 2014). These brain structures support many language and cognitive processes, as demonstrated throughout this book, and also appear to subserve emotional processing and emotional regulation (e.g., Damasio, 1998; Davidson, 2004; Lindquist et al., 2012; Ochsner et al., 2012; Phan et al., 2002; Wager et al., 2008). Denkova et al. (2013) specifically point out that operations linked to these brain structures—including language processing (Hagoort, 2005; Poldrack et al., 1999), controlled retrieval (Badre & Wagner, 2007), competition resolution (Thompson-Schill et al., 1999), information integration (Fuster, 2002), and response inhibition (Aron et al., 2004)—likely interact with the processing of internally triggered emotions underlying certain disorders of emotion.

Indeed, impaired emotional states such as depression and anxiety have been shown to disrupt cognitive function and result in information processing biases with a reduced ability to disengage from negative information and/or deficient cognitive performance (Crocker et al., 2013). These may include hyperfocus on processing negative materials in depression (Gotlib & Joormann, 2010; Levin et al., 2007) or heightened preference to processing threat information in anxiety (Bar Haim et al., 2007; Cisler et al., 2009; McNally, 1998; Sass et al., 2010). Some have associated these patterns with impaired attention control at different stages of information processing whereby anxiety affects orienting to stimuli and depression affects elaborative processing (e.g., Williams et al., 1997).

In recent years, important neural correlates of these emotion-cognition links have been identified (e.g., Chiew & Braver, 2011; Dolcos et al., 2011; Gray, 2004; Levin et al., 2007; Miller, 2010; Ochsner et al., 2012; Pessoa, 2008, 2009; Phelps, 2006). These include neural networks implicating the prefrontal cortex, cingulate, amygdala, striatum, hypothalamus, hippocampus, insula, and parietal structures (e.g., Miller et al., 2013). These findings are being used to design treatment regimens that ameliorate adverse effects of negative emotions on cognitive performance (e.g., Carrig et al., 2009; Fu et al., 2012; Miller et al., 2007). The assumption underlying these studies is that neural systems are flexible by nature and can be modified in response to input, with measurable metabolic, physiological, cellular, or structural brain changes (Crocker et al., 2013). This approach is completely aligned with our view of neural multifunctionality of language functions in the course of aphasia recovery.

However, a person need not be diagnosed with "psychopathology" in order to exhibit the effects of altered emotional state on cognitive performance. Some have found, for example, that poor attentional control, negative affect, and reduced parasympathetic tone as measured by heart-period variability predicted high trait anxiety in healthy college students (Healy, 2010). A relationship between prefrontal neural function and cognitive performance has been reported in studies of healthy adults with no emotional deficits in whom changes in affect were induced, for example, through threatening and nonthreatening situations (e.g., Thayer et al., 2009; Williams et al., 2009). In these studies, individual differences in the regulation of biomarkers of the autonomic nervous system (ANS)—such as heart-rate variability—were linked to performance on tasks of executive functions and prefrontal brain activation, where poorer physiological regulation was associated with greater decrements in cognitive and neural functioning (e.g., Gianaros et al., 2004; Lane et al., 2008; 2009; Nugent et al., 2007, 2008). Based on these findings, Thayer and colleagues (2009) proposed a neurovisceral model in which heart-rate variability serves as an index to the integrity of the neural networks—consisting of the central autonomic network and the rostral limbic system— that subserve goal-directed behaviors. Comparable claims have been made in relation to other ANS measures, such as pupillometric measures (e.g., Granholm & Steinhauer, 2004). This neurovisceral system is illustrated in Figure 6.1.

EMOTION-LANGUAGE/COGNITION-BRAIN INTERLINKS

Over the past decade, evidence for emotion-cognition-brain interdependencies has begun accumulating, promoting our understanding of how depression and anxiety affect brain structure and cognitive function (Crocker et al., 2013). Behavioral and neuroimaging studies of the effects of depression and anxiety on speech/language performance among nonaphasic persons are limited. There is some indirect evidence, however, that depressed persons have reduced performance on verbally mediated tasks assessing verbal fluency, verbal working memory, and planning (e.g., Levin et al., 2007; Snyder, 2013; Yee, 1995). To the best of our knowledge, neuroimaging correlates of these effects have not been explored.

Effects of anxiety on linguistic functioning, in contrast, have been studied extensively among nonaphasic persons, especially stutterers (e.g., Alm, 2004; Caruso et al., 1994; Doruk et al., 2008; Lundgren, Helm-Estabrooks, & Klein, 2010; Ozdemir et al., 2010; Palasik et al., 2009; Peters & Hulstijn, 1984; Weber & Smith, 1990), persons with psychogenic voice and speech disorders (Aronson, 1985; Cox, 1986; Sapir & Aronson, 1990), second-language learners (e.g., Duxbury & Tsai, 2010; Horwitz, 2001; MacIntyre,

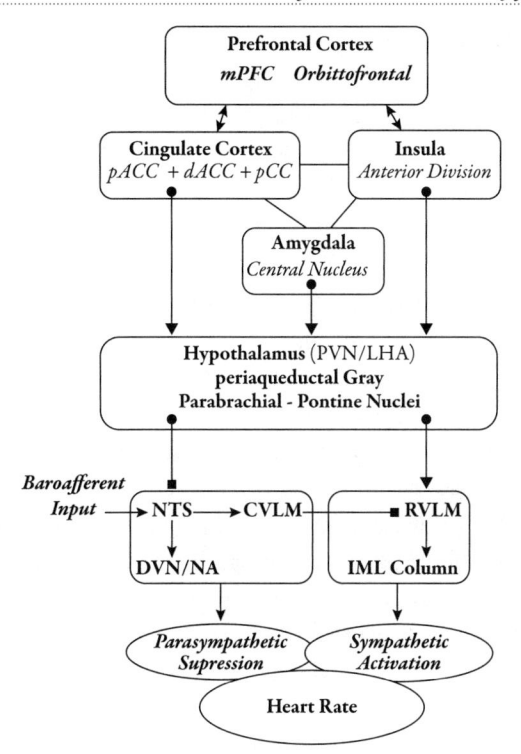

6. The Role of Emotion in Recovery from Aphasia 151

FIGURE 6.1 Neurovisceral model underlying goal-directed behavior. A composite schematic diagram showing the pathways by which the prefrontal cortex might influence control of heart rate. The prefrontal, cingulate, and insula cortices form an interconnected network with bidirectional communication with the amygdala. The amygdala is under tonic inhibitory control via prefrontal vagal pathways to intercalated cells in the amygdala. The activation of the central nucleus of the amygdala (CeA) inhibits the nucleus of the solitary tract (NTS: solid square), which in turn inhibits inhibitory caudal ventrolateral medullary (CVLM) inputs to the rostral ventrolateral medullary (RVLM) sympathoexcitatory neurons (solid square) and simultaneously inhibits vagal motor neurons in the nucleus ambiguus (NA) and the dorsal vagal motor nucleus (DVN). In addition, the CeA can directly activate the sympathoexcitatory neurons in the RVLM. The net effect of pharmacological blockade of the prefrontal cortex would be a disinhibition of the CeA, leading to disinhibition of medullary cardioacceleratory circuits and an increase in heart rate

Source: From Thayer, J. F., Hansen, A. L., Saus-Rose, E., & Johnson, B. H. (2009). Heart rate variability, prefrontal neural function, and cognitive performance: the neurovisceral integration perspective on self-regulation, adaptation, and health. *Annals of Behavioral Medicine, 37*(2), 141–153. Reprinted by permission from Springer [Annals of Behavioral Medicine], copyright 2009.

1995, 2002; MacIntyre & Gardner, 1994; Scovel, 1978), and persons faced with the task of public speaking (e.g., Behnke & Carlile, 1971; Bodie, 2010; Bosch et al., 2009; Carillo et al., 2001; Davidson, Marshall, Tomarken, & Henrique, 2000; Lam et al., 2009). Although the behavioral and neural mechanisms underlying these anxiety effects may be somewhat different for each of these groups, they seem to share two features. First, at a behavioral level, these people typically demonstrate limited command of the full range of speech/language systems available to native speakers and are therefore at increased risk of a communication breakdown. Second, at a psychophysiological level, they show changes in levels of biomarkers of stress reactivity, implicating the hypothalamo-pituitary-adrenal (HPA) axis, such as salivary cortisol, and autonomic nervous (ANS) system, such as heart rate, when asked to perform a language task (but see Dimberg & Thunberg, 2007; Gramer & Saria, 2007; Stone et al., 2001). For example, preparation for public speaking among healthy adults induces heightened electrodermal and cardiovascular responses during the anticipation of speech period (Kreibig, 2010). The exploration of these effects among persons with aphasia has begun receiving increased attention over the past 5 years and is discussed later in the chapter.

Given the paucity of evidence that speaks to *emotion-language-brain* interdependencies, we turn to studies examining the neural correlates of depression or anxiety-related effects on executive functions (Levin et al., 2007; Snyder, 2013), which, as pointed out in Chapter 3, closely interact with language and share some of the same neural substrates. In some of these studies, adverse effects of depression and anxiety on executive functions have been attributed to the presence of the psychopathology (e.g., Eysenck et al., 2007; Williams et al., 2000). In others, impaired cognitive control has been found to persist even after symptoms of the psychopathology improved (e.g., Austin et al., 2001), suggesting that executive functions may play a role in both onset and possible relapse of such emotional deficits (Crocker et al., 2013).

Depressed persons often show problems with inhibitory control of negative information, with expressed difficulty disengaging from it during task performance (e.g., Goeleven et al., 2006). They may, however, also show general impairment, intentionally ignoring distracting information regardless of its emotional valence (Gotlib & Joorman, 2010; Snyder, 2013). These problems have been linked to reductions in working memory of task-irrelevant information as well as poor attention switching to meet task goals (e.g., Banich et al., 2009; Joorman, 2010; Joorman & Gotlib, 2008).

Similarly, individuals with anxiety have been shown to have set-shifting problems (e.g., Airaksinen et al., 2005; Johnson, 2009) and working memory deficits (e.g., Derakshan & Eysenck, 1998; Eysenck et al., 2005; MacLeod & Donnelan, 1993), especially in highly stressful situations (Eysenck et al., 2007). These findings have led to the development of an anxiety-executive function model, termed the *attentional control model*, according to which anxiety leads to worry-based deficits in executive functions, thus adversely affecting central attention processes with impaired inhibition and shifting abilities (Eysenck et al., 2007). The deficit results from an imbalance between top-down and bottom-up attention processes, where impaired top-down control gives rise to hyperfocus on bottom-up stimulus-based processing (Derakshan & Eysenck, 2009; Eysenck & Derakshan, 2011). We return to this idea later in the chapter, when we discuss a comparable proposal put forth by Cahana-Amitay et al. (2011), who developed a worry-based framework for aphasic language performance, termed "linguistic anxiety."

The neural underpinnings of these depression- and anxiety-related impairments of executive functions have been associated with hypoactivation of the dorsolateral prefrontal cortex (DLPFC) as well as the dorsal and rostral anterior cingulate cortex (d- and r-ACC) (e.g., Bishop, 2007; 2008; Engels et al., 2007; 2010; Herrington et al., 2010; Silton et al., 2011). In addition, persons with comorbid depression and anxious arousal, when performing tasks evaluating executive functions, have been shown to have left-lateralized decreased activation in these brain structures (Engels et al., 2010). The DLPFC and ACC networks have been associated with processes integrating emotions, executive functions, and motivation (Gray, 2004; Gray et al., 2002; Pessoa, 2008, 2009; Spielberg et al., 2012a,b). Similar findings have been reported in studies using resting-state methods, where depressed individuals were found to have changes in intrinsic connectivity in the default mode network, salience network, and central executive network (e.g., Manoliu et al., 2014).

Depression and Anxiety After Stroke

Diagnoses of depression and anxiety following stroke are typically based on clinical definitions, such as those stated in the *Diagnostic and Statistic Manual of Mental Disorders*. For example, in the fourth edition, text revision (American Psychiatric Association, 2000), the definition of poststroke depression was stated as follows: "mood disorder due to stroke with depressive features for two weeks or more, including at least four of the following depressed mood features: changed appetite/weight, disrupted sleep, decreased interest or pleasure, psychomotor agitation or retardation, poor energy, feelings of worthlessness or inappropriate guilt, concentration problems, and suicidal thoughts." For anxiety, the definition was: "state of excessive worrying present for a period of at least 6 months, accompanied by at least three of the following symptoms: restlessness, irritability, low energy, poor concentration, increased muscle tension, poor sleep."

However, clinical assessment of these emotional states in patients with stroke remains a challenge (for a recent review, see D'Aniello et al., 2014; Hayhow, Brockman, & Starkstein, 2014). In the acute stage, their onset is often missed (Bogousslavsky, 2003; Chemerinski & Levine, 2006; Paolucci, 2008; Sagen et al., 2009, 2010), and they may remain undiagnosed in the chronic stage (Åström, Adolefsson, & Asplund, 1993; De Wit et al., 2008; Clarke & Currie, 2009; Sagen et al., 2009). As a result, there is some disagreement as to how common these conditions are following stroke. For poststroke depression, figures range from 5% to 60% (Barker-Collo, 2007; Chemerinski & Levine, 2006; Code & Herrmann, 2003; De Wit et al., 2008; Fure et al., 2006; Hackett et al., 2005; House et al., 1990; Johnson et al., 2006; Kauhanen, et al., 1999; Lipsey et al., 1985; Small & Llano, 2009; Starkstein & Robinson, 1988; Townend et al., 2007), although the consensus is that about one third of stroke survivors experience depression (e.g., Fure et al., 2006; Hackett et al., 2005; Hilari et al., 2010; Shahripour & Donnan, 2014). The figures for poststroke anxiety are more consistent, ranging from 14% to 25% (Åström, 1996; Barker-Collo, 2007; Burvill et al., 1995; Leppavouri et al., 2003; Sagen et al., 2010; Shahripour & Donnan, 2014).

The debate regarding what symptoms reliably reflect poststroke depression and anxiety also plagues experimental research in exploring their effects (Chemerinski & Levine, 2006). The utility of the clinical criteria mentioned above has been questioned because of the inclusion of symptoms that are not unique to depression or anxiety—such as weight loss, poor appetite, or insomnia (Chemerinski & Levine, 2006; Herrmann & Wallesch, 1993). Additionally, certain neurological symptoms, such as altered facial expressions or changes in motor speech and prosody, could be mislabeled as depression (Code & Herrmann, 2003; Code & Muller, 1992; Stern, 1999).

Moreover, studies rarely use comparable or standardized assessment tools, scales, questionnaires, and baseline measures, challenging the generalizability of the reported findings (Code & Herrmann, 2003; Frankel, 2008; Herrmann & Wallesch, 1993; Robinson, 2006). Furthermore, statistical analyses often fail to control for variables such as personality traits or coping styles, confounding the patterns observed (Cohen, 1998; Greenop, Almeida, Hankey, van Bockxmeer, & Lautenschlager, 2009). Interestingly, a recent language intervention study exploring the relationship between the effects of mood, personality traits, and cognitive functioning on treatment-based changes in language functioning has demonstrated a unique contribution of personality differences (which the authors termed "affectivity") on treatment outcome (Votruba et al., 2013).

Nonetheless, poststroke depression and anxiety have been reported to negatively affect self-agency and personality (Mukheriee et al., 2006), motivation (Santos et al., 2006), physical and cognitive function such as logical thinking, nonverbal problem solving, verbal memory, visual memory, attention, executive functions, and psychomotor speed (Berg et al., 2001; Carota et al., 2005; Herrmann et al., 1998; Kauhanen et al., 1999; Nannaetti et al., 2005; Robinson, 2006; Sagen et al., 2010; Sharpe et al., 1994). These adverse effects have been linked to neurological, psychological, and psychosocial factors (Code & Hermann, 2003; Cohen, 1998; Gainotti, 1997; Thomas & Lincoln, 2008).

From a psychological and psychosocial perspective, poststroke depression and anxiety have been viewed as secondary outcomes of the need to adapt to life with disability (Code & Herrmann, 2003; Herrmann & Wallesch, 1993; Robinson, 2006). This adaptation involves a growing dependence on others for the performance of activities of daily living (Åström et al., 1993; Kotila et al., 1998; Neau et al., 1998; Parikh et al., 1987; Primeau, 1988; Sinyor et al., 1986). Persons who do not adapt well show increased problems engaging in social interactions and often suffer from social isolation, stigmatization, and marginalization (Code & Herrmann, 2003; Herrmann & Wallesch, 1993;Mukheriee et al., 2006), which impede and even prevent physical, cognitive, and functional recovery (Bogousslavsky, 2003; Chemerinski & Levine, 2006; Chemerinski et al., 2001; Clarke & Currie, 2009; Gusev & Bogolepova, 2009; Masskulpan et al., 2008; Neau et al., 1998; Pohjasvaara et al., 1998, 2001; Singh et al., 2000). Among some stroke survivors, these emotional states have been correlated with increased risk of mortality (Bogousslavsky, 2003; Gainotti et al., 1999; Linden et al., 2007; Morris et al., 1993; Shimoda & Robinson, 1998; Townend et al., 2007a).

From a brain perspective, some have argued that poststroke depression and anxiety are primary consequences of damage to brain structures in the left hemisphere (Beblo et al., 1999; Castillo et al., 1993; Herrmann et al., 1993, 1995; House et al., 1990; Lauterbach et al., 1997; Morris et al., 1995; Robinson, 2003, 2006; Starkstein & Robinson, 1988; Starkstein et al., 1990; Terroni et al., 2011; Vataja et al., 2004), especially to structures implicating prefrontal cortex and the basal ganglia (e.g., Tang et al., 2011). However, findings of left-lateralized neuroanatomical correlates have not been reported systematically (e.g., Sharpe et al., 1990; Sinyor et al., 1986). Some have found right hemisphere correlates, particularly when both conditions are comorbid (e.g., Shahripour & Donnan, 2014). Others have argued that these emotional states are independent of one another and do not share the same etiology (Shimoda & Robinson, 1998) or the same neural substrates (Castillo et al., 1993; Starkstein et al., 1990). This statement needs to be qualified by the fact that the study of poststroke anxiety remains limited in scope (Sagen et al., 2010). This mixed picture appears to suggest that a wide array of brain structures is associated with poststroke depression and anxiety (e.g., Hackett et al., 2014), including but perhaps not limited to limbic areas, paralimbic structures such as the ventral lateral frontal cortex, the polar temporal cortex and basal ganglia (e.g., Spalletta et al., 2006).

At a physiological level, limbic and frontal brain structures in the healthy brain mediate the interpretation of emotional information and regulate the body's stress responses through biomarkers of the ANS and the HPA axis (Abreu et al., 2009; McEwen & Gianaros, 2010; Seeman et al., 2010). In the short-term, this psychophysiological reactivity is assumed to contribute to successful goal attainment, such as task performance or social engagement (Chrousos, 2009). However, long-term, chronic activation of biomarkers of stress reactivity can lead to physiological dysregulation and result in neurocognitive changes (McEwen, 2007; McEwen & Gianaros, 2010; McEwen & Stellar, 1993).

In the general stroke population, changes in the ability to regulate stress responses have been linked to the development of emotional deficits following stroke (e.g., Bao, Meynen, & Swaab, 2008; Brown & Harris, 1978; Fava & Kendler, 2000; Hewitt, Flett, & Mosher, 1992; Kendler et al., 1999). Such dysregulation has been found to adversely affects motor skills, cognitive function (Franceschini et al., 2001), prognosis, and mortality rate (e.g., Christensen et al., 2004; Marklund et al., 2004). The specific consequences such dysregulation might have for aphasia are discussed below.

ALTERED EMOTIONS IN APHASIA

Clearly an important component of emotional wellbeing following stroke is anchored in a person's capacity to engage in human interaction (Code, Hemsley, & Herrmann, 1999; Code & Herrmann, 2003; Code, 2010). This ability is forever changed in persons with aphasia (Tanner, 2003). Persons with aphasia often suffer emotionally devastating effects on the quality of their communicative experience as a result of their compromised linguistic skills (e.g., Cahana-Amitay et al., 2011). Such impaired communication alters functionality across a wide range of social domains, which may interfere with the extent to which persons with aphasia can optimally adapt to successful/failed attempts to meet their needs, goals, and concerns. Consistent mismatches between expected and actual progress towards a given goal can adversely affect their emotional state.

Early aphasia studies have linked emotional problems among persons with aphasia to heightened awareness of disorder/disability, unrealistic expectations of recovery, lack of acceptance of condition by friends and family, and discouraging or disrespectful feedback from caregivers and clinicians (e.g., Darley, 1975; Skelly, 1975; Swindell & Hammons, 1988). However, the systematic study of the emotional aftermath of aphasia has been sporadic. Much of this research has focused on exploring symptoms of depression, painting a mixed picture concerning the relationship between depression, its treatment, and the impact it might have on restoring language and cognitive function in aphasia (e.g., Code, 2003; 2010; Laures-Gore & DeFife, 2013). Studies exploring other emotional states in aphasia have not been conducted systematically (Cahana-Amitay et al., 2011), but there is a small number of studies that explored whether persons with aphasia show dysregulated stress reactivity (e.g., Cahana-Amitay, Oveis, Sayers, 2013; Laures et al., 2003; Laures-Gore, 2012; Laures-Gores et al., 2010; Laures-Gore, Hamilton, & Matheny, 2007; 2007).

Depression and Aphasia

Persons with aphasia are more likely to develop poststroke depression than nonaphasic stroke survivors (De Ryck et al., 2013; Laska et al., 2007; Small & Llano, 2009). Carota et al. (2001) described the initial frustration, depression, and anger observed in aphasia in the acute stage as a "reflex behavior" in the form of a "catastrophic reaction" specific to this population. They found that the manifestation of this extreme emotional distress (a "catastrophic reaction") was brought about repeatedly in the context of language testing, where the patient began to sob—producing angry gestures, phrases, and sounds often directed at the examiner—and then "refused to carry on with any language procedure or even with simple conversation" (Carota et al., 2001, p. 1902). Such behavior does not typically persist, but approximately two thirds of depressed aphasic patients continue to experience a steady decline in mood concomitant with impaired functionality across a range of cognitive, behavioral, and social domains, leading to reduced life participation as well as communicative and social isolation (Code, 2003; Code & Muller, 1992; Friedland & McColl, 1987; Gainotti, 1997; Herrmann & Wallesch, 1989; Taylor Sarno, 1993, 1997), thus severely compromising their quality of life (Code & Herrmann, 2003; Hilari & Byng, 2009; Hilari et al., 2010). Kauhanen et al. (1999, 2000), for example, found that of the aphasic patients they studied, 58% suffered minor depression and 12% suffered major depression at 3 months poststroke, compared with 25% minor and 35% major at 12 months, suggesting an increase in the incidence of major depression over time.

Most cases of depression in aphasia have been reported for nonfluent patients (Benson, 1973; Robinson & Benson, 1981; Robinson, 2006; Starkstein & Robinson, 1988). However, in all likelihood this observation underestimates the occurrence of depression in aphasia, since most studies typically exclude patients who lack the language comprehension skills that would enable them to participate in the verbal assessments usually used for diagnosing depression (Bugarski et al., 2009; Code & Herrmann, 2003; Robinson, 2006; Starkstein & Robinson, 1988; Stern, 1999; Townend et al., 2007).

To bypass this problem, Ghika-Schmid et al. (1999) and Bogousslavsky (2003) developed an emotional behavioral index describing patients' poststroke behavior—in terms of sadness, withdrawal, aggressivity, passivity, disinhibition, denial, and adaptation—which does not necessitate verbal communication. An additional measure proposed for assessing depression in chronic aphasia is the Aphasic Depression Rating Scale (ADRS), a nine-item scale based on the Hamilton Depression Rating Scale (Benaim et al., 2004) which has been found to be superior to the more widely used Visual Mood Analog Scale, a visual self assessment evaluation scale (Benaim et al., 2010). However, Townend et al. (2007, 2007a), who reviewed 60 studies of aphasic persons with poststroke depression, found that only 37% of the studies included persons with severe aphasia and only 48% used adaptive diagnostic measures of depression (e.g., the use of informants, clinical observation, modification of questions in interviews, modification of the timing of interviews, and the use of visual analogue scales), suggesting that current studies on depression in aphasia might not reflect the full extent of the problem (Spencer et al., 1997; Yu et al., 2004).

NEURAL AND PSYCHOSOCIAL FACTORS

Although poor language performance in aphasia has been linked to depression (Åström, 1993; Carota et al. 2001, 2005; Code & Herrmann, 2003; Kauhanen, 1999, 2000; Palomaki et al., 1999; Small & Llano, 2009), such that degree of emotional distress is associated with severity of communication deficit (e.g., Thomas & Lincoln, 2008), findings from such studies are somewhat inconclusive (Berg et al., 2001, 2003; Fedoroff et al., 1991; Hilari et al., 2010; Morris et al., 1990; Spalletta et al., 2002), leaving the nature of the relationship between the two conditions underdetermined (Bugarski et al., 2009).

Some researchers have suggested that depression and aphasia simply represent two common but independent sequelae of stroke, which might co-occur because of the proximity of the damaged neural networks in the left hemisphere, especially the frontal cortex and basal ganglia regions, associated with each condition (Bolla-Wilson et al., 1989; Bugarski, 2009; Carota et al., 2001; Castillo et al., 1993; Robinson, 2006; Sapir & Aronson, 1990; Starkstein et al., 1990; Starkstein & Robinson, 1988). Comorbidity of aphasia and depression has been observed even in crossed aphasia, where the affected patient showed reversed lateralization for both language and emotion (in the form of a catastrophic reaction) (Berthier & Starkstein, 1994).

Others have argued that it is aphasia itself that brings about depression as a reaction to the loss of the ability to speak (Benson, 1973, 1979; Gainotti, 1972; Sapir & Aronson, 1990; Tanner & Gerstenberger, 1988). However, this suggestion has been challenged (see Starkstein & Robinson, 1988, for a detailed review), the most convincing argument being the presence of the catastrophic reaction in mild-to-moderate fluent (posterior) aphasia, and the observation that awareness of one's impairment is not a prerequisite for experiencing depression. As pointed out by Bogousslavsky (2003), sadness can develop even in patients who are unaware of their condition (Starkestein et al., 1990). Support for this latter argument comes from a recent study in which poststroke perceived stress was found to be associated with the onset of depression among persons with aphasia and right hemisphere damage (Laures-Gore & DeFife, 2013).

Nonetheless, some researchers still entertain the possibility of a causal relationship between aphasia and depression. Bugarski et al. (2009), for example, found a significant and selective association between language and depression in persons with mild aphasia; they speculated that given the centrality of speech in our lives, "even mild deficits in language function, which can be manifested in various ways (e.g., difficulty naming objects, articulation, repeating phrases, etc.), present a stress for a given person and in this very manner bring on a depressive reaction" (p. 486).

Poststroke depression in aphasia can be viewed as "reactive" if the time course associated with its progression is taken into account (Code & Herrmann, 2003; Gainotti, 1997; Hemsley & Code, 1996; Herrmann et al., 1993; Herrmann & Wallesch, 1993; Starkstein & Robinson, 1988). There seems to be a trade-off between the predictive values of neurological versus psychological and psychosocial factors for the occurrence of depression in aphasia depending on how far along the patient is poststroke (Code & Herrmann, 2003). In the acute stages, the lesion characteristics best predict the onset of depression, whereas in the chronic phase, psychological aspects become increasingly and possibly equally important (Code & Herrmann, 2003; Herrmann & Wallesch, 1993; Starkstein & Robinson, 1988). One of the most significant and lingering psychosocial problems reported for depressed persons with chronic aphasia concerns altered responsibilities, functions, and roles within the family setting (Hemsley & Code, 1996; Herrmann & Wallesch, 1989; Santos et al., 1999; Wahrborg, 1991). These changes have been found to be particularly devastating for families dealing with the aftermath of aphasia, where the constant battle with the loss of functional communication leads to greater psychosocial dysfunction in both patient and spouse (Artes & Hoops, 1976; Christensen and Anderson, 1989; Herrmann, 1997; Kinsella & Duffy, 1979; Malone et al., 1970; Zraik & Boone, 1991).

Herrmann and Wallesch (1993) proposed a model to capture the progression of poststroke depression that identifies three distinct points in time that differentiate between the acute and chronic stages. In the first 3 months poststroke, patients experience "primary" depression as a direct consequence of structural and biochemical changes to the brain, unrelated to the feeling of loss or degree of depression. Six months into the chronic stage, "secondary" depression appears in reaction to the psychosocial, cognitive, and functional changes brought about by the stroke, especially in people who either initially denied the consequences of the stroke or were hoping for a more rapid recovery process. "Tertiary" depression then develops while transitioning from outpatient care, where patients are faced with the need to reintegrate into society and reclaim their prestroke social roles. The severity of secondary and tertiary depression in persons with chronic aphasia has been linked to the social value patients assigned to language premorbidly (Benson, 1973; Bugarski, 2009; Code & Herrmann, 2003; Starkestein & Robinson, 1988; Wahrborg, 1991) and to their coping skills in adjusting to a life with a language disorder and its impact on their ability to interact in the community (Code & Muller, 1992; Friedland, & McColl, 1987; Hemsley & Code, 1996; Taylor Sarno, 1993, 1997). Such adjustment has been argued to involve a grieving process (Tanner & Gerstenberger, 1988) in which patients experience a sequence of emotions that include denial, anger, bargaining, depression, and acceptance, all necessary for emotional recovery from the loss of person, self, and object. However, Code and Herrmann (2003) correctly point out that such an interpretation falls short of describing the dynamic nature of the course of depression in aphasia and of explaining its neurobiological basis.

The idea that the progression of depression in aphasia is time-sensitive finds support in a study examining predictors of poststroke psychological distress in aphasic and nonaphasic stroke survivors (Hilari et al., 2010). Stroke severity accounted for most of the variance at baseline, but loneliness and low satisfaction with one's social network did so at 6 months poststroke. Interestingly, aphasia was not found to predict psychological distress at any point in this study, but at 3 months poststroke patients with aphasia were found to be significantly more likely to experience psychological distress compared with nonaphasic patients (93% and 50%, respectively). It is not clear why this pattern failed to recur at 6 months; possibly it was because of sample size, as the authors themselves indicate. In addition, the findings concerned only patients who were able to self-report depression/distress on the different measures used in the study, once again limiting observations to persons with nonfluent aphasia and mild to moderate fluent aphasia.

DEPRESSION AND APHASIA: RECOVERY AND INTERVENTION EFFECTS

Much as in the general stroke population, depression in persons with aphasia adversely affects aphasia recovery (Code & Muller, 1992; Code & Herrmann, 2003; Herrmann & Wallesch, 1993; Robinson et al., 1986), since these patients have lower rates of recovery (Fucetola et al., 2006; Sinyor et al., 1986; Starkstein & Robinson, 1988) and greater cognitive impairment (Kauhanen et al., 1999; Starkstein & Robinson, 1988). This may be attributable to interdependencies found among mood and motivation and physical, cognitive, and language performance, which worsen in the face of emotional imbalance (Code et al., 1999) but significantly improve in the presence of emotional well-being (Code & Muller, 1992; Hemsley & Code, 1996; Oatley & Johnson-Laird, 1987; Tucker, 1981).

The range of factors affecting rehabilitation outcome for depressed persons with aphasia remains underdetermined (Code, 2001), especially in light of the considerable individual variability that patients demonstrate (Code & Herrmann, 2003; Hemsley & Code, 1996). Evidence of the efficacy of aphasia treatment comes from psychological-behavioral interventions for aphasic persons with depression, in which reliance on language abilities is not central to treatment participation, as the focus of the intervention is to enhance activity level and occurrence of pleasant events (Grober et al., 1993). Such studies often exclude participants with severe aphasia, limiting the generalizability of the results to persons with mild aphasia (e.g., Mitchell et al., 2009). Findings suggest that greater language impairment among persons with aphasia at baseline is associated with poorer mood enhancement (e.g., Thomas & Lincoln, 2006), but benefits can be observed up to 6 months postintervention (Thomas et al., 2012). In a large sample of over 100 aphasic participants, significant mood improvements were reported for persons who received behavioral therapy versus those who received language treatment alone as measured by self-reported mood and self-esteem as well as observer-rated mood (Thomas et al., 2012).

In addition, aphasia pharmacotherapy has provided some insight into the effects of biological interventions targeting depression for aphasia treatment (Beversdorf, 2007; Bullain et al., 2007; Code and Herrmann, 2003; Hermann and Wallesch, 1993; Llano & Small, 2009). The potential usefulness of different pharmacological agents for poststroke depression in aphasia has long been recognized (Lipsey et al., 1984; Reding et al., 1986; Sapir & Aronson, 1990; Solomonovici et al., 1962; Starkstein & Robinson, 1988; Voinescu & Gheorghita, 1978). However, systematic studies of how different drugs interact with mood changes and language performance in aphasia are rare (e.g., Cahana-Amitay, Albert, & Oveis, 2014), with mostly anecdotal reports on drug-induced mood effects in persons with aphasia (e.g., Bragoni et al., 2000; Gupta & Mlcoch, 1992).

Nonetheless, benefits from the use of the tricyclic nortriptyline (Lipsey et al., 1984), the serotonin reuptake inhibitor citalopram (Andersen et al., 1994; Rampello et al., 2004), the noreadrenergic reuptake inhibitor reboxetine (Rampello et al., 2004), and most recently escitalopram for the prevention of post troke depression (Robinson et al., 2008) have been reported. Since these interventions target different pathophysiological pathways that involve distinct neurotransmitter systems (cholinergic, noradrenergic, dopaminergic, or glutamatergic) (Beversdorf, 2007; de Boissezon et al., 2007; Bullain et al., 2007; Llano & Small, 2009), it is difficult to identify the specific mechanisms that might contribute to recovery of depressed aphasics. It is also difficult to predict the efficacy of a given drug for such patients, since different types of aphasia might show different pharmacotherapeutic sensitivities (Small & Llano, 2009). Still, the efficacy of pharmacotherapy for persons with aphasia is receiving increasing empirical support (e.g., Berthier, 2014), with some drugs demonstrating benefits in multiple cognitive domains such as attention and memory, which are often impaired in aphasia (Seniow et al., 2009). These findings may reflect the extent to which the neural substrates subserving aphasia recovery represent a system that is multifunctional in nature.

To alleviate the symptoms of depression and maximize the cooperation of depressed patients in the course of aphasia recovery, it has been argued that, in addition to use of antidepressants, electroconvulsive therapy (ECT) should be considered (Bullain et al., 2007). Such intervention might be efficacious, especially since there is some evidence that while pharmacotherapy is slow to affect a patient's depression, ECT is rapid in alleviating symptoms (Scott, 2010). In fact, ECT studies show that patients' depression improves upon therapy at no cost to other cognitive abilities (Kellner et al., 2010). Similar observations have been made with respect to repetitive transcranial magnetic stimulation (rTMS), a relatively noninvasive therapy for major depression (Matheson et al., 2010), which was approved by the FDA in 2008 for clinical use (Schönfeldt-Lecuona et al., 2010). rTMS might offer more direct benefits to aphasic patients, since it has also been found to improve language performance in persons with nonfluent aphasia (e.g., Devlin & Watkins, 2007; Hamilton et al., 2010; Martin et al., 2009; Naeser et al., 2005). Examining mood changes in depressed versus nondepressed aphasic patients undergoing rTMS treatment might help shed some light on this question.

Anxiety and Stress Reactivity in Aphasia

Some studies have explored the relationship between anxiety and motor speech functionality in aphasia (Heeschen et al., 1988; Luchsinger & Arnold, 1965; Masdeu et al., 1978; Ryalls, 1984; Sapir & Aronson, 1990), reporting patterns of dysphonia in patients with Broca's but not Wernicke's aphasia (Heeschen et al., 1988). However, little is known about the whether or not anxiety and its neurophysiological underpinnings affects language functions in aphasia other than the general claim that it impairs performance, especially among persons in whom comorbidity with depression is observed (Carota et al., 2001; Cohen, 1998; Gainotti, 1972, 1997; Sapir & Aronson, 1990; Starkstein et al., 1993).

MECHANISMS OF STRESS RESPONSES IN APHASIA

Cahana-Amitay et al. (2011) proposed a conceptual framework, which they termed *linguistic anxiety*, in which persons with aphasia are assumed to experience language as a stressor, which produces psychophysiological stress responses that alter (e.g., further impair) their language performance. This framework is reminiscent of models explaining the relationship between heightened anxiety and memory decline in healthy older adults (Coy et al., 2011; Kurosowa & Harackiewicz, 1995; Lachman & Agrigoroaei, 2012), where older adults' concerns about memory loss (Dixon, De Frias, & Maitland,

2001; Hultsch, Hertzog, Dixon, & Small, 1998; Lachman, 1991, 2000) result in subjective and psychophysiologic anxiety that impairs performance on memory tasks (Andreoletti, Veratti, & Lachman, 2006; Neupert, Miller, & Lachman, 2006).

The assumption is that persons with aphasia remain hyperfocused on the potential for language breakdown while engaged in a language task and that this concern is reinforced by an increased psychophysiological stress responses (Cahana-Amitay et al., 2011). This concern comes with a "cost," as it consumes some of the attention resources that would otherwise be allocated to supporting the performance of the language task at hand. In a state of *linguistic anxiety*, then, the attention resources that aphasic persons exert to suppress their anxiety compete with the resources necessary for processing task-relevant information, thus impairing their language performance. The greatest language performance decrements are expected when processing of linguistic stimuli involves inhibition of competing targets, the presence of which increases the attentional demands on task performance (Cahana-Amitay, Albert, & Oveis, 2014).

Cahana-Amitay et al.'s (2011) proposal is in line with the Eysenck et al.'s (2007) attentional control model, referred to earlier in the chapter, in which anxiety is argued to lead to worry-based deficits in executive functions. Cahana-Amitay and colleagues suggest a tight link between linguistic anxiety and attentional dysfunction in aphasia (e.g., Cahana-Amitay, Albert, & Oveis, 2014). This idea is supported by findings indicating, for example, that executive functions, such as working memory capacity, in part mediate the relationship between anxiety and cognitive performance (e.g., Owens et al., 2012). A potential neural correlate of this neurofunctional integration is the anterior cingulate (Yamasaki, LaBar, & McCarthy, 2002).

Importantly, while anxiety-induced increased psychophysiological stress reactivity can exacerbate language impairment, there is evidence that it may also positively contribute to language performance. Early aphasia studies demonstrated that sufficiently heightened anxiety among aphasic persons improved their motivation and task performance (Darley 1972, 1975; Luria, 1963, 1970; Shill, 1979; Wepman, 1951, 1953). This pattern might reflect the Yerkes-Dodson law (1908), which has linked successful task performance to levels physiological arousal, with poor performance being observed in relation to either insufficient or excessive arousal levels (Cahana-Amitay et al., 2011). From a brain perspective, this inverse U-shaped phenomenon is nontrivial, as there is emerging evidence that engagement of biomarkers of stress, such as those that underlie anxiety, contributes to neural plasticity in the limbic system (e.g., Sapolsky, 2003) and so may affect aphasia rehabilitation outcomes. Figure 6.2 depicts the potential consequences of hypo- and hyperneurovisceral reactivity on language performance in aphasia.

Findings regarding psychophysiological stress responses among persons with aphasia come from a series of studies by Laures-Gore and colleagues, who reported increased perceived stress and/or changes in levels of salivary cortisol, a biomarker of psychophysiological stress reactivity on the HPA axis (Laures-Gore, 2012; Laures et al., 2003, 2007, 2010; Laures-Gore, Hamilton, & Matheny, 2007). In these studies, greater self-perceived stress was consistently negatively associated with language performance among persons with aphasia (e.g., Laures et al., 2007; Laures-Gore, Hamilton, & Matheny, 2007), but the relative contribution of HPA axis stress reactivity to language performance showed a mixed picture.

For example, when Laures and colleagues (2003) examined changes in levels of salivary cortisol in response to a vigilance task among persons with aphasia, they found low levels of reactivity but higher afternoon baseline cortisol levels. In a subsequent study, Laures et al. (2007) compared cortisol levels obtained in response to the performance of linguistic versus nonlinguistic tasks, predicting increased activity among persons with aphasia to the linguistically demanding tasks. However, they found a muted cortisol response to the language task among the aphasic but not the control participants, in whom a gradual return to baseline levels was observed. No differences in cortisol levels at baseline were observed at this time. To account for this pattern, the authors suggested that persons with aphasia demonstrate chronic HPA axis hypoactivation, commonly observed in stress-related disorders (e.g., Fries et al., 2005; Heim et al., 2000). While such an account is reasonable, it fails to explain why it uniquely affected the linguistic task (Cahana-Amitay et al., 2011).

Interestingly, there are persons with aphasia in whom cortisol levels increase in response to performance of a language task, demonstrating a moderate association between measures of word productivity in discourse and elevated cortisol levels (Laures-Gore et al., 2010). These findings suggest that once the HPA axis stress reactivity mechanism is engaged, it can help persons with aphasia persist throughout a task, thus ameliorating task performance possibly through increased arousal. This interpretation is not only in line with the Yerkes-Dodson law (1908) (see Figure 6.2) but also consistent with Laures et al.'s (2003) claim that increased arousal among persons with aphasia is associated with increase in task demands (see Chapter 4).

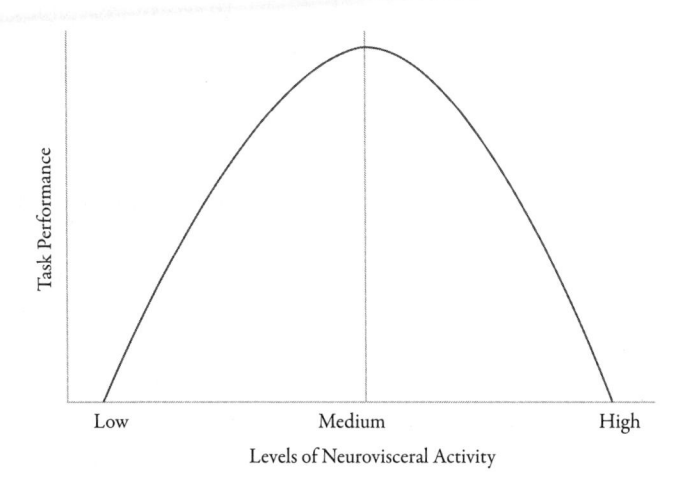

FIGURE 6.2 Anxiety-induced changes in biomarkers of neurovisceral activity and language performance in aphasia. Leftmost shows hypoactivation; rightmost shows hyperactivation

Less evidence exists regarding the role of biomarkers of ANS functions in aphasic language performance. In their vigilance task study, Laures et al. (2003) found mild changes in blood pressure among the aphasic participants. In a recent case study, Cahana-Amitay et al. (2013) explored whether changes in psychophysiologic reactivity were differentially related to performance on linguistic and nonlinguistic tasks under two different anxiety conditions—low and high. Anxiety was induced, following the Trier social stress test anxiety induction design, in which participants are instructed to prepare a public speech (Kirschbaum, Pirke, & Hellhammer, 1993). The authors examined measures of skin conductance and heart rate and found greater physiological reactivity in response to the linguistic tasks compared to the nonlinguistic tasks in the high-anxiety condition, providing preliminary support for their proposed framework of linguistic anxiety in aphasia.

TARGETING PSYCHOPHYSIOLOGICAL STRESS REACTIVITY IN APHASIA TREATMENT

As pointed out in Cahana-Amitay et al. (2011), if psychophysiological stress reactivity accounts in part for some of the language variability observed among persons with aphasia, the identification of biomarkers associated with impaired language performance could shed light on the mechanisms underlying adaptation and neural reorganization during aphasia recovery (see also Hula & McNeil, 2008). Because of the considerable variability in salivary cortisol levels observed among persons with aphasia (e.g., Laures-Gore, 2012), it is difficult to determine its specific contribution to language performance and aphasia recovery. In a recent study, Laures-Gore (2012) explored this question by comparing aphasic to right hemisphere participants. She predicted that the aphasic but not right hemisphere participants would have higher levels of baseline afternoon salivary cortisol and that these would decline over time (a 3-month period). Findings indicated that cortisol levels at baseline were not significantly higher in the aphasic group, with levels remaining steady throughout the study, and no association with language (naming) gains. Cortisol levels of the participants with damage to the right hemisphere also remained unchanged, although they did show an association between better language performance and reduced levels of afternoon salivary cortisol.

The potential role of ANS biomarkers to language performance in aphasia recovery has been explored more directly in stress-reduction studies. These include studies exploring the use of complementary alternative medicine (CAM) therapies such as acupuncture (Jianfei et al., 1988; Zhajun, 1989), hypnosis (Maganiello, 1986; Thompson et al., 1986), relaxation training (Ince, 1968; Marshall & Watts, 1976; Murray & Ray, 2001; Yesavage, 1984), biofeedback (Katz et al., 1999; McNeil et al., 1976), nature-based therapy (NBT; reviewed in Lundgren, 2004), and, more recently, unilateral nostril breathing (Shisler Marshall et al., 2014). The most systematic results come from mindfulness and relaxation studies, whose benefits have been documented among stroke survivors, patients with traumatic brain injury, and patients with dementia (Laures & Shisler, 2004; Lundgren, 2006; Marshall & Laures-Gore, 2008; Murray & Kim, 2004). This technique requires the retention of attentional focus on stimulus or muscle activity while suppressing competing input (mental or sensory), thus enhancing physiological responses that counter those associated with high levels of stress (Murray & Kim, 2004). Such techniques have been shown to improve language performance in persons with aphasia when used as an adjunctive therapy to conventional language interventions (Murray, 2008; Murray & Ray, 2001, 2004). For example, in a case study by Murray and Ray (2001), a person with chronic aphasia showed language gains upon administration of relaxation therapy prior to syntactic stimulation. In another study, Shisler Marshall et al. (2014) demonstrated reductions in levels of anxiety (self-reported) and gains in language performance following a 10-week unilateral nostril breathing intervention. Interestingly, attention measures did not show a comparable change over time.

Additional evidence suggesting that the targeting of ANS biomarkers among persons with aphasia might enhance their language performance comes from a small number of pharmacotherapy studies investigating the effects of beta-adrenergic blocking agents on language performance in this population (reviewed in Cahana-Amitay et al., 2011, 2014). Findings indicate that beta-blocking agents such as propranolol improve language performance among persons with aphasia, as measured, for example, by naming performance (e.g., Beversdorf et al., 2007; Tanaka et al., 2006, 2007, 2009, 2010). Tanaka et al. (2006, 2009) specifically explored whether improved language performance is related to measurable changes in the function of the ANS. They evaluated their participants' naming and auditory comprehension, heart rate, and self-reported mood at three time points and found improved language performance upon drug administration, with measurable physiological changes (reduction in heart rate).

Targeting dysregulated stress reactivity among persons with aphasia by manipulating their ANS responses might result in augmentation of their ability to attend to a given language task. The precise mechanism underlying these effects remains undetermined. Some have argued that these effects are similar to those observed in the amelioration of "performance anxiety," where the beta-blocking agent serves to reduce the autonomic response associated with the natural "fight or flight" response (such as increased heart rate) and so augments performance. Others have argued that these effects reflect modulation of signal-to-noise ratio in the cortex, which primarily increase efficiency of information processing (Hasselmo, Linster, Patil, Ma, & Cekic, 1997; Heilman, Nadeau, & Beversdorf, 2003). While the empirical validity of these explanations can be further explored in studies differentiating peripheral and central autonomic components in persons with and without aphasia (Cahana-Amitay et al., 2011), detailed psycholinguistic analyses of the types of errors affected by each pharmacological intervention might provide better insight into the linguistic, cognitive, and neural mechanism underlying these treatment effects (Cahana-Amitay et al., 2014).

In the absence of neuroimaging studies exploring the effects of such pharmacological interventions, it is difficult to predict which brain structures may underlie these treatment effects. However, we speculate that the inferior frontal gyrus might be a relevant candidate. Our proposal is based on a recent fMRI study of healthy adults designed to determine whether drug-induced alterations of noradrenergic signaling in the brain leads to changes in working memory and/or activation of specific brain structures (Becker et al., 2013). Results suggested that administration of propranolol induced a compensatory brain response in the inferior frontal region without impairing cognitive performance.

Studies exploring the influence of emotional changes among persons with aphasia on their language and cognitive functioning clearly lend support to the notion that "aphasia is a cross-disciplinary concern" (Code, 2001, p. 326), in which language breakdown cannot be viewed in isolation from its potential emotional underpinnings (Sapir & Aronson 1990). Although systematic neuroimaging studies exploring the neural underpinnings of depression in aphasia have yet to be conducted, evidence for the involvement of multiple biochemical pathways in the enhancement of performance among aphasic persons with depression speaks to a language recovery system that is multifunctional by nature. Similarly, observations about the putative relationship between psychophysiological mechanisms underlying anxiety and language functions, which point to an interplay between ANS and HPA axis biomarkers and psycholinguistic notions such as "linguistic anxiety" in aphasia, reflect a multifunctional approach to aphasia, where neurochemical changes in the brain are presumed to work in concert with coping styles and reactions to loss (Tanner, 2003) but also with the restitution of disrupted language function in aphasia. Thus examining the impact of emotional changes on language performance in aphasia is a critical step for uncovering the mechanisms associated with the reshaping of the neural circuitry underlying aphasia recovery.

References

Abreau, B. C., Zgaljardic, D., Borod, J. C., Seale, G., Temple, R. O., Ostir, G. V., & Ottenbacher, K. J. (2009). Emotional regulation, processing, and recovery after acquired brain injury. In K. Matsuka & C. Christiansen (Eds.), *Life balance: multidisciplinary theories and research* (pp. 223–240). Thorofare, NJ: Slack Incorporated; Bethesda, MD: AOTA Press.

Airaksinen, E., Larsson, M., & Forsell, Y. (2005). Neuropsychological functions in anxiety disorders in population-based samples: evidence of episodic memory dysfunction. *Journal of Psychiatric Research*, *39*(2), 207–214.

Alm, P. A. (2004). Stuttering, emotions, and heart rate during anticipatory anxiety: a critical review. *Journal of Fluency Disorders*, *29*, 123–133.

American Psychiatric Association. (2000). *Diagnostic and statistical manual of mental disorders* (4th ed., text rev.). Washington, DC: Author.

Andersen, G., Vestergaard, K., & Lauritzen, L. (1994). Effective treatment of poststroke depression with the selective serotonin reuptake inhibitor citalopram. *Stroke*, *25*(6), 1099–1104.

Andreoletti, C., Veratti, B. W., & Lachman, M. E. (2006). Age differences in the relationship between anxiety and recall. *Aging & Mental Health*, *10*, 265–271.

Aron, A. R., Robins, T. W., & Poldrack, R. A. (2004). Inhibition and the right inferior frontal cortex. *Trends in Cognitive Science*, *8*, 170–177.

Aronson, A. (1985). *Clinical voice disorders*. New York: Thieme.

Artes, R., & Hoops, R. (1976). Problems of aphasic and non-aphasic stroke patients as identified and evaluated by patients' wives. In Y. Lebrun & R. Hoops (Eds.), *Recovery in aphasics*. Amsterdam: Swets and Zeitlinger.

Åström, M. (1996). Generalized anxiety disorder in stroke patients. A 3-year longitudinal study. *Stroke*, *27*, 270–275.

Åström, M., Adolefsson, R., & Asplund, K. (1993). Major depression in stroke patients—a 3-year longitudinal study. *Stroke*, *24*(7), 976–982.

Atchley, R. A., Ilardi, S., & Enole, A. (2003). Hemispheric asymmetry in the processing of emotional content in word meanings: the effect of current and past depression. *Brain and Language*, *84(1)*, 105–119.

Austin, M. P., Mitchell, P., & Goodwin, G. M. (2001). Cognitive deficits in depression: possible implications for functional neuropathology. *The British Journal of Psychiatry*, *178*, 200–206.

Badre, D., & Wagner, A. D. (2007). Left ventrolateral prefrontal cortex and the cognitive control of memory. *Neuropsychologia*, *45*(13), 2883–2901.

Banich, M. T., Mackiewicz, K. L., Depue, B. E., Whitmer, A. J., Miller, G. A., & Heller, W. (2009). Cognitive control mechanisms, emotion and memory: a neural perspective with implications for psychopathology. *Neuroscience & Biobehavioral Reviews*, *33*(5), 613–630.

Bao, A. M., Meynen, G., & Swaab, D. F. (2008). The stress system in depression and neurodegeneration: focus on the human hypothalamus. *Brain Research Reviews*, *57*(2), 531–553.

Bar-Haim, Y., Lamy, D., Pergamin, L., Bakermans-Kranenburg, M. J., & van IJzendoorn, M. H. (2007). Threat-related attentional bias in anxious and nonanxious individuals: a meta-analytic study. *Psychological Bulletin*, *133*(1), 1–24.

Barker-Collo, S. L. (2007). Depression and anxiety 3 months post stroke: prevalence and correlates. *Archives of Clinical Neuropsychology*, *22*, 519–531

Beblo, T., Wallesch, C. W., & Herrmann, M. (1999). The crucial role of frontostriatal circuits for depressive disorders in the post-acute stage after stroke. *Neuropsychiatry, Neuropsychology, and Behavioral Neurology*, *12*, 234–246.

Becker, B., Androsch, L., Jahn, R. T., Alich, T., Striepens, N., Markett, S., … Hurlemann, R. (2013). Inferior frontal gyrus preserves working memory and emotional learning under conditions of impaired noradrenergic signaling. *Frontiers in Behavioral Neuroscience*, *7*, 197.

Behnke, R. R., & Carlile, L. (1971). Heart rate as an index of speech anxiety. *Speech Monographs*, *38*, 65–69.

Benaim, C., Cailly, B., Perennou, D., & Pelissier, J. (2004). Validation of the aphasic depression rating scale. *Stroke*, *35*(7), 1692–1696.

Benaim, C., Decavel, P., Bentabet, M., Froger, J., Pélissier, J., & Pérennou, D. (2010). Sensitivity to change of two depression rating scales for stroke patients. *Clinical Rehabilitation*, *24*(3), 251–257.

Benson, D. F. (1973). Psychiatric aspects of aphasia. *The British Journal of Psychiatry*, *123*, 555–566.

Benson, D. F. (1979). *Aphasia, alexia, and agraphia*. Edinburgh: Churchill-Livingstone.

Berenbaum, H., Raghavan, C., Le, H.-N., Vernon, L. L., & Gomez, J. J. (2003). A taxonomy of emotional disturbances. *Clinical Psychology: Science and Practice, 10*(2), 206–226.

Berg, A., Palomäki, H., Lehtihalmes, M., Lönnqvist, J., & Kaste, M. (2003). Poststroke depression an 18-month follow-up. *Stroke, 34*(1), 138–143.

Berg, A., Palomaki, H., Lehtihalmes, M., Lonqvist, J., & Kaste, M. (2001). Post stroke depression in acute phase after stroke. *Cerebrovascular Disease,12*, 14–20.

Berthier, M. L. (2014). Cognitive enhancing drugs in aphasia: a vote for hope. *Aphasiology, 28*(2), 128–132.

Berthier, M. L., & Starkstein, S. E. (1994). Catastrophic reaction in crossed aphasia. *Aphasiology, 8*(1), 89–95.

Beversdorf, D. Q. (2007). Pharmacotherapy of aphasia. *Journal of Head Trauma Rehabilitation, 22*(1), 65–66.

Beversdorf, D. Q., Sharma, U. K., Phillips, N. N., Notestine, M. A., Slivka, A. P., Friedman, N. M., ... Hillier, A. (2007). Effect of propranolol on naming in chronic Broca's aphasia with anomia. *Neurocase, 13*, 256–259.

Bishop S. J. (2007). Neurocognitive mechanisms of anxiety: an integrative account. *Trends in Cognitive Sciences, 11*, 307–316.

Bishop S. J. (2008). Neural mechanisms underlying selective attention to threat. *Annals of the New York Academy of Sciences, 1129*, 141–152.

Bodie, G. D. (2010). A racing heart, rattling knees, and ruminative thoughts: defining, explaining, and treating public speaking anxiety. *Communication Education, 59*(1), 70–105.

Bogousslavsky, J. (2003). William Feinberg lecture 2002. Emotions, mood and behavior after stroke. *Stroke, 34*, 1046–1050.

de Boissezon, X., Peran, P., de Boysson, C., & Démonet, J. F. (2007). Pharmacotherapy of aphasia: myth or reality? *Brain and language, 102*(1), 114–125.

Bolla-Wilson, K., Robinson, R. G., Starkstein, S. E., Boston, J., & Price, T. R. (1989). Lateralization of dementia of depression. *American Journal of Psychiatry, 146*(5), 627–634.

Borod, J. C., Bloom, R. L., Brickman, A. M., Nakhutina, L., & Curko, E. A. (2002). Emotional processing deficits in individuals with unilateral brain damage. *Applied Neuropsychology, 9*(1), 23–26.

Bosch, J. A., de Geus, E. J., Carroll, D., Goedhart, A. D., Anane, L. A., van Zanten, J. J., ... Edwards, K. M. (2009). A general enhancement of autonomic and cortisol responses during social evaluative threat. *Psychosomatic Medicine, 71*(8), 877–885.

Bragoni, M., Altieri, M., Di Piero, V., Padovani, A., Mostardini, C., & Lenzi, G. (2000). Bromocriptine and speech therapy in non-fluent chronic aphasia after stroke. *Neurological Sciences, 21*(1), 19–22.

Brown, G. W., & Harris, T. (1978). Social origins of depression: a reply. *Psychological Medicine, 8*(4), 577–588.

Bugarski, V., Semnic, M., & Slankamenac, P. (2009). Relationship between depressive symptoms and cognitive status in acute ischemic stroke. *Psihologija, 42*(4), 479–489.

Bullain, S. S., Chriki, L. S., & Stern, T. A. (2007). Aphasia: associated disturbances in affect, behavior, and cognition in the setting of speech and language difficulties. *Psychosomatics, 48*(3), 258–264.

Burvill, P. W., Johnson, G. A., Jamrozik, K. D., Anderson, C. S., Stewart-Wynne, E. G., Byng, S., & Black, M. (1995). What makes a therapy? Some parameters of therapeutic intervention in aphasia. *European Journal of Disorders of Communication, 30*(3), 303–316.

Cahana-Amitay, D., Albert, M. L., Pyun, S. B., Westwood, A., Jenkins, T., Wolford, S., & Finley, M. (2011). Language as a stressor in aphasia. *Aphasiology, 25*(2), 593–614.

Cahana-Amitay, D., Albert, M. L., & Oveis, A. (2014). Psycholinguistics of aphasia pharmacotherapy: Asking the right questions. *Aphasiology, 28*(2), 133–154.

Cahana-Amitay, D., Oveis, A. C., & Sayers, J. S. (2013). Feeling anxious can affect language performance in chronic aphasia: a case report. *Procedia—Social and Behavioral Studies, 94*, 149–150.

Carillo, E., Moya-Albiol, L., González-Bono, E., Salvador, A., Ricarte, J., & Gómez-Amor, J. (2001). Gender differences in cardiovascular and electrodermal responses to public speaking task: the role of anxiety and mood states. *International Journal of Psychophysiology, 42*(3), 253–264.

Carota, A., Berney, A., Aybek, S., Iaria, G., Staub, F., Ghika-Schmid, F., … Bogousslavsky, J. (2005). A prospective study of predictors of poststroke depression. *Neurology, 64*(3), 428–433.

Carota, A., Rossetti, A. O., Karapanayiotides, T., & Bogousslavsky, J. (2001). Catastrophic reaction in acute stroke: A reflex behavior in aphasic patients. *Neurology, 57*, 1902–1905.

Carrig, M. M., Kolden, G. G., & Strauman, T. J. (2009). Using functional magnetic resonance imaging in psychotherapy research: a brief introduction to concepts, methods, and task selection. *Psychotherapy Research, 19*(4–5), 409–417

Caruso, A. J., Chodzko-Zajko, W. J., Bidinger, D. A., & Sommers, R. K. (1994). Adults who stutter: responses to cognitive stress. *Journal of Speech and Hearing Research, 37*, 746–754.

Castillo, C. S., Starkstein, S., Fedoroff, P. J., Thomas, T. R., & Robinson, R. G. (1993). Generalized anxiety disorder after stroke. *The Journal of Nervous Mental Disease, 181*, 2.

Cato, A. M., Crosson, B., Gocay, D., Soltysik, D., Wierenga, C., Gopinanth, K., … Briggs, R. (2004). Processing words with emotional connotation: an fMRI study of time course and laterality in rostral frontal and retrosplenial cortices. *Journal of Cognitive Neuroscience, 16*(2), 167–177.

Cato Jackson, M. A., & Crosson, B. (2006). Emotional connotation of words: Role of emotion in distributed semantic systems. *Progress in Brain Research, 156*, 205–216.

Chemerinski, E., & Levine, S. R. (2006). Neuropsychiatric disorders following vascular brain injury. *Vascular Brain Injury, 73*(7), 1006–1014.

Chemerinski, E., Robinson, R. G., & Kosier, J. T. (2001). Improved recovery in activities of daily living associated with remission of poststroke depression. *Stroke, 32*, 113–117.

Chen, Y., Garcia, G. E., Huang, W., & Constantini, S. (2014). The involvement of secondary neuronal damage in the development of neuropsychiatric disorders following brain insults. *Frontiers in Neurology, 5*, 22.

Chiew, K. S., & Braver, T. S. (2011). Positive affect versus reward: emotional and motivational influences on cognitive control. *Frontiers in Psychology, 2*, 279.

Christensen, H., Boysen, G., & Johannsen, H. H. (2004). Serum-cortisol reflects severity and mortality in acute stroke. *Journal of Neurological Sciences, 217*, 175–180.

Christensen, J. M., & Anderson, J. D. (1989). Spouse adjustment to stroke: aphasic versus nonaphasic partners. *Journal of Communication Disorders, 22*(4), 225–231.

Chrousos, G. P. (2009). Stress and disorders of the stress system. *Nature Reviews Endocrinology, 5*(7), 374–381.

Cisler, J. M., Bacon, A. K., & Williams, N. L. (2009). Phenomenological characteristics of attentional biases toward threat: a critical review. *Cognitive Therapy and Research, 33*(2), 221–234.

Citron, F.M.M. (2012). Neural correlates of written emotion word processing: a review of recent electrophysiological and hemodynamic neuroimaging studies. *Brain and Language, 122*, 211–226. doi: 10.1016/j.bandl.2011.12.007

Clarke, D. M., & Currie, K. C. (2009). Depression, anxiety and their relationship with chronic diseases: a review of the epidemiology, risk, and treatment evidence. *The Medical Journal of Australia, 190*(7), S54–S60.

Code, C. (2001). Multifactorial processes in recovery from aphasia: developing the foundations for a multileveled framework. *Brain and Language, 77*(1), 25–44.

Code, C. (2003). The quantity of life for people with chronic aphasia. *Neuropsychological Rehabilitation, 13*, 365–378.

Code, C. (2010). Aphasia. In J. Damico, N. Muller, & M. J. Ball (Eds.), *The handbook of language and speech disorders* (pp. 317–336). Oxford, UK: Wiley-Blackwell.

Code, C., Hemsley, G., & Herrmann, M. (1999). The emotional impact of aphasia. *Seminars in Speech and Language, 20*, 19–31.

Code, C., & Herrmann, M. (2003). The relevance of emotional and psychosocial factors in aphasia to rehabilitation. *Neuropsychological Rehabilitation, 3*(1/2), 109–132.

Code, C., & Muller, D. J. (1992). *The Code-Muller protocols: assessing perceptions of psychosocial adjustment to aphasia and related disorders.* London: Whurr.

Cohen, M. R. (1998). Expression of anxiety and depression in a case of subcortical motor aphasia. *Neurorehabilitation, 11*(3), 255–260.

Cox, M. (1986). The psychologically maladjusted stutterer. In K. St Louis (Ed.), *The atypical stutterer: principles and practices of rehabilitation* (pp. 93–122). Orlando, FL: Academic Press.

Coy, B., O'Brien, W. H., Tabaczynski, T., Northern, J., & Carels, R. (2011). Associations between evaluation anxiety, cognitive interference and performance on working memory tasks. *Applied Cognitive Psychology, 25*(5), 823–832.

Crocker, L. D., Heller, W., Warren, S. L., O'Hare, A. J., Infantolino, Z. P., & Miller, G. A. (2013). Relationships among cognition, emotion, and motivation: implications for intervention and neuroplasticity in psychopathology. *Frontiers in Human Neuroscience, 7*, 261.

Crosson, B., Cato, M. A., Sadek, J., Radonovich, K., Gökçay, D., Bauer, R., ... Briggs, R. (2002). Semantic monitoring of words with emotional connotation during fMRI: contribution of left-hemisphere limbic association cortex. *Journal of the International Neuropsychological Society, 8*, 607–622.

Crosson, B., Radonovich, K., Sadek, J. R., Gökçay, D., Bauer, R.M., Fischler, I. S., ... Briggs, R. W. (1999). Left-hemisphere processing of emotional connotation during word generation. *NeuroReport, 10*, 2449–2455.

D'Aniello, G. E., Scarpina, F., Mauro, A., Mori, I., Castelnuovo, G., Bigoni, M., ... Molinari, E. (2014). Characteristics of anxiety and psychological well-being in chronic post-stroke patients. *Journal of the Neurological Sciences, 338*(1–2), 191–196.

Damasio, A. R. (1998). Emotion in the perspective of an integrated nervous system. *Brain Research Reviews, 26*(2), 83–86.

Darley, F. L. (1972). The efficacy of language rehabilitation in aphasia. *Journal of Speech and Hearing Disorders, 37*, 3–21.

Darley, F. L. (1975). Treatment of acquired aphasia. In W. J. Friedlander (Ed.), *Advances in neurology* (Vol. 7). New York: Raven Press.

Davidson, R. J. (2004). What does the prefrontal cortex "do" in affect: perspectives on frontal EEG asymmetry research. *Biological Psychology, 67*(1–2), 219–234.

Davidson, R. J., Marshall, J. R., Tomarken, A. J., & Henriques, J. B. (2000). While a phobic waits: regional brain electrical and autonomic activity in social phobics during anticipation of public speaking. *Biological Psychiatry, 47*(2), 85–95.

De Ryck, A., Brouns, R., Fransen, E., Geurden, M., Van Gestel, G., Wilssens, I., ... Engelborghs, S. (2013). A prospective study on the prevalence and risk factors of poststroke depression. *Cerebrovascular Diseases Extra, 3*(1), 1–13.

De Wit, L., Putman, K., Baert, I., Lincoln, N. B., Angst, F., Bevens, H., ... Feys, H. (2008). Anxiety and depression in the first six months after stroke: a longitudinal multicentre study. *Disability & Rehabilitation, 30*(24), 1858–1866

Demaree, H. A., Everhart, D. E., Youngstrom, E. A., & Harrison, D. W. (2005). Brain lateralization of emotional processing: historical roots and a future incorporating "dominance." *Behavioral and Cognitive Neuroscience Reviews, 4*(1), 3–20.

Denkova, E., Dolcos, S., & Dolcos, F. (2013). The effect of retrieval focus and emotional valence on the inferior frontal cortex activity during autobiographical recollection. *Frontiers in Behavioral Neuroscience, 7*, 192.

Derakshan, N., & Eysenck, M. W. (1998). Working memory capacity in high trait-anxious and repressor groups. *Cognition and Emotion, 12*, 697–713

Derakshan, N., & Eysenck, M. W. (2009). Anxiety, processing efficiency, and cognitive performance: new developments from attentional control theory. *European Psychologist, 14*, 168–176

Devlin, J. T., & Watkins, K. E. (2007). Stimulating language: insights from TMS. *Brain, 130*(3), 610–622.

Dimberg, U., & Thunberg, M. (2007). Speech anxiety and rapid emotional reactions to angry and happy facial expressions. *Scandinavian Journal of Psychology, 48*(4), 321–328.

Dixon, D.J.H., De Frias, C. M., & Maitland, S. B. (2001). Memory in midlife. In M. E. Lachman (Ed.), *Handbook of midlife development* (pp. 248–278). New York: Wiley.

Dolcos, F., Iordan, A. D., & Dolcos, S. (2011). Neural correlates of emotion–cognition interactions: a review of evidence from brain imaging investigations. *Journal of Cognitive Psychology, 23*(6), 669–694

Dolcos, F., Kragel, P., Wang, L. H., & McCarthy, G. (2006). Role of the inferior frontal cortex in coping with distracting emotions. *Neuroreport, 17*, 1591–1594.

Doruk, A., Turkbay, T., Yelboga, Z., Ciyiltepe, M., Iyisoy, A., Sutcigil, L., & Ozsahin, A. (2008). Autonomic nervous system imbalance in young adults with developmental stuttering. *Bulletin of Clinical Psychopharmacology, 18*, 274–281.

Duxbury, J. G., & Tsai, L. (2010). The effects of cooperative learning on foreign language anxiety: a comparative study of Taiwanese and American universities. *International Journal of Instruction, 3*(1), 3–18.

Engels, A. S., Heller, W., Mohanty, A., Herrington, J. D., Banich, M. T., Webb, A. G., & Miller, G. A. (2007). Specificity of regional brain activity in anxiety types during emotion processing. *Psychophysiology, 44*(3), 352–363.

Engels, A. S., Heller, W., Spielberg, J. M., Warren, S. L., Sutton, B. P., Banich M. T., & Miller, G. A. (2010). Co-occurring anxiety influences patterns of brain activity in depression. *Cognitive, Affective, and Behavioral Neuroscience, 10*(1), 141–156.

Eysenck, M. W., & Derakshan, N. (2011). New perspectives in attentional control theory. *Personality and Individual Differences, 50*, 955–960

Eysenck, M. W., Derakshan, N., Santos, R., & Calvo, M. G. (2007). Anxiety and cognitive performance: attentional control theory. *Emotion, 7*(2), 336–353.

Eysenck, M. W., Payne, S., & Derakshan, N. (2005). Trait anxiety, visuospatial processing, and working memory. *Cognition and Emotion, 19*(8), 1214–1228

Fava, M., & Kendler, K. S. (2000). Major depressive disorder. *Neuron, 28*(2), 335–341.

Fedoroff, J. P., Lipsey, J. R., Starkstein, S. E., Forrester, A., Price, T. R., & Robinson, R. G. (1991). Phenomenological comparisons of major depression following stroke, myocardial infarction or spinal cord lesions. *Journal of Affective Disorders, 22*(1), 83–89.

Franceshini, R., Tenconi, G.L., Zoppoli, F., & Barreca, T. (2001). Endocrine abnormalities and outcome of ischaemic stroke. *Biomedicine & Pharmacotherapy, 55*(8), 458–465.

Frankel, T. (2008). Conversation intelligence after stroke: a drug trial. Doctoral dissertation. Johannesburg: University of Witwatersrand. Available at: witsetd.wits.ac.za:8080/dspace/.../1/PhD%20introductory%20pages.pdf

Friedland, J., & McColl, M. (1987). Social support and psychosocial dysfunction after stroke: buffering effects in a community sample. *Archives of Physical Medicine and Rehabilitation, 68*(8), 475–480.

Fries, E., Hesse, J., Hellhammer, J., & Hellhammer, D. H. (2005). A new view on hypocortisolism. *Psychoneuroendocrinology, 30*(10), 1010–1016.

Fu, C. H., Steiner, H., & Costafreda, S. G. (2012). Predictive neural biomarkers of clinical response in depression: a meta-analysis of functional and structural neuroimaging studies of pharmacological and psychological therapies. *Neurobiology of Disease, 52*, 75–83

Fucetola, R., Connor, L. T., Perry, J., Leo, P., Tucker, F. M., & Corbetta, M. (2006). Aphasia severity, semantics, and depression predict functional communication in acquired aphasia. *Aphasiology, 20*(5), 449–461.

Fure, B., Wyller, T. B., Engedal, K., & Thommessen, B. (2006). Emotional symptoms in acute ischemic stroke. *International Journal of Geriatric Psychiatry, 21*(4), 382–387.

Fuster, J. M. (2002). Frontal lobe and cognitive development. *Journal of Neurocytology, 31*, 373–385.

Gainotti, G. (1972). Emotional behavior and hemispheric side of the lesion. *Cortex, 8*, 41–55.

Gainotti, G. (1997). Emotional, psychological, and psychosocial problems of aphasic patients: an introduction. *Aphasiology, 11*, 635–650.

Gainotti, G., Azzoni, A., & Marra, C. (1999). Frequency, phenomenology and anatomical-clincial correlates of major post-stroke depression. *British Journal of Psychiatry, 175*, 163–167.

Ghika-Schmid, F., Van Melle, G., Guex, P., & Bogousslavsky, J. (1999). Subjective experience and behavior in acute stroke: the Lausanne emotion in acute stroke study. *Neurology, 52*(1), 22–22.

Gianaros, P. J., Van Der Veen, F. M., & Jennings, J. R. (2004). Regional cerebral blood flow correlates with heart period and high-frequency heart period variability during working-memory tasks: implications for the cortical and subcortical regulation of cardiac autonomic activity. *Psychophysiology, 41*(4), 521–530.

Goeleven, E., De Readt, R., Baert, S., & Koster, E.H.W. (2006). Deficient inhibition of emotional information in depression. *Journal of Affective Disorders, 93*, 149–157.

Goldstein, K. (1942). *Aftereffects of brain injuries in war: their evaluation and treatment.* New York: Grune & Stratton.

Goldstein, K. (1948). *Language and language disturbances: aphasic symptom complexes and their significance for medicine and theory of language.* New York: Grune & Stratton.

Goldstein, K. (1959). Functional disturbances in brain damage. In S. Arieti (Ed.), *American handbook of psychiatry* (pp. 770–794). New York: Basic Books.

Gotlib, I. H., & Joormann, J. (2010). Cognition and depression: current status and future directions. *Annual Review of Clinical Psychology, 6*, 285–312.

Gramer, M., & Saria, K. (2007). Effects of social anxiety and evaluative threat on cardiovascular responses to active performance situations. *Biological Psychology, 74*(1), 67–74.

Granholm, E., & Steinhauer, S. R. (2004). Pupillometric measures of cognitive and emotional processes. *International Journal of Psychophysiology, 52*(1), 1–6.

Gray, J. R. (2004). Integration of emotion and cognitive control. *Current Directions in Psychological Science, 13*, 46–48.

Gray, J. R., Braver, T. S., & Raichle, M. E. (2002). Integration of emotion and cognition in the lateral prefrontal cortex. *Proceedings of the National Academy of Sciences of the United States of America, 99*, 4115–4120.

Greenop, K. R., Almeida, O. P., Hankey, G. J., van Bockxmeer, F., & Lautenschlager, N. T. (2009). Premorbid personality traits are associated with post-stroke behavioral and psychological symptoms: a three-month follow-up study in Perth, Western Australia. *International Psychogeriatrics, 21*, 1063–1071.

Grober, S., Hibbard, M. R., Gordon, W. A., Stein, P. N., & Freeman A. (1993). The psychotherapeutic treatment of post-stroke depression with cognitive behavioural therapy. In W. A. Gordon (Ed.), *Advances in stroke rehabilitation* (pp. 215–241). Andover, Massachusetts: Andover Medical Publishers.

Gupta, S. R., & Mlcoch, A. G. (1992). Bromocriptine treatment of nonfluent aphasia. *Archives of Physical Medicine and Rehabilitation, 73*(4), 373–376.

Gusev, E. I., & Bogolepova, A. N. (2009). Depressive disorders in stroke patients. *Neuroscience and Behavioral Physiology, 39*(7), 639–643.

Hackett, M. L., Yapa, C., Parag, V., & Anderson, C. S. Frequency of depression after stroke. A systematic review of observational studies. *Stroke, 36*(6), 1330–1340.

Hackett, M. L., Köhler, S., O'Brien, J. T., & Mead, G. E. (2014). Neuropsychiatric outcomes of stroke. *The Lancet Neurology, 13*(5), 525–534.

Hagoort, P. (2005). On Broca, brain, and binding: a new framework. *Trends in Cognitive Science, 9*, 416–423.

Hamilton, R. H., Sanders, L., Benson, J., Faseyitan, O., Norise, C., Naeser, M., ... Coslett, H. (2010). Stimulating conversation: enhancement of elicited propositional speech in a patient with chronic non-fluent aphasia following transcranial magnetic stimulation. *Brain and Language, 113*(1), 45–50.

Hasselmo, M. E., Linster, C., Patil, M., Ma, D., & Cekic, M. (1997). Noradrenergice suppression of synaptic transmission may influence cortical signal-to-noise ratio. *Journal of Neurophysiology, 77*(6), 3326–3339.

Havas, D. A., Glenberg, A. M., & Rinck, M. (2007). Emotion simulation during language comprehension. *Psychonomic Bulletin and Review, 14*(3), 436–441.

Hayhow, B., Brockman, S., & Starkstein, S. E. (2014). Post-stroke depression. In T. A. Schweizer & L. Macdonald (Eds.), *The behavioral consequences of stroke*. New York: Springer.

Healy, B. (2010). The effect of attentional control and heart-period variability on negative affect and trait anxiety. *The Journal of General Psychology, 137*(2), 140–150.

Heeschen, C., Ryalls, J., & Hagoort, P. (1988). Psychological stress in Broca's versus Wernicke's aphasia. *Clinical Linguistics & Phonetics, 2*, 309–316.

Heilman, K. M., Nadeau, S. E., & Beversdorf, D. O. (2003). Creative innovation: possible brain mechanisms. *Neurocase, 9*(5), 369–379.

Heim, C., Ehlert, U., & Hellhammer, D. (2000). The potential role of hypocortisolism in the pathophysiology of stress-related bodily disorders. *Psychoneuroendocrinology, 25*, 1–35.

Hemsley, G., & Code, C. (1996). Interactions between recovery in aphasia, emotional and psychosocial factors in subjects with aphasia, their significant others and speech pathologists. *Disability and Rehabilitation, 18*(11), 567–584.

Herrington, J. D., Heller, W., Mohanty, A., Engels, A. S., Banich, M. T., Webb, A. G., & Miller, G. A. (2010). Localization of asymmetric brain function in emotion and depression. *Psychophysiology, 47*, 442–454.

Herrmann, M. (1997). Studying psychosocial problems in aphasia: some conceptual and methodological considerations. *Aphasiology, 11*(7), 717–725.

Herrmann, M., Bartels, C., Schumacher, M., & Wallesch, C.W. (1995). Poststroke depression: is there a patho-anatomical correlate for depression following the post-acute stage of stroke? *Stroke, 26*, 850–856.

Herrmann, M., Bartels, C., & Wallesch, C. W. (1993). Depression in acute and chronic aphasia—symptoms, pathoanatomico-clinical correlations, and clinical implications. *Journal of Neurology, Neurosurgery, and Psychiatry, 56*, 672–678.

Herrmann, M., & Wallesch, C. W. (1993). Depressive changes in stroke patients. *Disability & Rehabilitation, 15*(2), 55–66.

Herrmann, N., Black, S. F., Lawrence, J., Szekely, C., & Szalai, J. P. (1998). The Sunnybrook stroke study: a prospective study of depressive symptoms and functional outcomes. *Stroke, 29*, 618–624.

Hewitt, P. L., Flett, G. L., & Mosher, S. (1992). The perceived stress scale: factor structure and relation to depression symptoms in a psychiatric sample. *Journal of Psychopathology and Behavioral Assessment, 14*(3), 247–257.

Hilari, K., Northcott, S., Roy, P., & Marshall, J. (2010). Psychological distress after stroke and aphasia: the first six months. *Clinical Rehabilitation, 24*, 181–190.

Holt, S. K., Lynn, S. K., & Kuperberg, G. R. (2009). Neurophysiological correlates of comprehending emotional meaning in context. *Journal of Cognitive Neuroscience, 21*(11), 2245–2262.

Horwitz, E. K. (2001). Language anxiety and achievement. *Annual Review of Applied Linguistics, 21*, 112–126.

House, A., Dennis, M., Warlow, C., Hawton, K., & Molyneaux, A. (1990). Mood disorders after stroke and their relation to lesion location—A CT scan study. *Brain, 113*, 1113–1129.

Hula, W. D., & McNeil, M. R. (2008). Models of attention and dual-task performance as explanatory constructs in aphasia. *Seminars in Speech and Language, 29*(3), 169–87.

Hultsch, D. F., Hertzog, C., Dixon, R. A., & Small, B. J. (1998). *Memory change in the aged.* New York: Cambridge University Press.

Ince, L. (1968). Desensitization with an aphasic patient. *Behavioral Research and Therapy, 6*, 235–237.

Jianfei, C., Meifang, Y., & Jia, W. (1988). Hemorrheological study on the effect of acupuncture in treating cerebral infarction. *Journal of Traditional Chinese Medicine, 8*(3), 167–172.

Johnson, D. R. (2009). Emotional attention set-shifting and its relationship to anxiety and emotion regulation. *Emotion, 9*, 681–690.

Johnson, J. L., Minarik, P. A., Nyström, K. V., Bautista, C., & Gorman, M. J. (2006). Poststroke depression incidence and risk factors: an integrative literature review. *Journal of Neuroscience Nursing, 38*(4), 316–327.

Joormann, J. (2010). Cognitive inhibition and emotion regulation in depression. *Current Directions in Psychological Science, 19*, 161–166.

Joormann, J., & Gotlib, I. H. (2008). Updating the contents of working memory in depression: interference from irrelevant negative material. *Journal of Abnormal Psychology, 117*, 182–192.

Katz, W., Bhardawaj, S., & Carstens, B. (1999). Electromagnetic articulatography treatment for an adult with Broca's aphasia and apraxia of speech. *Journal of Speech, Language, and Hearing Research, 42*(6), 1355–1366.

Kauhanen, M. L., Korpelainen, J. T., Hiltunen, P., Brusin, E., Mononen, H., Maatta, R., … Myllyla, V. V. (1999). Poststroke depression correlates with cognitive impairment and neurological deficits. *Stroke, 30*, 1875–1880.

Kauhanen, M. L., Korpelainen, J. T., Hiltunen, P., Määttä, R., Mononen, H., Brusin, E., … Myllylä, V. V. (2000). Aphasia, depression, and non-verbal cognitive impairment in ischaemic stroke. *Cerebrovascular Diseases, 10*(6), 455–461.

Kellner, C. H., Knapp, R., Husain, M. M., Rasmussen, K., Sampson, S., Cullum, M., … Petrides, G. (2010). Bifrontal, bitemporal and right unilateral electrode placement in ECT: randomised trial. *The British Journal of Psychiatry, 196*(3), 226–234.

Kinsella, G. J., & Duffy, F. D. (1979). Psychosocial readjustment in spouses of aphasic patients. *Scandinavian Journal of Rehabilitation Medicine, 11*, 129–132.

Kirschbaum, C., Pirke, K. M., & Hellhammer, D. H. (1993). The "Trier social stress test"—a tool for investigating psychobiological stress responses in a laboratory setting. *Neuropsychobiology, 28*(1–2), 76–81.

Kissler, K., Herbert, C., Peyk, P., & Junghofer, M. (2007). Early cortical responses to emotional words during reading. *Psychological Science, 18*(6), 475–480.

Kotila, M., Numminen, H., Waltimo, O., & Kaste, M. (1998). Depression after stroke: results from the Finnstroke Study. *Stroke, 29*(2), 368–372.

Kotz, S. A., & Friederici, A. D. (2003). Electrophysiology of normal and pathological language processing. *Journal of Neurolinguistics, 16*, 43–58.

Kousta, S.-T., Vinson, D. P., & Vigliocco, G. (2009). Emotion words, regardless of polarity, have a processing advantage over neutral words. *Cognition, 112*(3), 473–481.

Kozak, M. J., & Miller, G. A. (1982). Hypothetical constructs versus intervening variables: a reappraisal of the three-systems model of anxiety assessment. *Behavioral Assessment, 4*, 347–358.

Kreibig, S. D. (2010). Autonomic nervous system activity in emotion: a review. *Biological Psychology, 84*, 394–421.

Kurosowa, K., & Harackiewicz, J. M. (1995). Test anxiety, self-awareness, and cognitive interference: a process analysis. *Journal of Personality, 63*(4), 931–951.

Lachman, M. E. (1991). Perceived control over memory aging: developmental and intervention perspectives. *Journal of Social Issues, 47*(4), 159–175.

Lachman, M. E. (2000). Promoting a sense of control over memory aging. In L. Backman, R. D. Hill, & A. Stigdotter-Neely (Eds.), *Cognitive rehabilitation in old age* (pp. 106–120). New York: Oxford University Press.

Lachman, M. E., & Agrigoroaei, S. (2012). Low perceived control as a risk factor for episodic memory: the mediational role of anxiety and task interference. *Memory & Cognition, 40*, 287–296.

Lam, S., Dickerson, S. S., Zoccola, P. M., & Zaldivar, F. (2009). Emotion regulation and cortisol reactivity to a social-evaluative speech task. *Psychoneuroendocrinology, 34*(9), 1355–1362.

Landis, T. (2006). Emotional words: what's so different from just words? *Cortex, 42*(6), 823–830.

Landis, T., Graves, R., & Goodglass, H. (1983). Semantic paralexia: a release of right hemisphere function from left hemispheric control? *Neuropsychologia, 21*, 359–364.

Lane, R. D., McRae, K., Reiman, E. M., Chen, K., Ahren, G. L., & Thayer, J. F. (2009). Neural correlates of heart rate variability during emotion. *Neuroimage, 44*, 213–222.

Lane, R. D., Weidenbacher, H., Fort, C. L., Thayer, J. F., & Allen, J.J.B. (2008). Subgenual anterior cingulate (BA25) activity covaries with changes in cardiac vagal tone during affective set shifting in healthy adults. *Psychosomatic Medicine, 70*, A-42.

Lang, P. J. (1968). Fear reduction and fear behavior: problems in treating a construct. Paper presented at thr Research in Psychotherapy Conference, American Psychological Association, Chicago.

Laska, A. C., Martensson, B., Kahan, T., von Arbin, M., & Murray, V. (2007). Recognition of depression in aphasic stroke patients. *Cerebrovascular Diseases, 24*(1), 74–79.

Laures-Gore, J. S. (2012). Aphasia severity and salivary cortisol over time. *Journal of Clinical and Experimental Neuropsychology, 34*(5), 489–496.

Laures-Gore, J. S., & DeFife, L. C. (2013). Perceived stress and depression in left and right hemisphere post-stroke aphasia. *Neuropsychological Rehabilitation, 23*(6), 783–797.

Laures-Gore, J. S., DuBay, M., Duff, M. C., & Buchanan, T. W. (2010). Identifying behavioral measures of stress in individuals with aphasia. *Journal of Speech, Language, and Hearing Research, 53*(5), 1394–1400.

Laures, J. S., Odell, K., & Coe, C. (2003). Arousal and auditory vigilance in individuals with aphasia during a linguistic and nonlinguistic task. *Aphasiology, 17*(12), 1133–1152.

Laures, J. S., & Shisler, R. (2004). Complementary and alternative medicine in the treatment of adult neurogenic communication disorders: a review. *Disability and Rehabilitation, 26*(6), 315–325.

Lauterbach, E. C., Jackson, J. G., Wilson, A. N., Dever, G. E., & Kirsh, A. D. (1997). Major depression after left posterior globus pallidus lesions. *Neuropsychiatry, Neuropsychology, and Behavioral Neurology, 10*, 9–16.

Leppavuori, A., Pohjasvaara, T., Vataja, R., Kaste, M., & Erkinjuntti, T. (2003). Generalized anxiety disorders three to four months after ischemic stroke. *Cerebrovascular Diseases, 16*(3), 257–264.

Levin, R. L., Heller, W., Mohanty, A., Herrington, J. D., & Miller, G. A. (2007). Cognitive deficits in depression and functional specificity of regional brain activity. *Cognitive Therapy and Research, 31*, 211–233.

Linden, T., Bloomstand, C., & Skoog, I. (2007). Depressive disorders after 20 months in elderly stroke patients: a case control study. *Stroke, 38*(6), 1860–1863.

Lindquist, K. A., Wager, T. D., Kober, H., Bliss-Moreau, E., & Feldman Barrett, L. (2012). The brain basis of emotion: A meta-analytic review. *Behavioral and Brain Sciences, 35*, 121–202.

Lipsey, J. R., Robinson, R.G. Pearlson, G.D., Rao, K., & Price, T. R. (1984). Nortriptylinetreatment of post-stroke depression: a double-blind study. *Lancet, 1*(8372), 297–300.

Lipsey, J. R., Robinson, R. G., Pearlson, G. D., Rao, K., & Price, T. R. (1985). The dexamethasone suppression test and mood following stroke. *American Journal of Psychiatry, 142*, 318–323.

Luchsinger, R., & Arnold, G. E. (1965). *Voice, speech, and language. clinical communicology: its physiology and pathology.* Belmont, CA: Wadsworth.

Lundgren, K., Helm-Estabrooks, N., & Klein, R. (2010). Stuttering following acquired brain damage: a review of the literature. *Journal of Neurolinguistics, 23*(5), 447–454.

Lundgren, K. (2004). Nature-based therapy: its potential as a complementary approach to treating communication disorders. *Seminars in Speech and Language, 25*(2), 121–31.

Lundgren, K. (2006). Complementary and alternative treatment of aphasia. Presented at the Canadian Association of Speech-Language Pathologists and Audiologists; Winnipeg, Manitoba.

Luria, A. (1963). *Restoration of function after brain injury.* New York: MacMillan.

Luria, A. (1970). *Traumatic aphasia: its syndromes, psychology, and treatment.* The Hague: Mouton.

MacIntyre, P. D. (1995). How does anxiety affect second language learning? A reply to Sparks and Ganschow. *The Modern Language Journal, 79*(1), 90–99.

MacIntyre, P. D. (2002). Motivation, anxiety and emotion in second language acquisition. *Individual Differences and Instructed Language Learning, 2*, 45–68.

MacIntyre, P.D., & Gardner, R. C. (1994). Methods and results in the study of anxiety and language learning: a review of the literature. *Language Learning, 41*(1), 85–117.

MacLeod C., & Donnelan, A. M. (1993). Individual differences in anxiety and the restriction of working memory capacity. *Personality and Individual Differences, 15*, 163–173

Maddock, R. J., & Buonocore, M. H. (1997). Activation of left posterior cingulate gyrus by the auditory presentation of threat-related words: an fMRI study. *Psychiatry Research, 75*(1), 1–14.

Maddock, R. J., Garrett, A. S., & Buonocore, M. H. (2003). Posterior cingulate cortex activation by emotional words: fMRI evidence from valence decision task. *Human Brain Mapping, 18*, 30–41.

Magnaniello, A. (1986). Hypnotherapy in the rehabilitation of a stroke victim: a case study. *American Journal of Clinical Hypnosis, 29*, 64–68.

Malone, R. L., Ptacek, P. H., & Malone, M. S. (1970). Attitudes expressed by families of aphasics. *British Journal of Communication Disorders, 5*, 174–179.

Manoliu, A., Meng, C., Brandl, F., Doll, A., Tahmasian, M., Scherr, M., ... Sorg, C. (2014). Insular dysfunction within the salience network is associated with severity of symptoms and aberrant inter-network connectivity in major depressive disorder. *Frontiers in Human Neuroscience, 7*, 930. doi: 10.3389/fnhum.2013.00930

Marklund, N., Peltonen, M., Nilsson, T. K., & Olsson, T. (2004). Low and high circulating cortisol levels predict mortality and cognitive dysfunction early after stroke. *Journal of Internal Medicine, 256*, 15–21.

Marshall, R., & Watts, M. (1976). Relaxation training: Effects of communicative ability of aphasic adults. *Archives of Physical Medicine and Rehabilitation, 57*, 464–467.

Marshall, R.J.S., & Laures-Gore, J. (2008). A single subject study of unilateral nostril breathing in aphasia. Poster presented at the Annual Meeting of the International Neuropsychological Society; Hawaii.

Martin, P. I., Naeser, M. A., Ho, M., Doron, K. W., Kurland, J., Kaplan, J., ... Pascual-Leone, A. (2009). Overt naming fMRI pre-and post-TMS: two nonfluent aphasia patients, with and without improved naming post-TMS. *Brain and Language, 111*(1), 20–35.

Masdeu, J. C., Schoene, W. C., & Funkenstein, H. (1978). Aphasia following infarction of the left supplementary motor area. *Neurology, 28*, 1220

Masskulpan, P., Riewthong, K., Diapratham, P., & Kiptniratsaikul, V. (2008). Anxiety and depressive symptoms after stroke in nine rehabilitation centers. *Journal of Medical Association Thailand, 91*(10), 1595–1602.

McEwen, B. S. (2007). Physiology and neurobiology of stress and adaptation: central role of the brain. *Physiological Reviews, 87*, 873–904.

McEwen, B., & Gianaros, P. J. (2010). Central role of the brain in stress and adaptation: links to socioeconomic status, health, and disease. *Annals of the New York Academy of Sciences, 1186*, 190–222.

McEwen, B. S., & Stellar, E. (1993). Stress and the individual. Mechanisms leading to disease. *Archives of Internal Medicine, 153*(18), 2093–2101.

McNally, R. J. (1998). Information-processing abnormalities in anxiety disorders: implications for cognitive neuroscience. *Cognition and Emotion, 12*(3), 479–495.

McNeil, M., Prescott, T., & Lemme, M. (1976). An application of electromygraphic biofeedback to aphasia/apraxia treatment. *Clinical Aphasiology Conference Proceedings*, 151–171.

Miller, G. A. (2010). Mistreating psychology in the decades of the brain. *Perspectives on Psychological Science, 5*, 716–743.

Miller, G. A., Crocker, L. D., Spielberg, J. M., Infantolino, Z. P., & Heller, W. (2013). Issues in localization of brain function: the case of lateralized frontal cortex in cognition, emotion, and psychopathology. *Frontiers in Integrative Neuroscience, 7*, 2. 10.3389/fnint.2013.00002.

Miller, G. A., Elbert, T., Sutton, B. P., & Heller, W. (2007). Innovative clinical assessment technologies: challenges and opportunities in neuroimaging. *Psychological Assessment, 19*(1), 58–73.

Miller, G. A. (2010). Mistreating psychology in the decades of the brain. *Perspectives on Psychological Science, 5*, 716–743.

Mitchell, A. J., Vaze, A., & Rao, S. (2009). Clinical diagnosis of depression in primary care: a meta-analysis. *The Lancet, 374*(9690), 609–619.

Morris, P. L., Robinson, R. G., & Raphael, B. (1990). Prevalence and course of depressive disorders in hospitalized stroke patients. *The International Journal of Psychiatry in Medicine, 20*(4), 349–364.

Morris, P.L.P., Robinson, R. G., Andrzejewski, P., Samuels, J., & Price, T. R. (1993). Association of depression with 10 year poststroke mortality. *American Journal of Psychiatry, 150*, 124–129.

Morris, P.L.P., Robinson, R. G., Raphael, B., & Hopwood, M. J. (1995). Lesion location and poststroke depression. *Journal of Neuropsychiatry, 8*, 399–403.

Mukheriee, D., Levin, R. L., & Heller, W. (2006). The cognitive, emotional, and social sequelae of stroke: psychological and ethical concerns in post-stroke adaptation. *Topics in Stroke Rehabilitation, 13*(4), 26–35.

Murray, L. L. (2008). The application of relaxation training approaches to patients with neurogenic disorders and their caregivers. *Perspectives on Neurophysiology and Neurogenic Speech and Language Disorders, 18*, 90–98.

Murray, L. L., & Kim, H. Y. (2004). A review of select alternative treatment approaches for acquired neurogenic disorders: relaxation therapy and acupuncture. *Seminars in Speech and Language, 25*(2), 133–149.

Murray, L., & Ray, H. (2001). A comparison of relaxation training and syntax stimulation for chronic nonfluent aphasia. *Journal of Communication Disorders, 34*, 87–113.

Naeser, M. A., Martin, P. I., Nicholas, M., Baker, E. H., Seekins, H., Helm-Estabrooks, N., ... & Pascual-Leone, A. (2005). Improved naming after TMS treatments in a chronic, global aphasia patient–case report. *Neurocase, 11*(3), 182–193.

Nannaetti, L., Paci, M., Pasquini, J., Lombardi, B., & Taiti, P. G. (2005). Motor and functional recovery in patients with post-stroke depression. *Disability and Rehabilitation, 27*(4), 170–175.

Neau, J. P., Ingrand, P., Mouille-Brachet, C., Rosier, M. P., Couderq, C., Alvarez, A., & Gil, R. (1998). Functional recovery and social outcome after cerebral infarction in young adults. *Cerebrovascular Disease, 8*, 296–302.

Neupert, S. D., Miller, L. S., & Lachman, M. E. (2006). Physiological reactivity to cognitive stressors: variations by age and socioeconomic status. *International Journal of Aging & Human Development, 62*, 221–235.

Niedenthal P. M. (2007). Embodying emotion. *Science, 316*, 1002–1005. doi: 10.1126/science.1136930

Nugent, A. C., Bain, E. E., Thayer, J. F., Sollers, J. J., & Drevets, W. C. (2007). Sex differences in the neural correlates of autonomic arousal: a pilot PET study. *The International Journal of Psychophysiology, 80*(3), 182–191.

Nugent, A. C., Bain, E. E., Sollers, J. J., Thayer, J. F., & Drevets, W. C. (2008). Alterations in neural correlates of autonomic control in females with major depressive disorders. *Psychosomatic Medicine, 70*, A-99.

Oatley, K., & Johnson-Laird, P. N. (1987). Towards a cognitive theory of emotions. *Cognition and Emotion, 1*(1), 29–50.

Ochsner, K. N., Silvers, J. A., & Buhle, J. T. (2012). Functional imaging studies of emotion regulation: a synthetic review and evolving model of the cognitive control of emotion. *Annals of the New York Academy of Science, 1251*, E1–E24.

Ofek, E., & Pratt, H. (2005). Neurophysiological correlates of subjective significance. *Clinical Neurophysiology*, *116*(10), 2354–2362.

Ofek, E., Purdy, S.C., Ali, G., Webster, T., Gharahdaghi, N., & McCann, C. M. (2013). Processing of emotional words after stroke: an electrophysiological study. *Clinical Neuropsychology*, *124*(9), 1771–1778.

Ortigue, S., Michel, C. M., Murray, M. M., Mohr, C., Carbonnel, S., & Landis, T. (2004). Electrical neuroimaging reveals early generator modulation to emotional words. *NeuroImage*, *21*, 1242–1251.

Owens, M., Stevenson, J., Hadwin, J. A., & Norgate, R. (2012). When does anxiety help or hinder cognitive test performance? The role of working memory capacity. *British Journal of Psychology*, *105*(1), 92–101.

Ozawa, S., Matsuda, G., & Hiraki, K. (2014). Negative emotion modulates prefrontal cortex activity during a working memory task: a NIRS study. *Frontiers in Human Neuroscience*, *8*, 46. doi: 10.3389/fnhum.2014.00046

Ozdemir, B., Doruk, A., Celik, C., Amasyali, B., Ciyiltepe, M., & Ozcan, C. (2010). Evaluation of autonomic nervous system function with tilt table testing in young adults with persistent developmental stuttering. *Bulletin of Clinical Psychopharmacology*, *20*(1), 45–49.

Palasik, S., Irani, F., & Goberman, A. M. (2009). Trait and state anxiety in people who stutter and people who do not stutter. *Perspectives on Fluency and Fluency Disorders*, *19*, 99–105.

Palomäki, H., Kaste, M., Berg, A., Lönnqvist, R., Lönnqvist, J., Lehtihalmes, M., & Hares, J. (1999). Prevention of poststroke depression: 1 year randomised placebo controlled double blind trial of mianserin with 6 month follow up after therapy. *Journal of Neurology, Neurosurgery & Psychiatry*, *66*(4), 490–494.

Paolucci, S. (2008). Epidemiology and treatment of post-stroke depression. *Neuropsychiatric Disease and Treatment*, *4*(1), 145–154.

Parikh, R. M., Lipsey, J. R., Robinson, R. G., & Price, T. R. (1987). A two-year longitudinal study of post-stroke mood disorders: dynamic changes in correlates of depression at one and two years. *Stroke*, *18*, 579–584.

Pessoa, L. (2008). On the relationship between emotion and cognition. *Nature Reviews Neuroscience*, *9*(2), 148–158

Pessoa, L. (2009). How do emotion and motivation direct executive control? *Trends in Cognitive Sciences*, *13*(4), 160–166

Peters, H. F., & Hulstijn, W. (1984). Stuttering and anxiety: the difference between stutterers and nonstutterers in verbal apprehension and physiologic arousal during the anticipation of speech and nonspeech tasks. *Journal of Fluency Disorders*, *9*, 67–84.

Phan, K. L., Wager, T., Taylor, S. F., & Liberzon, I. (2002). Functional neuroanatomy of emotion: a meta-analysis of emotion activation studies in PET and fMRI. *Neuroimage*, *16*, 331–348.

Phelps, E. A. (2006). Emotion and cognition: insights from studies of the human amygdala. *Annual Review of Psychology*, *57*, 27–53

Pohjasvaara, T., Erkinjuntti, T., Vataja, R., & Kaste, M. (1998). Correlates of dependent living 3 months after ischemic stroke. *Cerebrovascular Disease*, *8*, 259–266.

Pohjasvaara, T., Vataja, R., Leppavuori, A., Kaste, M., & Erkinjuntti, T. (2001). Depression is an independent predictor of poor long-term functional outcome post-stroke. *European Journal of Neurology*, *8*, 315–319.

Poldrack, R. A., Wagner, A. D., Prull, M. W., Desmond, J. E., Glover, G. H., & Gabrieli, J. D. (1999). Functional specialization for semantic and phonological processing in the left inferior prefrontal cortex. *Neuroimage, 10*, 15–35.

Primeau, F. (1988). Post-stroke depression: a critical review of the literature. *Canadian Journal of Psychiatry, 33*, 757–765.

Rampello, L., Chiechio, S., Nicoletti, G., Alvano, A., Vecchio, I., Raffaele, R., & Malaguarnera, M. (2004). Prediction of the response to citalopram and reboxetine in post-stroke depressed patients. *Psychopharmacology, 173*(1–2), 73–78.

Reding, M. J., Orto, L. A., Winter, S. W., Fortuna, I. M., Di Ponte, P., & McDowell, F. H. (1986). Antidepressant therapy after stroke: a double-blind trial. *Archives of Neurology, 43*(8), 763–765.

Robinson, R. G. (2006). *The clinical neuropsychiatry of stroke* (2nd ed.). New York: Cambridge University Press.

Robinson, R. G., & Benson, D. F. (1981). Depression in aphasic patients: frequency, severity, and clinical-pathological correlations. *Brain and Language, 14*(2), 282–291.

Robinson, R. G., Bolla-Wilson, K., Kaplan, E., Lipsey, J. R., & Price, T. R. (1986). Depression influences intellectual impairment in stroke patients. *The British Journal of Psychiatry, 148*(5), 541–547.

Robinson, R. G., Jorge, R. E., Moser, D. J., Acion, L., Solodkin, A., Small, S. L., ... Arndt, S. (2008). Escitalopram and problem-solving therapy for prevention of poststroke depression: a randomized controlled trial. *JAMA, 299*(20), 2391–2400.

Robinson, R. G. (2003). Poststroke depression: prevalence, diagnosis, treatment, and disease progression. *Biological Psychiatry, 54*, 376–587.

Roseman, I. J. (2008). Structure of emotions. Motivations and emotivations: approach, avoidance, and other tendencies in motivated and emotional behavior. In A. Elliot (Ed.), *Handbook of approach and avoidance motivation* (pp. 343–366). New York: Psychology Press.

Ryalls, J. (1984). Some acoustic aspects of CVC utterances in aphasia. *Phonetica, 41*, 103–111.

Sagen, U., Arnstein, F., Moum, T., Morland, T., Vik, T. G., Nagy, T., & Dammen, T. (2010). Early detection of patients at risk for anxiety, depression, and apathy after stroke. *General Hospital Psychiatry, 32*(1), 80–85.

Sagen, U., Vik, T. G., Moum, T., Morland, T., Finset, A., & Dammen, T. (2009). Screening for anxiety and depression after stroke: comparison of the hospital anxiety and depression scale and the Montgomery and Asberg depression rating scale. *Journal of Psychosomatic Research, 67*(4), 325–332.

Santos, C. O., Caeiro, L., Ferro, J. M., Albuquerque, R., & Figueira, M. L. (2006). Anger, hostility, and aggression in the first days of acute stroke. *European Journal of Neurology, 13*(4), 351–358.

Santos, M. E., Farrajota, M. L., Castro-Caldas, A., & De Sousa, L. (1999). Problems of patients with chronic aphasia: different perspectives of husbands and wives? *Brain Injury, 13*(1), 23–29.

Sapir, S., & Aronson, A. (1990). The relationship between psychopathology and speech and language disorders in neurogenic patients. *Journal of Speech and Hearing Disorders, 55*(3), 503–509.

Sapolsky, R. M. (2003). Stress and plasticity in the limbic system. *Neurochemical Research, 28*(11), 1735–1742.

Sarno, M. T. (1997). Quality of life in aphasia in the first post-stroke year. *Aphasiology, 11*(7), 665–679.

Sarno, M. T. (1997). Quality of life in aphasia in the first post-stroke year. *Aphasiology, 11*(7), 665–679.

Sass, S. M., Heller, W., Stewart, J. L., Silton, R. L., Edgar, J. C., Fisher, J. E., & Miller, G. A. (2010). Time course of attentional bias in anxiety: emotion and gender specificity. *Psychophysiology, 47*(2), 247–259.

Schönfeldt-Lecuona, C., Cardenas-Morales, L., Freudenmann, R. W., Kammer, T., & Herwig, U. (2010). Transcranial magnetic stimulation in depression—lessons from the multicentre trials. *Restorative Neurology and Neuroscience, 28*(4), 569–576.

Scott, A. I. (2010). Electroconvulsive therapy, practice and evidence. *The British Journal of Psychiatry, 196*(3), 171–172.

Scovel, T. (1978). The effect of affect on foreign language learning: a review of the anxiety research. *Language Learning, 28*(1), 129–142.

Seeman, T., Epel, E., Gruenewald, T., Karlamangla, A., & McEwen, B. S. (2010). Socioeconomic differentials in peripheral biology: cumulative allostatic load. *Annals of the New York Academy of Sciences, 1186*, 223–239.

Seniów, J., Litwin, M., Litwin, T., Leśniak, M., & Członkowska, A. (2009). New approach to the rehabilitation of post-stroke focal cognitive syndrome: effect of levodopa combined with speech and language therapy on functional recovery from aphasia. *Journal of the Neurological Sciences, 283*(1), 214–218.

Shahripour, R. B., & Donnan, G. A. (2014). The long-term management of stroke. In B. Norrving (Ed.), *Oxford textbook of stroke and cerebrovascular disease*. Oxford, UK: Oxford University Press.

Sharpe, M., Hawton, K., House, A., Molyneux, A., Sandercock, P., Bamford, J., & Warlow, C. (1990). Mood disorders in long-term survivors of stroke: associations with brain lesion location and volume. *Psychological Medicine, 20*(4), 815–828.

Sharpe, M., Hawton, K., Seagroatt, V., Bamford, J., House, A., Molyneux, A., ... Warlow, C. (1994). Depressive disorders in long-term survivors of stroke. Associations with demographic and social factors, functional status, and brain lesion volume. *The British Journal of Psychiatry, 164*, 380–386.

Shill, M. (1979). Motivational factors in aphasia therapy: research suggestions. *Journal of Communication Disorders, 12*, 503–517.

Shimoda, K., & Robinson, R. G. (1998). Effect of anxiety disorder on impairment and recovery from stroke. *The Journal of Neuropsychiatry and Clinical Neurosciences, 10*, 34–40.

Shisler Marshall, R., Basilakos, A., Williams, T., & Love-Myers, K. (2014). Exploring the benefits of unilateral nostril breathing practice post-stroke: attention, language, spatial abilities, depression, and anxiety. *The Journal of Alternative and Complementary Medicine, 20*(3), 185–194.

Silton, R. L., Heller, W., Engels, A. S., Towers, D. N., Spielberg, J. M., Edgar, J. C., ... Miller, G. A. (2011). Depression and anxious apprehension distinguish frontocingulate cortical activity during top-down attentional control. *Journal of Abnormal Psychology, 120*, 272–285.

Singh, A., Black, S. E., Hermann, N., Leibovitch, F. S., Ebert, P. L., Lawrence, J., & Szalai, J. P. (2000). Functional and neuroanatomical correlations in post stroke depression: the Sunnybrook Stroke Study. *Stroke, 31*, 637–644.

Sinyor, D., Amato, P., Kaloupek, D. G., Becker, R., Goldenberg, M., & Coopersmith, H. (1986). Post-stroke depression: relationships to functional impairment, coping strategies, and rehabilitation outcome. *Stroke, 17,* 1102–1107.

Sinyor, D., Jacques, P., Kaloupek, D. G., Becker, R., Goldenberg, M., & Coopersmith, H. (1986). Poststroke depression and lesion location: an attempted replication. *Brain, 109*(3), 537–546.

Skelly, M. (1975). Re-thinking stroke: aphasia patients talk back. *American Journal of Nursing, 75*(7), 1140–1142.

Small, S., & Llano, D. (2009). Biological approaches to aphasia treatment. *Current Neurology and Neuroscience Reports, 9*(6), 443–450.

Snyder, H. R. (2013). Major depressive disorder is associated with broad impairments on neuropsychological measures of executive function: a meta-analysis and review. *Psychological Bulletin, 139,* 81–132.

Solomonovici, A., Fradis, A., Mixaliescu, L., & Sevastopol, M. (1962). Tratamental cu imipramine in afaziile de origine vasulara. *Studii si Cercetari de Neurologie, 7,* 257–263.

Spalletta, G., Bossu, P., Ciaramella, A., Bria, P., Caltagirone, C., & Robinson, R. G. (2006). The etiology of poststroke depression: a review of the literature and a new hypothesis involving inflammatory cytokines. *Molecular Psychiatry, 11*(11), 984–991.

Spencer, K. A., Tompkins, C. A., & Schulz, R. (1997). Assessment of depression in patients with brain pathology: the case of stroke. *Psychological Bulletin, 122*(2), 132.

Spielberg, J. M., Miller, G. A., Warren, S. L., Engels, A. S., Crocker, L. D., Banich M. T., … Heller, W. (2012a). A brain network instantiating approach and avoidance motivation. *Psychophysiology, 49*(9), 1200–1214.

Spielberg, J. M., Miller, G. A., Warren, S. L., Engels, A. S., Crocker, L. D., Sutton, B. P., & Heller, W. (2012b). Trait motivation moderates neural activation associated with goal pursuit. *Cognitive, Affective, & Behavioral Neuroscience, 12,* 308–322.

Starkstein, S. E., & Robinson, R. G. (1988). Aphasia and depression. *Aphasiology, 2*(1), 1–20.

Starkstein, S. E., Cohen, B. S., Fedoroff, P., Parikh, P., Price, T. R., & Robinson, R. G. (1990). Relationship between anxiety disorders and depressive disorders in patients with cerebrovascular injury. *Archives of General Psychiatry, 47*(3), 246–251.

Starkstein, S. E., Fedoroff, J. P., Price, T. R., Leiguarda, R., & Robinson, R. G. (1993). Catastrophic reaction after cerebrovascular lesions: frequency, correlates, and validation of a scale. *Journal of Neuropsychiatry & Clinical Neurosciences, 5,* 189–194.

Stern, R. A. (1999). Assessment of mood states in aphasia. *Seminars in Speech & Language, 20,* 33–51.

Stone, A. A., Schwartz, J. E., Smyth, J., Kirschbaum, C., Cohen, S., Hellhammer, D., & Grossman, S. (2001). Individual differences in the diurnal cycle of salivary free cortisol: a replication of flattened cycles for some individuals. *Psychoneuroendocrinology, 26*(3), 295–306.

Swindell, C. S., & Hammons, J. (1988). Poststroke depression: neurologic, physiologic, diagnostic, and treatment implications. *Journal of Speech, Language, and Hearing Research, 34,* 325–333.

Tanaka, Y., Albert, M. L., Hujita, F., Nonaka, C., & Oka T. (2006). Beta-blocker improves language output in aphasia. Presented at American Neurological Association 131th Annual Meeting; Chicago.

Tanaka, Y., Albert, M. L., Fujita, K., Nonaka, C., Miyazaki, M., & Yokoyama, E. (2009). Autonomic nervous system and aphasia. Presented at the Neurobiology of Language Conference; Chicago.

Tanaka, Y., Cahana-Amitay, D., Albert, M., Fujita, K., Chieko, N., & Miyazaki, M. (2010). Treatment of anxiety in aphasia. *Procedia-Social and Behavioral Sciences, 6*, 252–253.

Tang, L., Ge, Y., Sodickson, D. K., Miles, L., Zhou, Y., Reaume, J., & Grossman, R. I. (2011). Thalamic resting-state functional networks: disruption in patients with mild traumatic brain injury. *Radiology, 260*(3), 831–840.

Tanner, D. (2003). Eclectic perspectives on the psychology of aphasia. *Journal of Allied Health, 32*(4), 256–260.

Tanner, D. C., & Gerstenberger, D. L. (1988). The grief response in neuropathologies of speech and language. *Aphasiology, 2*(1), 79–84.

Taylor Sarno, M. (1993). Aphasia rehabilitation: psychological and ethical considerations. *Aphasiology, 7*, 321–334.

Terroni, L., Amaro, E., Iosifescu, D. V., Tinone, G., Sato, J. R., Leite, C. C., ... Fráguas, R. (2011). Stroke lesion in cortical neural circuits and post-stroke incidence of major depressive episode: a 4-month prospective study. *The World Journal of Biological Psychiatry, 12*(7), 539–548.

Thayer, J. F., Hansen, A. L., Saus-Rose, E., & Johnson, B. H. (2009). Heart rate variability, prefrontal neural function, and cognitive performance: the neurovisceral integration perspective on self-regulation, adaptation, and health. *Annals of Behavioral Medicine, 37*(2), 141–153.

Thomas, S. A., & Lincoln, N. B. (2006). Factors relating to depression after stroke. *The British Journal of Clinical Psychology, 45*(Pt1), 49–61.

Thomas, S. A., & Lincoln, N. B. (2008). Predictors of emotional distress after stroke. *Stroke, 39*, 1240–1245.

Thomas, S. A., Walker, M. F., Macniven, J. A., Haworth, H., & Lincoln, N. B. (2012). Communication and Low Mood (CALM): a randomized controlled trial of behavioural therapy for stroke patients with aphasia. *Clinical Rehabilitation, 27*(5), 398–408.

Thompson, C., Hall, H., & Sison, C. (1986). Effects of hypnosis on imagery training on naming behavior in aphasia. *Brain & Language, 28*, 141–153.

Thompson-Schill, S. L., D'Esposito, M., & Kan, I. P. (1999). Effects of repetition and competition on activity in the left prefrontal cortex during word generation. *Neuron, 23*, 513–522.

Townend, B. S., Whyte, S., Desborough, T., Crimmins, D., Markus, R., Levi, C., & Sturm, J. W. (2007). Longitudinal prevalence and determinants of early mood disorder post-stroke. *Journal of Clinical Neuroscience, 14*, 429–434

Townend, E., Brady, M., & McLaughlan, K. (2007a). A systematic evaluation of the adaptation of depression diagnostic methods for stroke survivors who have aphasia. *Stroke, 38*, 3076–3083.

Tucker, D. M. (1981). Lateral brain function, emotion, and conceptualization. *Psychological Bulletin, 89*(1), 19–46.

Vataja, R., Leppävuori, A., Pohjasvaara, T., Mäntylä, R., Aronen, H. J., Salonen, O., ... Erkinjuntti, T. (2004). Poststroke depression and lesion location revisited. *Journal of Neuropsychiatry and Clinical Neurosciences, 16*(2), 156–162.

Voinescu, I., & Gheorghita, N. (1978). Adjuvant drug therapy with psychologopedic rehabilitation of aphasic patients. *Neurologie et Psychiatrie, 16*(3), 155–161.

Votruba, K. L., Rapport, L. J., Whitman, R. D., Johnson, A., & Langenecker, S. (2013). Personality differences among patients with chronic aphasia predict improvement in speech-language therapy. *Topics in Stroke Rehabilitation, 20*(5), 421–431.

Wager, T. D., Barrett, L. F., Bliss-Moreau, E., Lindquist, K., Duncan, S., Kober, H., ... Mize, J. (2008). The neuoimaging of emotion. In M. Lewis, J. M. Haviland-Jones, & L. F. Barrett, (Eds.), *Handbook of emotion* (pp. 249–227). New York: Guilford.

Währborg, P. (1991). *Assessment & management of emotional reactions to brain damage & aphasia*. San Diego, CA: Singular.

Weber, C. M., & Smith, A. (1990). Autonomic correlates of stuttering and speech assessed in a range of experimental tasks. *Journal of Speech and Hearing Research, 33*, 690–706.

Wepman, J. M. (1951). *Recovery from aphasia*. New York: Ronald.

Wepman, J. M. (1953). A conceptual model for the processes involved in recovery from aphasia. *Journal of Speech and Hearing Disorders, 18*, 4–13.

Williams, J.M.G., Watts, F. N., MacLeod, C., & Mathews, A. (1997). *Cognitive psychology and emotional disorders* (2nd ed.). Chichester, UK: Wiley.

Williams, P. G., Suchy, Y., & Rau, H. K. (2009). Individual differences in executive functioning: implications for stress regulation. *Annals of Behavioral Medicine, 37*(2), 126–140.

Williams, R. A., Hagerty, B. M., Cimprich, B., Therrien, B., Bay, E., & Oe, H. (2000). Changes in directed attention and short-term memory in depression. *Journal of Psychiatric Research, 34*(3), 227–238.

Yamasaki, H., LaBar, K. S., & McCarthy, G. (2002). Dissociable prefrontal brain systems for attention and emotion. *Proceedings of the National Academy of Sciences, 99*(17), 11447–11451.

Yee, C. M. (1995). Implications of the resource allocation model for mood disorders. In G. A. Miller (Ed.), *The behavioral high-risk paradigm in psychopathology* (pp. 271–288). New York: Springer.

Yerkes, R. M., & Dodson, J. D. (1908). The relation of strength of stimulus to rapidity of habit formation. *Journal of Comparative Neurology and Psychology, 18*(5), 459–482.

Yesavage, J. A. (1984). Relaxation and memory training in 39 elderly patients. *American Journal of Psychiatry, 141*(6), 778–781.

Yu, L., Liu, C. K., Chen, J. W., Wang, S. Y., Wu, Y. H., & Yu, S. H. (2004). Relationship between post-stroke depression and lesion location: a meta-analysis. *The Kaohsiung Journal of Medical Sciences, 20*(8), 372–380.

Zhanjun, Z. (1989). Efficacy of acupuncture in the treatment of post stroke aphasia. *Journal of Traditional Chinese Medicine, 9*(2), 87–89.

Zraik, R. L. & Boone, D. R. (1991). Spouse attitude toward the person with aphasia. *Journal of Speech and Hearing Research, 34*, 123–128.

7

Praxis in Recovery from Aphasia

Introduction

In this chapter we wish to add a new piece to the neural multifunctionality edifice we have been carefully assembling here, which points to a language system subserved by intricately connected neural networks that jointly mediate multiple cognitive and emotional functions, all of which play a role in the recovery of language functions in aphasia. Specifically we will consider the extent to which voluntary control of motor systems, termed in the literature *praxis*, contributes to the neural and behavioral changes associated with the recovery of language functions in aphasia. The motivation for this exploration is anchored in the simple but well-established observation that persons with aphasia often exhibit disruption of motor functions—*apraxia*—which interferes with interpretation and/or execution of intended actions (e.g., Arbib, 2006; Buxbaum & Kalenine, 2010; Buxbaum, Kyle, & Menon, 2005; Cubelli, Marchetti, Boscolo, & Della Sala, 2000; De Renzi & Luchelli, 1988; Duffy & Duffy, 1981; Fazio et al., 2009; Feyereisen & Seron, 1982; Gainotti & Lemmo, 1976; Geschwind, 1965; Hickok & Peoppel, 2000; Heilman & Rothi, 1997; 2003; Heilman, Rothi, & Valenstein, 1982; Iacoboni & Wilson, 2006; Kertesz & Hooper, 1982; Kimura & Archibald, 1974; Kobayashi & Ugawa, 2013; Liepmann, 1908; Pazzaglia, Smania, Corato, & Aglioti, 2008; Papagano, Della Salla, & Basso, 1993; Roy & Square, 1985; Saygin, Wilson, Dronkers, & Bates, 2004; Tranel, Kemmerer, Adolphs, Damasio, & Damasio, 2003; Wang & Goodglass, 1992).

Much like the other nonlinguistic domains discussed in previous chapters, the question of whether deficits in praxis are independent of or integral to the language impairments observed in aphasia remains a matter of debate (Roby-Brami, Hermsdörfer, Roy, & Jacobs, 2012). Papagano, Della Salla, and Basso (1993), for example, demonstrated a double dissociation between aphasia and apraxia, lending support to the notion that their co-occurrence is merely a result of their shared arterial blood supply. Others have argued for an opposite view, whereby language and praxis share the same neuroanatomical-functional organization and that the occurrence of deficits in one or both simply reflects natural interindividual variability in brain structure and function (Iacoboni & Wilson, 2006). Other proposals have suggested tying both functions through different mechanisms, including, for example, a global communicative or semantic system (Duffy & Duffy, 1981) or a left hemisphere-based control of complex sequencing (Feyereisen & Seron, 1982; Kimura, 1977; Kimura & Archibald, 1974; Kobayashi & Ugawa, 2013). Regardless of the exact characteristics of these proposals, cumulative evidence suggests that the neural correlates of language and praxis are strongly left-lateralized and that they intersect in certain important ways, at least among some persons with aphasia (Roby-Brami et al., 2012).

Although most observations about the relationship between language and praxis have been based on analyses of their dysfunction in the brain, we first review evidence of their interdependencies in the intact brain, using findings from healthy adults and in some cases from animal studies. We describe the putative link among action recognition, repetition, imitation, gestural communication, and vocalizations; these are commonly observed in motor learning (e.g., Bradshaw & Nettleton, 1982; Corballis, 2003; Steele & Uomini, 2009), which has fueled the call to integrate systems of motor control and language in the brain (e.g., Gentilucci & Dalla Volta, 2008; Roby-Brami et al., 2012; Steele, Ferrari, & Fogassi, 2012). Specifically, we introduce the debate surrounding the idea that mirror neurons serve as the neural foundation upon which action and language are integrated in the brain (e.g., Arbib, 2010; Hickok, 2009; Pulvelmüller & Fadiga, 2010).

We then describe deficits associated with praxis, most commonly known as apraxia, and their neurobehavioral manifestations among persons with aphasia. Specifically we present evidence that speaks to the disruption of pantomiming (Buxbaum et al., 2005), tool use (Goldenberg & Spatt, 2009), gesture imitation and recognition (Buxbaum et al., 2005; Ochipa, Rothi, & Heilman, 1994), and utilization of the conceptual knowledge underlying actions and tools (Buxbaum & Saffran, 2002; Buxbaum, Vermonti, & Schwartz, 2000; De Renzi & Luchelli, 1988; Myung et al., 2010) in apraxia. We discuss theoretical accounts that have proposed to liken these deficits to aphasic language impairments and consider whether these presumed similarities reflect damage to a shared left-lateralized neural system (Binder et al., 1997; De Renzi, 1989; Goodglass & Kaplan, 1963; Heilman and Rothi, 1997; 2003; Kertesz & Ferro, 1984; Kertesz, Ferro, & Shewan, 1984; Kobayashi & Ugawa, 2013; Papagno, Della Sala, & Basso, 1993). Drawing on research addressing both semantic and conceptual knowledge, we will show that contemporary accounts of impaired voluntary control of movement indicate that the neural substrates underlying praxis and language in aphasia represent the activation of dynamic brain networks in which complex motor and linguistic processes interact, reflecting what we argue to be neural multifunctionality in recovery from aphasia (Buxbaum et al., 2005; Frey, 2008).

We conclude with a consideration of how insights about motor-linguistic integration have been used to guide current practices in aphasia rehabilitation. We present treatment studies that call for combining gesture in aphasia treatment on the assumption that preserved abilities, such as gesture, can serve as crossmodal adjunctive method to reestablish language use through the activation of all available neural networks that support language function (e.g., Rose, 2013). We also analyze the opposing view, which discourages gesture use in aphasia treatment on the assumption that impaired language use in aphasia can be reshaped through strategic, repetitive, intensive learning in which nonuse of nonverbal communication, together with the use of residual language abilities, is thought to behaviorally stimulate neuronal activity in perilesional areas (Berthier & Pulvermüller, 2011). As in previous chapters, we also review neuroimaging findings that attest to treatment-induced neural changes. We close with comments about the relevance of these findings to our concept of neural multifunctionality.

Praxis, Language, and the Brain

We refer to *praxis* as the ability to perform meaningful or coordinated movements under voluntary control (e.g., Arbib, 2006; Kertesz & Hooper, 1982; Schnider, Hanlon, Alexander, & Benson, 1997). Other researchers have ascribed this ability to left hemispheric dominance, as evidenced in studies of pantomime (Buxbaum et al., 2005), tool use (Goldenberg & Spatt, 2009), gesture imitation (Buxbaum et al., 2005; Nelissen et al., 2010; Ochipa et al., 1994), and conceptual knowledge about action and tools (De Renzi & Luchelli, 1988).

The literature on praxis draws a distinction between *simple* and *complex* motor movements, discussed mostly in the context of the study of tool use (recently reviewed in Roby-Brami et al., 2012). These studies suggest that simple tool use, such as using a stick to obtain food, is an extension of limb movement (e.g., Arbib, Bonaiuto, Jacobs, & Frey, 2009; Cardinali et al., 2009) and involves sensorimotor integration in the dorsal stream of visual processing for action control (Frey, 2007; Iriki, Tanaka, & Iwamura, 1996; Jacobs, Danielmeier, & Frey, 2010; Obayashi et al., 2001; Rizzolat & Luppino, 2001; Umilta et al., 2008). Complex tool use, in contrast, reflects a transformation of hand movements into new mechanical actions (Johnson-Frey, 2003), which also requires the use of semantic knowledge about the tool and its functional features (Hodges, Bozeat, Lambon Ralph, Patterson, & Spatt, 2000) and therefore also implicates the ventral stream, mostly neural networks in the left temporal, parietal, and frontal cortices (Johnson-Frey, 2004; Lewis, 2006). These neural networks engage in processes associated with object recognition, semantic storage, contextual information, and the agent's intention, suggesting that praxis and language are intimately intertwined (Creem & Proffitt, 2001; Frey, 2007, 2008; Randerath, Li, Goldenberg, & Hermsdörfer, 2009).

Claims about the interconnectivity of praxis and language systems have emerged in part from studies of the relationship between gesture and language. Behavioral findings point to a reciprocal relationship between the two, with evidence demonstrating effects of arm gestures on sentence comprehension (Glenberg & Kaschak, 2002; Zwaan & Taylor, 2006), as well as effects of action-related semantic knowledge on movement planning (Fischer, 2003; Gentilucci, Benuzzi, Bertolani, Daprati, & Gangitano, 2000; Glover, Rosenbaum, Graham, & Dixon, 2004). In many of these studies, motor control of gesture is construed as an affordance process that helps to determine the availability of an object for future interactions, rendering gesturing a primitive means for expressing communicative meanings (Gentilucci & Dalla Volta, 2008). From a brain perspective, this process involves—based on the goals of the individual and the features of the object—the analysis of an object as a set of affordances within the dorsal stream, its recognition in the ventral stream, and selection of the appropriate affordance in the prefrontal cortex (Arbib, 2006).

The symbolic meaning encoded in manual gestures has been taken by many to reflect an evolutionary path from motor control to language functions, which have converged on shared left-specialized neural circuits (Arbib, 2005, 2006; Corballis, 2002, 2003; Fogassi & Ferrari, 2007; Gentilucci & Corballis, 2006; Hewes, 1973; Rizzolatti & Arbib, 1998). The study of tool use has been particularly instrumental in the development of this point of view, the assumption being that the neural substrates underlying complex gesturing are inseparable from those associated with tool use and establishment of contralateral hand preference (e.g., Bradshaw & Nettleton, 1982; Frey, 2008; Gibson & Ingold, 1993; Roby-Brami et al., 2012). This assumption has been supported by ontogenetic findings from early child development studies, which show that the ability to manipulate complex objects in response to complex commands coincides with development of aspects of grammar mediated by Broca's region (Greenfield, 1991).

Indeed, some researchers have suggested that the principles underlying the behavioral components of complex tool use, especially nested actions, are reminiscent of the hierarchical organization governing language structures, such as sentence embedding (Steele et al., 2012). This view reflects a more general motor approach to language processing according to which the hierarchical, temporal, and spatial organization of praxis (mediating action goals, sequencing, and embodiment of tools) mirrors the organizational principles of language (Arbib, 2010; Pulvermüller & Fadiga, 2010), discussed later in the chapter.

COGNITIVE MECHANISMS UNDERLYING GESTURE-LANGUAGE INTERLINKS

Gentilucci and Dalla Volta (2008) reviewed a series of studies exploring the relationship between gesture and language, all of which seemed to suggest that both functions comprise a unitary communication system. For example, they described an experiment in which the coupling of meaningful and meaningless arm gestures with words has been shown to affect word pronunciation (as measured by pitch and vocal spectra) only when meaningful gestures were performed. The baseline values for the pronunciation measures were obtained from words produced with no accompanying arm gestures in both conditions. Based on these and similar findings, they concluded that the meaning borne by gestures is core and inextricable from mechanisms of speech production.

Several researchers have proposed that gesture and language converge onto "idea units," representing the contribution of two modalities to a single communication system generating a given thought (e.g., Kendon, 1980; McNeill, 1992). In this context, McNeill (1992) proposed a left-to-right gesture continuum (based on Kendon's [1980] earlier classification), which proceeds such that the obligatory production of speech with gesture declines on the one hand and the linguistic properties and social regulation encoded in gestures increase on the other. The progression along the continuum is as follows: (1) gesticulation, or cospeech gestures, in which speech must accompany gesture, as gesture is insufficient to express meaning independently; (2) pantomimes, in which gestures can be combined to express a sentence-like idea and so do not require speech; (3) emblems, in which standard linguistic meaning, such as "thumbs up," is expressed with some degree of gesture regularity, and (4) sign language of the deaf, which is a full-fledged linguistic system. The production of these different gesture types is assumed to rely on distinct but interrelated cognitive processes, where aspects of thought are assumed to be represented through linguistic and/or spatial gestural units (de Ruiter, 2000; Rose, 2013).

However, the precise details of the mechanisms by which gesture and language interact remain underdetermined. There is considerable variability among proposals regarding this presumed interdependence, ranging from gestures as a reflection of levels of arousal in speech (Dittman, 1972), gestures as a marker of communicative intention (Kendon, 1980; McNeill, 1992), gestures as a source of competition for processing resources (Feyereisen, 1997), and gestures as facilitators of word production (e.g., Butterworth & Hadar, 1989; Hadar et al., 1998a; Krauss & Hadar, 1999; Levelt, Richardson, & La Heij, 1985).

An important proposal in this regard is the "lexical gesture" model, which argues that gestures provide ancillary support to language during temporary disruptions (as in cases of word-finding problems) (Hadar et al., 1998b; Krauss & Hadar, 1999). In this model, gesture serves as the imagistic basis upon which conceptualization of a message is formed. The spatial dynamic features of the image are converted into abstract representations of temporospatial properties of movement, which are processed in a motor planner that executes the gesture. The gesture-based features of the concept are thought to prime the lexical features of the target word and thus facilitate its retrieval. This model, however, does not specify the level(s) at which the gestural and word processing interact, although the proposal implies a direct route between gesture and phonological processing (Krauss, Chen, & Grossman, 2000). Despite its underspecificity, this model has served as the basis for some aphasia intervention studies—to which we return later in the chapter—where the contribution of gestures to naming performance has been explored (e.g., Rose, 2013).

There is good evidence that gesturing supports aspects of word production, as restriction of gesturing among healthy adults has been shown to increase dysfluencies for items representing spatial content (Morsella & Krauss, 2004; Rauscher, Krauss, & Chen, 1996) and to decrease successful resolution of tip-of-the-tongue states (Frick & Guttentag, 1998; Pyers et al., 2010). Interestingly, reliance on gesturing during failed lexical retrieval attempts has been linked to performance on tasks assessing auditory working memory, such that persons with poorer auditory memory appear to rely more on gesturing to resolve tip-of-the-tongue situations than those with better auditory memory (Pyers et al., 2010). These findings suggest that the role of gesture in language performance cannot be divorced from additional higher-order cognitive abilities, such as memory, as we would predict in a language system that is neurally multifunctional.

In summary, as Rose (2013) points out, the picture emerging from these various proposals, while incomplete, indicates that gesture and language processing are cognitively linked, both in terms of the meanings they express and in their temporal coordination (Kendon, 1980; Morrel-Samuels & Kraus, 1992). They comprise a multimodal communication system (Kita et al., 2007; McNeill, 2005) that serves to (1) promote the expression of meaning (Melinger & Levelt, 2004), (2) support occasional word-finding difficulties (Krauss et al., 2000), and (3) facilitate thinking for speaking under high processing demands (Kita & Davies, 2009). What these accounts leave unaddressed is the question of how these cognitive mechanisms map onto the brain.

NEURAL MECHANISMS UNDERLYING LANGUAGE-PRAXIS INTERCONNECTIONS

One account of how praxic and linguistic information might be integrated in the brain is the perceptual symbol systems theory, or cognitive embodiment (e.g., Barsalou, 1999). In this framework, the semantic representation of an object is assumed to comprise visual and functional characteristics of the object as well as sound and motor features associated with it. In broader terms, an embodied view of language processing assumes a direct interaction among perceptual, motor, and higher cognitive processes such as language and thought (Jirak, Menz, Buccino, Borghi, & Binkofski, 2010). In such as system, then, perceptual and conceptual processes are presumed to rely on shared neurocognitive mechanisms, where the same neural circuits supporting perception are also recruited for the performance of conceptual tasks. Such a view would explain, for example, why speed of lexical processing is reduced in a lexical decision task only when the target word and its prime share object manipulation features (e.g., "typewriter" and "piano") (e.g., Myung, Blumstein & Sedivy, 2006).

A more extreme stance in an attempt to elucidate the neural underpinnings of praxis-language interconnections is the motor theory of speech perception (Fowler, 1986; Liberman & Mattingly, 1985; Liberman et al., 1967). In this framework, the neural foundation for processing speech sounds rests on motor representations underlying speech gestures rather than on auditory representations. Although one would be hard pressed to find proponents for this view in its strongest form, over the years it has sparked an intense interest in the exploration of the neural correlates of these presumed praxis-language links.

Proposals inspired by the motor theory of speech perception proliferated with the discovery of *mirror neurons* (Arbib, 2005, 2006; Fogassi & Ferrari, 2007; Fogassi & Lupino, 2005; Rizzolatti & Arbib, 1998; Rizzolatti & Craighero, 2004). In both animal and human studies, mirror neurons have been found to activate the same motor substrates during the execution *and* perception of an action (e.g., grasping), engaging in a process of "action understanding." However, as Hickok (2009) points out, the literature has been unclear about what this process exactly involves. Notions such as action recognition, action differentiation, internal description of action, appropriate action selection, and assessment of action outcome have all been invoked to define the process (Hickok, 2009). At present, although a uniform definition has yet to be proposed, many studies have attempted to capture the idea that an observed action serves as the foundation for the planning of future behaviors.

In studies on macaques, action understanding has been argued to implicate mirror neurons in the ventral premotor area and the inferior parietal lobule, also known as the F5 region (Arbib, 2005; Gallese, Fadiga, Fogassi, & Rizzolatti, 1996; Rizzolatti, Fadiga, Gallese, & Fogassi, 1996). In human studies, these neurons have been identified in brain structures within the left frontoparietal network, especially Brodmann's area (BA) 44 (e.g., Buccino et al., 2001; Fogassi et al., 2005; Rozzi, Ferrari, Bonini, Rizzolatti, & Fogassi, 2008) and the ventral premotor cortex BA 6 (Morin & Grezes, 2008). The exploration of how mirror neurons give rise to praxis-language interlinks in humans is rooted in the homology between the premotor macaque F5 and human Broca's speech area (Arbib, 2006; Rizzolatti & Arbib, 1998). In what follows, we will focus on findings concerning the human brain.

Specifically in humans, the left parietal and premotor structures have been found to be activated during observations of transitive actions, which refer to movements directed towards an object, and intransitive actions, which reflect internally generated communicative gestures (Bohlhalter et al., 2009; Buccino et al., 2001, 2004; Johnson-Frey, Funnell, Gerry, & Gazzaniga, 2005; Hermsdörfer, Terlinden, Mühlau, Goldenberg, & Wohlschläger, 2007). For example, in a neuroimaging study of healthy adults, Bohlhalter and colleagues (2009) compared patterns of neural activation in response to pantomiming transitive ("show me X") and intransitive ("wave goodbye") gestures in both hands and found strong activation of the left premotor cortex for intransitive gestures regardless of which hand performed the action. They attributed this pattern to the communicative meaning typically expressed by this class of gestures.

Thus mirror neurons have been argued to mediate action understanding by matching action execution with observation, reflecting a rudimentary communication mechanism

(Fadiga et al., 1995; Rizzolatti, Fogassi, & Gallese, 2001). Pulvelmüller & Fadiga (2010) have proposed that mirror neurons represent an intention-driven system harnessing motor regions in service of language perception at the neuronal level. In this system, the motor regions match stimulus features with the actions that give rise to these features; they feed this information into the auditory cortex through the arcuate fasciculus to augment the perceptual saliency of the sensory stimulus. Their proposal fits nicely with Iacoboni and Wilson's (2006) ideas about the neural underpinnings of imitation, according to which Broca's area mediates action goals, the superior temporal lobe supports higher-order descriptions of the percept, and the inferior parietal lobe subserves somatosensory feedback. From an evolutionary perspective, then, the mirror neuron system provides a potential mechanism for understanding the transition from processing of primitive gestural communication via gesture recognition and imitation to action understanding through language (Arbib, 2010; Roby-Brami et al., 2012).

Importantly, Arbib (2010) has pointed out that action understanding cannot be strictly reliant on activation mirror neurons, as evidenced, for example, in the differences in neural activation of the inferior frontal gyrus in response to a video of a person moving his lips as if he were speaking, a monkey smacking his lips, and a dog barking (Buccino et al., 2004). Assuming that the participants understood all three actions, the contribution of mirror neurons was observed only for the human lip-reading and monkey lip-smacking actions. Thus Arbib (2010) suggested assigning a complementary role for mirror neurons in action understanding, which are embedded in an integrated system of dorsal and ventral neural pathways and regard words as articulatory actions independent of their meanings. In this system, perceptual schemas are processed in the dorsal pathway in relation to motor schemas for motor control while the ventral pathway mediates planning and decision making. The execution of the intended action relies on the variables defined in the dorsal pathway.

Indeed, the neural basis of motor speech perception has been associated with neural networks known to mediate language functions—for example, in a neuroimaging study of healthy adults by Fridriksson et al. (2008), who explored whether observation of speech movements (nonsense syllables) and nonspeech motor movements (of tongue, cheek, and lip) differentially activated cortical regions associated with speech functions. They found that speech movements activated frontal and temporal regions, whereas nonspeech movements engaged parietal regions, concluding that frontal brain regions play a crucial role in language-based action perception. These findings are consistent with related reports of an association between neural activation of Broca's area during lip reading (Calvert, Campbell, & Brammer, 2000; Campbell et al., 2001; Hall, Fussell, & Summerfield, 2005).

Several neuroimaging and transcranial magnetic stimulation (TMS)studies in healthy adults have reported specific patterns of motor activation in frontal brain structures during the processing of different types of linguistic information (e.g., Fogassi & Ferrari, 2007; Gentilucci & Corballis, 2006; Pulvelmüller & Fadiga, 2010; Rizzolatti &

Craighero, 2004). For example, a functional neuroimaging study of healthy adults engaged in movement of articulators to produce the speech sounds *t* and *p*, silent articulation of syllables containing these sounds, and listening to these syllables demonstrated across-task activation of tongue and lip motor regions (e.g., Fadiga, Fogassi, Pavesi, & Rizzolatti, 1995; Pulvelmüller, 2006). Relatedly, application of TMS to tongue and lip regions among healthy adults affected their phoneme discrimination abilities when phoneme-consonant syllables were presented against background noise, enhancing the identification of tongue sounds but slowing down recognition of lip sounds (D'Ausillio et al., 2009).

However, some neuroimaging studies comparing cortical responses to speech and nonspeech sounds have failed to reveal differential patterns of brain activation within the motor cortex associated with different sound types (Scott, McGettigan, & Eisner, 2009). Specifically, across 12 studies, no differences in peak neural activations within the left primary motor, supplementary motor, and premotor areas were found in response to speech sounds, distorted speech, emotional vocalizations, singing, animal vocalizations, tool sounds, sounds based on human actions, and music. Note that these findings may reflect methodological differences in neuroimaging techniques or acoustic measures rather than dispute the role of motor pathways in processing of speech sounds.

An example from the semantic system includes a study of healthy adults in whom neural activation of the same somatotopic areas in the premotor and motor cortices was observed during comprehension of action-related words referring to face, arm, leg, and movement of the related body parts (e.g., Hauk, Johnsrude, & Pulvelmüller, 2004). Comparable activation patterns were observed in a similar study in which the action words were presented in a sentential context (Tettamanti et al., 2005). Motor activation in response to lexical processing of such category-specific information has been found to be predominantly left-lateralized in frontal brain regions, as sham application of TMS to right hemisphere hand and leg areas failed to affect speed of processing of arm and leg words (Pulvermüller, Hauk, Nikulin, & Ilmoniemi, 2005). Some have argued, however, that the recruitment of neural regions to process category-specific semantic information is not unique to the motor cortex (Scott et al., 2009); such differentiation has been reported for neural activation of visual association areas in response to high- versus low-imageability words (Fiebach & Friederici, 2004; Wise et al., 2000).

Findings regarding the involvement of motor circuits in syntactic processing appear to be somewhat less clear (Arbib, 2006; Fiebach & Schubotz, 2006; Roy & Arbib, 2005). The underlying assumption in these studies is that the neural representation for syntactic processing has evolved from brain mechanisms that support intention-based action sequencing (Fogassi & Ferrari, 2007; Greenfield, 1991). Specifically, some have proposed that BA 44 mediates a domain-general function of hierarchical structuring, which, for actions, has emerged from earlier premotor functions of action control and action recognition (Pulvelmüller & Fadiga, 2010). Yet although neuroimaging studies of the healthy brain have demonstrated that Broca's area is associated with local syntactic computations (Fiebach & Schubotz, 2006; Friederici, 2006; see also Chapter 2) and although TMS studies of the healthy brain have shown that inhibition of BA 44 interferes with action sequencing (Clerget, Winderickx, Fadiga, & Olivier, 2009), evidence directly relating these two function has been based primarily on findings from persons with aphasia (Fazio et al., 2009).

A strong position against the idea that mirror neurons are involved in action understanding has been voiced in several publication, by Hickok and collaborators (Hickok, 2009, 2010; Lotto, Hickok, & Holt, 2008; Toni, de Lange, Noordzij, & Hagoort, 2008). The main criticisms point to several theoretical and empirical fallacies that have emerged from the animal, human, and clinical literature upon which this framework was founded. These include: (1) multiple definitions of the term action understanding, which we briefly mentioned earlier, (2) the not so clear-cut brain regions in which mirror neurons have been found in monkey brains, (3) mixed findings about the involvement of mirror neurons in action understanding among monkeys, (4) the accomplishment of action understanding via other types of neurons, (5) the degree to which the mirror neuron system can be generalized to the human brain, and (6) the questionable empirical validity of extending this system to the domain of speech perception. Moreover, Hickok and his collaborators note documented dissociations between action perception and action execution in clinical populations, as well as cases in which brain damage in the human homologues of the macaque F5 (i.e., BA 44/6) did not result in the expected behavioral patterns. We will return to this issue shortly, when we discuss the neuroanatomical correlates of apraxia among persons with aphasia. The ventral-dorsal speech perception model proposed by Hickok and Peoppel (2007), introduced in Chapter 2, continues to lead the pursuit of an alternative to the mirror neuron system.

A possible role for mirror neurons in action understanding was proposed by Mahon & Caramazza (2008) in their discussion of the framework of embodied cognition. Specifically they proposed that action-based concepts have an abstract representation that is independent of the sensorimotor systems. The activation of these abstract representations is sufficient for action recognition. Understanding the concept "basketball playing" does not require prior experience of playing the game. But when coupled with sensorimotor knowledge, such an abstract representation is enriched and even altered via specific sensorimotor associations within a relational context. The notion of basketball playing can be reshaped after attending a tournament or following participation in a basketball clinic, for example. Such sensorimotor knowledge also allows the prediction of subsequent actions and thus may influence action recognition from a top-down perspective. This proposal is reconcilable with Jirak et al.'s (2010) meta-analysis of neuroimaging studies of embodiment theory, in which language processing has been associated with activation of primary motor, supplementary motor, and premotor cortices. In addition, it has important clinical implications, as it suggests a certain degree of malleability in the mechanisms underlying action understanding that likely play a role in aphasia rehabilitation settings, as we discuss later in this chapter.

The controversy surrounding the involvement of motor circuits in speech perception has encouraged some researchers to consider a new role for the motor cortex in language processing—one that is not strictly associated with action understanding. For example, Scott, McGettigan, and Eisner (2009) have proposed that motor regions support the temporal coordination of turn-taking in conversation. Their proposal is based on the observation that people engage in what is known as *interactional synchrony*—in which unintentional action, posture, and gesture coordination is performed jointly by discourse participants (Condon & Ogston, 1967)—alongside alignment of conceptual and syntactic structures among participants (Garrod & Pickering, 2004; Pickering & Garrod, 2007). In this system, then, as the temporal lobe and its associated networks process acoustic and linguistic information to support the meaning of what is being said, the motor system engages in tracking speech rate and rhythm, including aspects of interactional synchrony. The latter include the listener's entrainment to the speech rate of the speaker at the level of the syllable so as to time subsequent output accurately. This hypothesis is appealing, but as the authors themselves point out, no neuroscientific evidence is currently available to support it.

Note that Scott, McGettigan, and Eisner (2009) suggest that the motor processing of synchronicity and timing is most likely also observed in domains other than language, as fMRI studies demonstrate sensorimotor activation in response to nonverbal noises of emotion, such as laughter (Warren et al., 2006) or music (Scott, 1998). Indeed, emotional meaning has been found to have an effect on rate of gesture recognition, with positive emotional primes (happy faces) slowing down recognition rate of open versus closed hand postures and those involving negative emotions (angry faces) showing the opposite pattern (slowing down of closed hand gestures) (Vicario & Newman, 2013). In addition, evidence for the integration of emotional, motor, and linguistic information has been found in a study using MRI, where the presentation of abstract emotional words, such as *dread*, but not of emotionally neutral items activated precentral cortical regions that typically respond to face and arm words (Mosely, Carota, Hauk, Mohr, & Pulvermüller, 2012). The authors interpreted this finding as evidence for dorsally mediated semantic binding of meanings associated with body-internal states. Once again we are witness to neural interconnectedness, which speaks to the need to assume a brain system that is multifunctional in nature.

Apraxia and Aphasia: Behavioral and Neural Correlates

Praxis that is impaired because of brain damage, better known as *apraxia*, involves an inability to execute and/or interpret purposeful skilled movements in the presence of preserved spontaneous mobility and normal comprehension of language (e.g., De Renzi, 1989; De Renzi Motti, & Nichelli, 1980; Goldenberg, 2009; Heilman and Rothi; 1997, 2003; Liepmann, 1920; Steinhal, 1871). Disrupted praxic functions may include poor pantomiming (Buxbaum et al., 2005), impaired tool use (Goldenberg & Spatt, 2009), incorrect gesture imitation and recognition (Buxbaum et al., 2005; Ochipa et al., 1994), and difficulties employing conceptual knowledge concerning actions and tools (Buxbaum et al., 2000; Buxbaum & Saffran, 2002; De Renzi & Luchelli, 1988; Myung et al., 2010). Indeed, in clinical assessment, it is not uncommon to see a brain-damaged person handle a knife as if it were a fork, incorrectly pantomime the act of hammering, or fail to imitate a salute.

However, despite the frequent occurrence of apraxia after stroke, the figures regarding its prevalence remain vague (Zwinkels, Geusgens, van de Sande, & van Heugten, 2004). Part of the problem has to do with the scarcity of standardized tests of the disorder (e.g., van Heugten, Dekker, Deelman, Stehmann-Saris, & Kinebanian, 1999), which is typically assessed through the evaluation of tool-based intransitive ("show me how to use a hammer") and communicative transitive gestures ("salute like a soldier"). Other tests include Schoppe's (1974) battery evaluating aiming, tapping, line following, and steadiness (e.g., Motomura, 1994). The extent to which these tests of apraxia correlate with performance on experimental tasks assessing motor control is unclear, however. For example, De Renzi and Luchelli (1988) showed that performance on tests evaluating tool and object properties through gesture selection and recognition correlated with each other but not with tests assessing ideomotor apraxia. Furthermore, performance on apraxia assessment batteries among persons with aphasia might sometimes be confounded by the presence of comprehension deficits affecting the ability to follow commands (Kobayashi & Ugawa, 2013).

Nonetheless, the observation that left hemisphere damage often leads to difficulties in the voluntary control of motor movements is undisputed (De Renzi et al., 1980; Liepmann, 1920; Steinhal, 1871). Indeed, Heilman and colleagues (1982) convincingly showed that lesions in certain regions of the left parietal lobe—the supramarginal gyrus and underlying white matter of the left parietal lobe—lead to difficulties in both recognizing and performing transitive tool-based gestures. Others have identified damage to Broca's region as a primary cause of apraxia of speech (Bates et al., 2003; Bonilha, Moser, Rorden, Baylis, & Fridriksson, 2006; Dronkers, 1996; Hillis et al., 2004; Ogar, Slama, Dronkers, Amici, & Gorno-Tempini, 2005; Schmid & Ziegler, 2006). These patterns do not suggest that the right hemisphere does not partake in aspects of motor control, whose role has been limited to the processing of concrete, context-dependent familiar movements such as intransitive symbolic gestures (e.g., Heath, Roy, Westwood, & Black, 2001; Rapcsak, Ochipa, Beeson, & Rubens, 1993; Stamenova, Roy, & Black, 2010).

Apraxia and aphasia frequently co-occur (Ajuriaguerra, Hécaen, & Angelergues, 1960; De Renzi et al., 1980), with some findings indicating correlations between the severity of motor disturbance and degree of language deficit (De Renzi, Pieczuro, & Vignolo, 1968; Kertesz & Ferro, 1984). Early work by Gainotti and Lemmo (1976) clearly indicates that some persons with aphasia have trouble recognizing and pantomiming symbolic gestures. In some cases, these difficulties have been taken to reflect a general cognitive disorder of asymbolia, adversely affecting symbol use and sign (e.g., Duffy & Duffy, 1981). However, in a more recent study, Saygin et al. (2004) compared the effects of nonverbal (pictorial) to verbal (written) cues on action recognition among persons with aphasia who showed difficulties primarily with verbal cues, thus challenging the argument of asymbolia as a source of their deficit.

Many have attributed the comorbidity of apraxia and aphasia to the neuroanatomical proximity of the two systems (De Renzi, 1989; Kertesz & Ferro, 1984), but the relationship between them remains, by and large, underdetermined (Kobayashi & Ugawa, 2013). Early work addressing this question suggested that apraxia and aphasia represent two independent neuropsychological syndromes (e.g., Binder et al., 1997; De Renzi, 1989), a claim largely based on the double dissociations reported between the two (e.g., Goodglass & Kaplan, 1963; Kertesz et al., 1984; Papagno et al., 1993). In a large study of 699 brain-damaged individuals with left hemisphere lesions, Papagno and colleagues found that 10 participants had apraxia without aphasia, while 149 had aphasia but not apraxia (Papagno et al., 1993). Additional evidence comes from studies of handedness, in which right-handedness has been associated with aphasia but not with apraxia (Kobayashi & Ugawa, 2013), although some would argue that the picture from the aphasia literature is not clear-cut (e.g., Knecht et al., 2000). Moreover, some symptoms exhibited by persons with apraxia, such as deficient mechanical reasoning, are not shown by persons with aphasia (e.g., Goldenberg & Hagmann, 1998).

However, as we will show below, newer studies indicate that the neural substrates underlying praxis and language in aphasia represent the activation of dynamic brain networks in which complex motor and linguistic processes interact, both drawing on semantic and conceptual knowledge (Buxbaum et al., 2005; Frey, 2008). We do not argue that this activation necessarily reflects the disruption of a unitary mechanism subserving praxic and linguistic functions; rather, we claim that it is indicative of the multifunctional properties of the neural networks implicated in aphasia recovery, evidenced time and again throughout this book.

THEORETICAL ACCOUNTS OF APRAXIA

Liepmann (1920) was the first to systematically relate functions of voluntary motor control with left hemisphere brain structures. He proposed that the left hemisphere in right-handed persons contains "movement formulas," which, when disrupted, can result in distinct behavioral patterns depending on lesion location. For example, he showed that damage to occipitoparietal regions results in impaired execution of complex sequential movements, which he termed *ideational apraxia*. Such poor motor control may involve omissions, transpositions, and/or additions of movements (Kobayashi & Ugawa, 2013).

When brain damage affects more anterior regions spanning parietal sensorimotor cortices, Liepmann (1920) identified deficiency in performance of on-command movements that can otherwise be executed successfully, which he named *ideomotor apraxia*. This type of apraxia is extremely common among persons with aphasia (Helm-Estabrooks, Albert, & Nicholas, 2014), in whom spatiotemporal features of movement—such as amplitude, trajectory, and timing—are often compromised during pantomiming and/ or imitation (Buxbaum, 2001; Koski, Iacoboni, & Mazziotta, 2002). For example, when asked to demonstrate the act of hair brushing, a patient might fail by aiming her hand toward her jaw in spite of routinely brushing her hair every morning.

A subset of persons with apraxia shows differentiation of automatized and voluntary motor control specifically affecting speech muscles (Wertz et al., 1984). This type of apraxia, known as *apraxia of speech*, involves impaired planning and manipulation of speech muscles in service of phoneme production without any muscle weakness during performance of automatic speech movements. The occurrence of apraxia of speech has been noted in developmental studies as well (Dewey, Roy, Square-Storer, & Hayden, 1988). The behavioral patterns observed in apraxia of speech include speech initiation difficulties, poor articulation with increasing word length, simplification of consonant clusters, phonemic substitutions, and highly preserved articulation of automatized speech (Bowman, Hodson, & Simpson, 1980; Johns & Darley, 1970; Wertz, 1985). Interestingly, the sparing of automatic perceptuomotor processing among persons with apraxia has been compared with the preservation of formulaic social expressions commonly observed in nonfluent aphasia (Hillis, 2007).

The presumed parallelism between apraxia and aphasia has inspired some researchers to seek theoretical accounts that might accommodate the behavioral expressions of both disorders. Geschwind (1965), for example, suggested that the behavioral manifestations of apraxia are a consequence of damage to the arcuate fasciculus, which disconnects frontal premotor brain structures and Wernicke's region and leads to impaired pantomiming or poor object use on command, much like the phonological and repetition deficits observed among persons with conduction aphasia (see Chapters 2 and 5).

Within this type of model, then, deficient gestural imitation in apraxia would be likened to impaired verbal repetition in aphasia, both of which derive from damage to the left supramarginal gyrus and planum temporale (Buchsbaum et al., 2011; Fridriksson et al., 2010). Furthermore, the frequent repositioning of the hand in relation to other body parts observed in ideomotor apraxia (Goldenberg & Hagmann, 1997) would be equated with the repeated approximations of correct word pronunciation ("conduite d'approche") typical of conduction of aphasia. A case study reported by Ochipa, Rothi, and Heilman (1994) speaks to the empirical validity of this proposal, as they documented impaired pantomiming of tool use in a person with conduction aphasia associated with a lesion in the inferior parietal lobule. Along these lines, cases of apraxia of speech have been argued to be indistinguishable from the types of speech errors persons with conduction aphasia exhibit (McNeill, Robin, & Schmidt, 2009).

Heilman and Rothi (1997, 2003) proposed an action semantic system model in which they laid out a mechanism that explicitly integrates motor and language processing. Their model consists of several modules with lexical and nonlexical routes. One module is an action input lexicon in which information regarding the physical properties of the perceived action, primarily visual features, is represented. This information is transmitted to an action output lexicon in which information relevant to the action to performed, mostly kinesthetic properties is represented. In addition, a nonlexical module engages visual processing of perceived gestures and enables the imitation of random or novel gestures, allowing for dissociations in patterns of apraxic deficits, such as impaired versus preserved gesture recognition.

Most theoretical models of apraxia draw to some extent on distinctions between *input* and *output* mechanisms. For example, Roy and Square (1985) proposed an action model consisting of two components: (1) a conceptual system, which represents semantic knowledge of tools, objects, and actions, and (2) a production system, which encodes the sensorimotor knowledge of an action and the perceptuomotor information necessary for its planning and execution. The action plan is first defined in the conceptual system based on context-independent knowledge of the semantics of actions and of action sequencing. The production system then implements a motor program that matches the action to the specific context and needs. Within this system, then, damage to the conceptual component would result in ideational apraxia, and disturbance of the production system would lead to ideomotor apraxia. Although this model fails to capture the entire range of apraxic behaviors, it nevertheless does address the potential neurocognitive links between apraxia and aphasia.

The idea that apraxia and aphasia share certain neurobehvioral characteristics, while appealing, is not fully supported by the literature discussing gestural communication in aphasia. Although in some studies impairments in gestural communication and language functions among apraxic persons with aphasia have been found to correlate with one another (Cicone, Wapner, Foldi, Zurif, & Gardner, 1979; McNeill, 1985), in other studies symbolic gesturing has been shown to be spared relative to language abilities, reflecting a possible dissociation between the two (Herrmann et al., 1988; Rousseaux, Daveluy, & Kozlowski, 2010). In fact, the ability to gesture with one or both hands in spontaneous conversation among apraxic persons with aphasia, especially during word-finding pauses, has been taken to reflect a right hemisphere-based compensatory mechanism for lexical retrieval deficits (Foundas et al., 1995).

Because persons with apraxia are typically better at performing communicative gestures (Buxbaum et al., 2007; Mozaz et al., 2002) and because impairment of gestural communication can result from both left and right hemisphere damage (Heath et al., 2001), it has been proposed that examination of transitive tool-based gestures offers a more direct window into the overlap between apraxia and aphasia (Roby-Brami et al., 2012). This idea seems particularly plausible, especially in light of the observation that impaired tool-based gestures and tool-related naming have both been associated with lesions to the left inferior frontal gyrus (e.g., Fazio et al., 2009; Goldenberg et al., 2007). Some have argued, though, that both gesture types represent a hierarchically organized motor system in which transitive gestures are harder to perform than intransitive communicative ones (Buxbaum et al., 2007; Heath et al., 2001; Mozaz et al., 2002), as no double dissociation between these gesture types has been documented among persons with brain damage (Carmo & Rumiati, 2009).

THE ROLE OF FRONTOPARIETAL NETWORKS IN APRAXIA AND APHASIA

It seems, then, that the shared neural foundation of apraxia and aphasia comprises neural networks widely distributed in the left hemisphere, implicating superior temporal, rostral inferior parietal, and ventral premotor cortices (e.g., Hickok & Peoppel, 2000; Johnson-Frey, 2004). In a recent paper, Kobayashi and Ugawa (2013) outlined the ways in which damage to the dorsal and ventral streams might result in parallel apraxic and aphasic behavioral patterns, as shown in Figure 7.1.

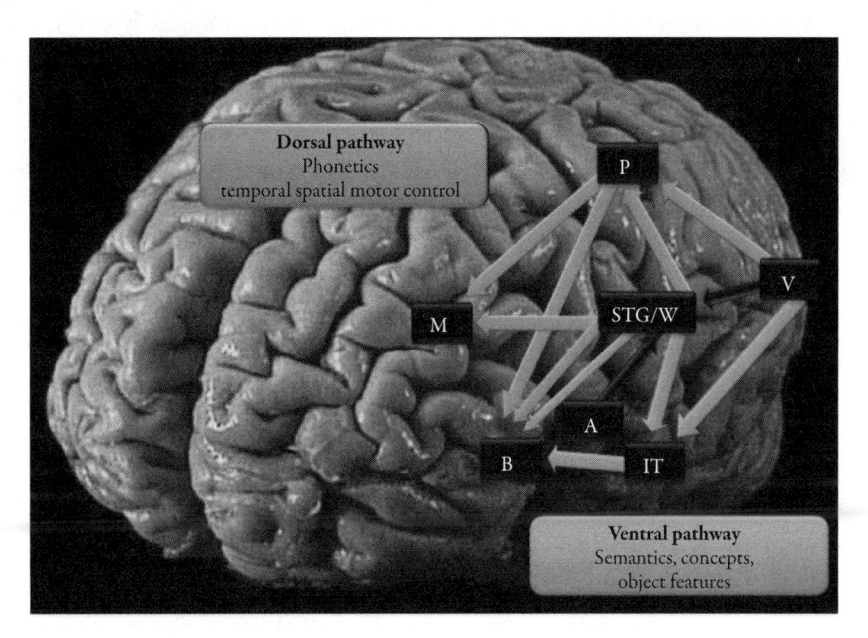

FIGURE 7.1 Neural parallels between apraxia and aphasia. The dorsal route (orange) comprises pathways from the parietal cortex (P) and posterior part of the superior temporal gyrus (STG/W) to the premotor area (M) and to Broca's area (B), connected via the arcuate/superior longitudinal fasciculus. The dorsal route may process phonetic information to produce verbal output without accessing word meaning. Word repetition may rely on this route, as evidenced by the phonemic paraphasia caused by damage to this pathway. The dorsal route may also be involved when guiding the hand to target objects via temporal spatial control combined with visual/tactile feedback. Damage to this route may impair gesture imitation. The ventral route (green) comprises pathways from the superior temporal gyrus (STG/W) to Broca's area (B) via the extreme capsule, and from the anterior part of the superior temporal gyrus (IT) to the frontal operculum via the uncinated fasciculus. Injury to the ventral pathway may result in sensory aphasia. It may also cause apraxia accompanied with difficulties with actual tool use (See color insert.)

A, auditory cortex; M, motor-related areas; V, visual cortex.

Source: From Kobayashi, S., & Ugawa, Y. (2013). Relationships between aphasia and apraxia. *Journal of Neurology and Translational Neuroscience, 2*(1), 1028, Figure 2. Reprinted under the Creative Commons Attribution License.

Findings in support of this functional neuronantomy have emerged from neuroimaging studies exploring observation and imitation of object-related actions among persons with apraxia (Buxbaum et al., 2005; Pazzaglia et al., 2008). In these studies deficient recognition of transitive gestures has been associated with two different neural regions: the left inferior parietal lobe and intraparietal sulcus (Buxbaum et al., 2005) and the left inferior frontal gyrus (Pazzaglia et al., 2008; Saygin et al., 2004; Tranel et al., 2003). Activation patterns in these different regions have been attributed to methodological differences among the tasks administered in these studies, with the tasks activating the parietal structures being more kinematic in nature and those inducing frontal activation requiring assessment of gesture goals. Such goal assessment likely engages other higher-order cognitive abilities, such as executive functions, which are known to be mediated by the same frontal neural structures (as discussed in Chapter 3).

Bringing executive functions into the current discussion is completely in line with our neural multifunctionality view of aphasia recovery. Apraxia, as measured by gesture demonstration (use of key, saw, toothbrush, spoon, hammer, etc.) and gesture imitation (blowing out candles, sticking out tongue, etc.) has indeed been associated with aphasia but also with deficits of memory, attention, and planning as measured by performance on tests such as letter cancellation, Raven's colored progressive matrices, trail making A and B, and the Tower of London (Zwinkles et al., 2004). In fact, some have argued that apraxic functions, measured by cube copying, are predictors of nonverbal abilities in persons with aphasia (Maeshima et al., 2002). The relationship between apraxia and higher-order cognitive abilities has also been considered in cases of apraxia of speech, where planning of the articulation of speech sounds has been associated with reduced memory spans and absence of phonological similarity effects and word length on span (Rochon, Caplan, & Waters, 1991; Waters, Rochon, & Caplan, 1992, see also Chapter 5).

Newer accounts of apraxia touch on this motor-language-cognition-brain interrelatedness more directly. Buxbaum (2001), for example, proposed a model in which gesture processing implicates memory-based sensorimotor representations of familiar gestures stored in the left inferior parietal lobule, where the ventral and dorsal stream meet to support the recognition and production of a given gesture. Roughly speaking, the ventral system, which purportedly houses the lexical semantic system, responds to the verbal command used to invoke the gesture, and the dorsal stream controls the execution of the gesture. This account could explain the selective impairment of voluntary compared with automatic motor processing in apraxia, as damage to the left inferior parietal lobule would interfere with the conceptual knowledge required for executing a command to grasp but would still allow grasping on the basis of physical properties alone. It also fits with the idea that the dorsal-ventral junction subserves the integration of object recognition, semantic storage, contextual information, and the agent's intention, as discussed previously in this chapter (e.g., Frey, 2007, 2008).

Impaired gestural praxis has been argued to involve deficient conceptual representation of skilled movement, in line with the cognitive embodiment framework (Buxbaum &

Saffran, 2002; Buxbaum et al., 2000; Myung et al., 2010). This claim is based on the behavioral observation that persons with apraxia compared with nonapraxic brain-damaged participants perform worse on tasks assessing semantic knowledge of tools, body parts, and object manipulation features (e.g., Buxbaum Saffran, 2002). It is also based on neuroanatomical findings suggesting that the frontoparietal lesions in persons with apraxia implicate the same brain structures associated with conceptual processing of object manipulation in the healthy brain (Boronat et al., 2005; Chao & Martin, 2000; Kellenbach, Brett, & Pattern, 2003).

In their study of apraxic persons, Myung and colleagues (2010) proposed that the motor problems in persons with apraxia reflect an *access deficit* to conceptual representations of skilled movement. They found differences between explicit and implicit processing of object manipulation information that speak to preserved motor knowledge. Specifically, when asked to assess the relationship between pictures of objects on the basis of object manipulation features, their apraxic participants showed systematic difficulties with explicit judgments of object relatedness; in contrast, they were able to use this knowledge during an eye-tracking experiment in which they spent longer times fixating on pictures with shared manipulation features compared to those with unrelated features, much like their nonapraxic counterparts.

THE RELEVANCE OF MIRROR NEURONS TO APHASIA

How do the findings described above tie in with mirror neuron-based theories of language functions? Recall that the mirror neuron framework supposes that Broca's region develops in relation to the mirror neuron system for grasping (e.g., Arbib, 2005), predicting a close relationship between motor disorders of praxis and aphasic language impairment whereby damage to the mirror neuron system would necessarily result in deficient speech perception in aphasia. This prediction, however, has encountered some serious empirical challenges (e.g., Hickok, 2009, 2010). These include findings pointing to (1) double dissociations between gesture production and gesture recognition in aphasia, (2) deficits in action understanding that do not implicate areas BA 44/6 within Broca's region, and (3) preservation of repetition abilities alongside severe comprehension problems in cases of mixed transcortical aphasia (Bougousslavsky et al., 1988; Geschwind et al., 1968), all of which call for the differentiation of speech motor and speech understanding functions.

Rejection of the mirror neuron framework in its strongest form would rule out any motor involvement in mediation of action perception. Thus, for example, although action naming has been found to be more vulnerable to frontal damage than object naming (Hillis, Tuffiash, Wityk, & Barker, 2002; Tranel, Adolphs, Damasio, & Damasio, 2001), this pattern does not seem to carry over to action comprehension (e.g., Hickok, 2009, 2010). A study by Hillis and colleagues demonstrated that in persons with aphasia in whom both action naming and action comprehension were deficient, brain damage also extended to temporal regions, whereas in those with intact action comprehension, lesions involved the precentral gyrus only (Hillis et al., 2002). This finding was confirmed in a later study by Rogalsky et al. (2011), who demonstrated that brain damage to frontoparietal structures spared speech perception among persons with aphasia (as measured by word comprehension and syllable discrimination tasks), while lesions that also involved temporal regions led to poor performance on measures of speech perception. These authors concluded that it was damage within temporal structures rather than deficits to the mirror neuron system that accounted for impaired speech perception.

Nonetheless, involvement of frontal brain structures in action-related deficits (e.g., Kemmerer & Tranel, 2003; Neininger & Pulvermüller, 2003; Saygin et al., 2004; Tranel et al., 2003) may reflect *impaired access* to action knowledge, as Hickok (2010) himself points out. As an example, he cited Saygin et al.'s (2004) study, in which perception of object relatedness was assessed through pictorial and linguistic stimuli, with results demonstrating lack of correlation between performances on both types of stimuli, each being associated with distinct neural substrates. Performance on the nonverbal tasks was correlated with lesions in the inferior frontal gyrus, whereas performance on the verbal tasks involved temporoparietal structures. Hickok concluded that given this modality-specific pattern, frontally mediated impairments in processing action information could not reflect deficits in action knowledge. This argument is reminiscent of the interpretation of apraxia as an access deficit to motor programming mentioned above (Myung et al., 2010) and represents a somewhat weakened objection to the presumption of involvement of mirror neurons in action perception.

The Role of Gesture (or Lack Thereof) in Aphasia Treatment

For approximately 40 years, the notion that arm and hand gestures can augment lexical retrieval in aphasia has guided aphasia rehabilitation practices (e.g., Rao, 1994; Rose, 2006, 2013; Rose et al., 2002; Skelly et al., 1974). Researchers have consistently demonstrated that the inclusion of gesture in aphasia treatment can result in language facilitation as measured, for example, by improved word finding, especially among persons with severe nonfluent aphasia (Code & Gaunt, 1986; Coelho, 1991; Conlon & McNeill, 1991; Hanlon et al., 1990; Hoodin & Thompson, 1983; Pashek, 1997; Ramsberger & Helm-Estabrooks, 1989; Raymer & Thompson, 1991). Thus coupling of gestures with phonologically based naming has been found to result in significant improvements in lexical retrieval among persons with aphasia (Lanyon & Rose, 2009; Pashek, 1997; Raymer & Thompson, 1991; Rose & Douglas, 2001). However, these effects may be sensitive to gesture type. For example, in a study by Rose et al. (2002), the use of iconic gestures but not of pointing, visualization, and cued articulation was associated with improved picture naming in a person with aphasia (enhanced phonological access), with long-term effects lasting up to 3 months, including generalization to novel stimuli in conversation.

Studies that combine gesture with verbal treatment components have been argued to reflect an approach to aphasia intervention focusing on the recruitment of preserved cognitive abilities as *compensatory mechanisms* in the face of language breakdown (Rothi, 1995), in line with Luria's (1972) notion of inter- and intrasystemic reorganization. These treatments harness preserved capacities—such as gesture, drawing, and in some cases reading, and writing—when spoken communication cannot be restored or as a crossmodal adjunct method to reestablish language use (Rose, 2013). Common protocols include promoting aphasics communicative effectiveness (Davis & Wilcox, 1985), copy and recall treatment (Beeson, Rising, & Volk, 2003), drawing treatment (Farias, Davis, & Harrington, 2006; Morgan & Helm-Estabrooks, 1987), gesture treatment (Rose, 2006), and multimodality aphasia treatment (Rose & Attard, 2011).

Some have proposed that these compensatory-based interventions can be more effective in treating persons with aphasia than those methods which target restoration of normal linguistic function (Rothi, 1995). However, findings from a study by Rodriguez, Raymer, and Rothi (2006), who contrasted two interventions representing these different approaches—a compensatory combined gestural/verbal therapy and a semantic-phonological restorative therapy—do not entirely support this claim. This study examined the effects of each method on verb retrieval among four participants and revealed no differences in treatment outcomes. Under both treatment protocols, benefits were observed only for the participant whose naming problems were phonologically based and affected trained verbs only. The authors interpreted these findings as evidence that verb treatment is more affected by the source and severity of naming deficit than by time postonset. The absence of any advantage to gesture-based treatment surprised the authors, who, given the presumed link between the neural networks associated with verb processing and action knowledge, had predicted greater benefits to this method (Druks, 2002). Interestingly, gesture training did lead to improved gesturing in two of the four participants, who had severe limb apraxia, thus augmenting their communicative capacity even in the absence of measurable language gains.

Importantly, not all persons with aphasia respond to treatments incorporating gestures (reviewed in Rose, 2013). Indeed, the efficacy of gesture as a therapeutic modality in aphasia treatment remains controversial. Some have argued that the incorporation of gestures into aphasia therapy discourages the use of verbal communication among patients, thus limiting the extent of their language recovery (Pulvermüller et al., 2001). This claim is supported by findings from studies using "constraint-induced movement therapy," an intervention developed to treat deficits in limb movement among stroke survivors (Taub, 2004). In this method, treatment limits the use of the less affected limb for approximately 90% of the day, intensively training movement of the more affected limb for up to 6 hours per day. The neural basis upon which this method rests is the principle of Hebbian plasticity (1949), according to which repeated coactivation of neurons during learning leads to correlational brain wiring (Kleim & Jones, 2008; see also Chapter 5).

With this rationale in mind, researchers have proposed to incorporate movement constraint into aphasia therapy, resulting in the development of several constraint-based protocols, including constraint-induced aphasia therapy (Pulvermüller et al., 2001), constraint-induced language therapy plus (Meinzer et al., 2005), constraint-induced language therapy (Maher et al., 2006), and intensive language action therapy (Berthier & Pulvermüller, 2011; Pulvermüller & Berthier, 2008). The major elements these protocols have in common include (1) *intensive training* spanning over 30 hours per week over a short period (usually 1 to 2 weeks); (2) *hierarchical response shaping* from simple to complex targets, according to participant's level of performance; (3) *response constraining* to spoken modality only, with explicit discouragement of nonverbal communication; and (4) embedding of language into an *action-based context*. These responses include both participant responses and clinician cues.

In later work, Pulvermüller & Berthier (2008) proposed two additional principles that further characterize constraint-based aphasia therapy; these are specifically grounded in neuroscientific evidence attesting to motor/sensory interdependencies in animals and humans, as described throughout this chapter. The first is the *behavioral relevance principle*, which states that the benefits of language use are maximized in an action-relevant context (i.e., when language use is clearly socially motivated). The second is the *focusing principle*, which speaks to the advantage of learned nonuse, also documented in animal and human motor retraining studies (Taub et al., 2006) where therapeutic gains are assumed to emerge when use of the residual language abilities, especially those that participants avoid, is encouraged.

Note that Pulvermüller and Berthier (2008) do not rule out the use of augmentative methods such as gesturing, but they suggest utilizing them only when participants reach a plateau. Rose (2013) has criticized this position, arguing instead that gestures are a viable primary target of language rehabilitation in aphasia. Specifically, she has proposed a *multimodality principle* according to which language practice affords greatest benefits in rich multimodal contexts that simulate real-life situations, which necessarily include naturally occurring gestures. Indeed, spontaneous gesture production in discourse is quite common among persons with aphasia, more so than among healthy adults (e.g., Ahlsén, 1991; Le May, David, Thomas, 1988; Lott, 1999, Pedelty, 1987; Sekine & Rose, 2013). Quantitative differences have been measured in terms of total number of gestures as well as ratio of gestures per 100 spoken words (e.g., Lott, 1999). Qualitative differences have involved the production of gesture types that seem to be unique to persons with aphasia, including pointing to objects in space, self-pointing, pantomiming, and letter gesturing (e.g., Sekine & Rose, 2013). These findings suggest that limiting gesture use among persons with aphasia might impede their communicative power, especially if gestures serve as ancillary support for lexical retrieval problems. In fact, some studies have demonstrated that training gesture does improve word production in persons with aphasia with deficient lexical retrieval (Caute et al., 2013; Maher et al., 2006; Marshall et al., 2012; Raymer et al., 2012).

Because constraint-based aphasia therapy restricts all interactions with the spoken modality, including cues provided by the clinician, Rose (2013) has also argued that it ignores the role of multimodal cueing in treatment. She maintains that such cueing is designed to activate all available neural networks that previously supported language functions so as to facilitate the reaccessing of linguistic information. Relatedly, the exclusion of nonverbal cues from treatment may limit the potential neural effects of interactional synchrony on enhancement of communicative meaning among codiscourse participants in clinical settings (for related comments, see Ahlsén, 2008). This limitation may explain why constraint-based therapies have failed to show consistent benefits for discourse abilities among persons with aphasia (Attard et al., 2013; Faroqui-Shah & Virion, 2009; Goral & Kempler, 2009; Maher et al., 2006; Szaflarski et al., 2008).

Nonetheless, evidence for the efficacy of constraint-based methods for improving language performance has been demonstrated in several language domains, including content information units, phrase length, confrontation naming, grammatical structure, verb generation in narrative context, and auditory comprehension (Barthel et al., 2008; Cherney et al., 2008; Cherney, Patterson, & Raymer, 2011; Kurland, Baldwin, & Tauer, 2010; Maher et al., 2006; Meinzer et al., 2005, 2008; Pulvermüller et al., 2001, 2005; Pulvermüller & Berthier, 2008; Richter, Miltner, & Straube, 2008; Szaflarski et al., 2008). Pulvermüller and colleagues (2001), for example, compared the effects of standard language therapy to those of constraint-based method on language functions of persons with aphasia; they demonstrated major gains in communicative effectiveness in everyday settings in response to the constraint-based but not the standard intervention. These improvements were measured in terms of scores on standardized language tests, participant self-ratings, and blinded-observer ratings of communicative effectiveness. It is important to note, though, that subsequent studies did not consistently replicate this finding, with considerable variability in responses to treatment (Attard et al., 2013; Breier et al., 2006; Faroqui-Shah, 2009; Szaflarski et al., 2008).

The assumption underlying constraint-based language therapies is that neurologically based language impairment in aphasia can be reshaped through strategic nonuse learning, which behaviorally stimulates neuronal activity in perilesional areas (Berthier & Pulvermüller, 2011). Accordingly, coupling this method with biological interventions that target preserved neural systems, such as pharmacotherapy, has been found to result in significant language gains (Berthier & Pulvermüller, 2011). Specifically, improved performance on standardized language tests, especially on naming tasks, has been observed in studies that combined constraint-induced language therapy with pharmacological interventions targeting glutamatergic neurotransmission. Some drugs (e.g., memantine), for example, are known to enhance processing efficiency of spared neural networks (Berthier & Pulvermüller, 2011; Berthier et al., 2009; Pulvermüller et al.,

2001; Pulvermüller & Berthier, 2008). In some cases, benefits have been documented in post-treatment follow-up (e.g., Berthier et al., 2009).

Recently comparable results have been reported in a study incorporating constraint-based aphasia intervention (CILT) into a transcranial magnetic stimulation (TMS) protocol designed to suppress neural activation in the right pars triangularis (Martin et al., in press). Administration of modified CILT immediately after TMS to two participants with chronic aphasia resulted in significant gains in picture naming and propositional speech at 1 to 2 months postintervention, with naming gains lasting longer (6 months in one participant and 16 months in the other). The authors acknowledge that a larger sham-controlled study would allow one to determine whether it is the TMS, modified CILT, or both that accounts for the results.

Neuroimaging and neurophysiological studies exploring the long-term effects of constraint-based language therapies have revealed that treatment-based neural changes are also observable in chronic stages of aphasia (Breier et al., 2006, 2007, 2009; Meinzer et al., 2004, 2008, 2010; Menke et al., 2009; Pulvermüller et al., 2005). These changes appear both perilesionally and bilaterally. For example, bilateral brain activation in superior temporal cortices, measured through magnetoencephalography, has been found to predict treatment-based language improvement among persons with chronic aphasia (Breier et al., 2006), although long-term effects seem to be left-lateralized (Breier et al., 2009). Relatedly, left-lateralized changes in brain activation, as measured by reduction in slow-wave activity, have been found to be a predictor of degree of treatment success (Meinzer et al., 2004). Based on these observations, Berthier and Pulvermüller (2011) concluded that neural structures in the left hemisphere brain play the critical role in recovery of language functions in aphasia, although the right hemisphere may also contributes to this process secondarily. Furthermore, these findings can be predicted from the action-perception networks, which are considered, by proponents of the mirror neuron framework, to be the basic building blocks of language processing in the brain (Pulvermüller & Berthier, 2008).

In this regard, it is interesting to note that success with constraint-based aphasia therapy has been demonstrated even among aphasic participants with comorbid apraxia of speech (AOS) (Kurland et al., 2012; Maher et al., 2006). Findings from a neuroimaging study of two participants with chronic, moderate-to-severe aphasia and AOS indicate that administration of constraint-induced aphasia therapy, as compared with the protocol promoting aphasics communicative effectiveness, resulted in greater naming speed and accuracy. Naming gains were associated with treatment-based changes in blood oxygenation level dependent (BOLD) activation in perilesional areas, further supporting the thesis of action-perception neural organization.

Others, however, have argued that persons with comorbid aphasia and AOS stand to benefit more from treatment that leverages implicit learning (see Chapter 5), free of overt verbal responses, than from protocols requiring speech production (David, Farias, & Baynes, 2009). Specifically, David and colleagues (2009) showed that covert rehearsal and subvocal articulation during tasks involving covert phoneme manipulation improved speech production in a person with mild aphasia and AOS, by engaging the neural networks associated with motor planning without taxing the speech production mechanism. According to Kurland and colleagues (2012), this finding can be easily incorporated into their constraint-induced protocol within the hierarchical cueing provided to participants. This idea is appealing but the potential results are unclear, often it is the introduction of "complex" material first that gives rise to treatment-induced benefits (e.g., Kiran, 2008; Thompson et al., 2003; see also Chapter 5).

The role of motor programming in promoting treatment-induced neural changes in the aphasic brain cannot be isolated from its interaction with other higher-order cognitive processes during aphasia recovery. To use Kurland et al.'s (2012) words: "At the level of brain function, this implies a well-tuned interaction between linguistic neural systems with motor and sensory circuits, as well as systems of memory, planning, and emotion" (p. S66). In Chapter 3, we reviewed an example of such an interaction in studies of intention treatment among persons with aphasia, which elucidated the relationship among motor planning, executive functions, and naming (e.g., Crosson, 2012; Crosson et al., 2007). Indeed, as Kurland et al. (2012) point out, naming in aphasia implicates a web of brain structures beyond Broca's regions including at least the following: (1) heteromodal cortices (Brodmann's area 37 and 39), which support phonological and lexical processing (e.g., De Leon et al., 2007; Fridriksson et al., 2010), (2) temporal cortices, which subserve concept and word retrieval (e.g., Schwartz et al., 2009), (3) sensorimotor networks, which mediate action understanding (e.g,. Pulvermüller & Fadiga, 2010); (4) hippocampal, fusiform gyrus and inferior parietal lobe structures, which engage memory systems (e.g., Meinzer et al., 2010; Menke et al., 2009), and (5) pre- and supplementary motor cortices and subcortical structures (basal ganglia, insula, putamen) that partake in executive functions (e.g., Baldo et al., 2006; Crosson, 2012). We argue that this interconnectivity represents a neurally multifunctional system that drives the reshaping of neural networks which support language functions in aphasia, accounting for much of the individual variability we observe in the course of aphasia recovery.

References

Ahlsén, E. (1991). Body communication and speech in a Wernicke's aphasic—a longitudinal study. *Journal of Communication Disorders, 24*, 1–12.

Ahlsén, E. (2008). Embodiment in communication—aphasia, apraxia and the possible role of mirroring and imitation. *Clinical Linguistics & Phonetics, 22*(4–5), 311–315.

de Ajuriaguerra J., Hécaen, H., & Angelergues, R. (1960). Les apraxies: variétés cliniques et latéralisation lésionelle. *Revue Neurologique, 102*, 566–594.

Arbib, M. A., Bonaiuto, J. B., Jacobs, S., & Frey, S. H. (2009) Tool use and the distalization of the end-effector. *Psychological Research, 73*, 441–462.

Arbib, M. A. (2005). Interweaving protosign and protospeech: further developments beyond the mirror. *Interaction Studies: Social Behavior and Communication in Biological and Artificial Systems, 6*, 145–171.

Arbib, M. A. (2006). Aphasia, apraxia and the evolution of the language-ready brain. *Aphasiology, 20*, 1125–1155.

Arbib, M. A. (2010). Mirror system activity for action and language is embedded in the integration of dorsal and ventral pathways. *Brain and Language, 112*, 12–24.

Attard, M., Rose, M., & Lanyon, L. (2013). The comparative effects of multimodality aphasia therapy-plus for severe chronic Broca's aphasia: which aspects contribute most? Aphasiology, *27*(1), 80–111.

Baldo, J. V., Schwartz, S., Wilkins, D., & Dronkers, N. (2006). Role of frontal versus temporal cortex in verbal fluency as revealed by voxel-based lesion symptom mapping. *Journal of the International Neuropsychological Society, 12*, 896–900.

Barsalou, L. W. (1999). Perceptual symbol systems. *Behavioral and Brain Sciences, 22*, 577–660.

Barthel, G., Meinzer, M., Djundja, D., & Rockstroh, B. (2008). Intensive language therapy in chronic aphasia: Which aspects contribute most? *Aphasiology, 22*(4), 408–421.

Bates, E., Wilson, S. M., Ayse, P. S., Dick, F., Sereno, M. I., Knight, R. T., & Dronkers, N. F. (2003). Voxel-based lesion-symptom mapping. *Nature Neuroscience, 6*(5), 448–450.

Beeson, P., Rising, K., &Volk, J. (2003). Writing treatment for severe aphasia. *Journal of Speech, Language, and Hearing Research, 46*, 1038–1060.

Berthier, M. L., Green, C., Lara, J. P., Higueras, C., Barbancho, M. A., Davila, G., & Pulvermuller, F. (2009). Memantine and constraint-induced aphasia therapy in chronic poststroke aphasia. *Annals of Neurology, 65*, 577–585.

Berthier, M. L., & Pulvermüller, F. (2011). Neuroscience insights improve neurorehabilitation of poststroke aphasia. *Nature Reviews Neurology, 7*, 86–97.

Binder, J. R., Frost, J. A., Hammeke, T. A., Cox, R. W., Rao, S. M., & Preito, T. (1997). Human brain language areas identified by functional magnetic resonance imaging. *Journal of Neuroscience, 17*, 353–362.

Bohlhalter, S., Hattori, N., Wheaton, L., Fridman, E., Shamim, E. A., Garraux, G., & Hallet, M. (2009). Gesture subtype-dependent left lateralization of praxis planning: an event-related fMRI study. *Cerebral Cortex, 19*, 1256–1262.

Bonilha, L., Moser, D., Rorden, C., Baylis, G. C., & Fridriksson, J. (2006). Speech apraxia without oral apraxia: can normal brain function explain the physiopathology? *Neuroreport, 17*, 1027–1031.

Boronat, C. B., Buxbaum, L. J., Coslett,H. B., Tang, K., Saffran, E. M., Kimberg, D. Y., & Detre, J. A. (2005). Distinctions between manipulation and function knowledge of objects: evidence from functional magnetic resonance imaging. *Cognitive Brain Research, 23*, 361–373.

Bogousslavsky, J., Van Melle, G., & Regli, F. (1988). The Lausanne Stroke Registry: analysis of 1,000 consecutive patients with first stroke. *Stroke, 19*, 1083–1092

Bowman, C. A., Hodson, B. W., & Simpson, R. K. (1980). Oral apraxia and aphasic misarticulations. *Clinical Aphasiology, 8*, 89–95.

Bradshaw, J. L., & Nettleton, N. C. (1982). Language lateralization to the dominant hemisphere: tool use, gesture and language in hominid evolution. *Current Psychology, 2*, 171–192.

Breier, J. I., Juranek, J., Maher, L.M., Schmadeke, S., Men, D., & Papanicolaou, A.C. (2009). Behavioural and neuropsychologic response to therapy for chronic aphasia. *Archives of Physical Medicine and Rehabilitation, 90,* 2026–2033.

Breier, J. I., Maher, L. M., Schmadeke, S., Hasan, K. M., & Papanicolaou, A. C. (2007) Changes in language-specific brain activation after therapy for aphasia using magneto-encephalography: a case study. *Neurocase, 13,* 169–177.

Breier, J. I., Maher, L.M., Noval, B., & Papanicolaou, A. C. (2006) Functional imaging before and after constraint-induced language therapy for aphasia using magnetoencephalography. *Neurocase, 12,* 322–331.

Buccino, G., Binkofski, F., Fink, G. R., Fadiga, L., Fogassi, L., Gallese, V., ... Freund, H. J. (2001). Action observation activates premotor and parietal areas in somatotopic manner: an fMRI study. *European Journal of Neuroscience, 13,* 400–404.

Buccino, G., Lui, F., Canessa, N., Patteri, I., Lagravinese, G., Benuzzi, F, ... Rizzolatti, G. (2004). Neural circuits involved in the recognition of actions performed by non-conspecifics: an fMRI study. *Journal of Cognitive Neuroscience, 16,* 114–126.

Buchsbaum, B. R., Baldo, J., Okada, K., Berman, K. F., Dronkers, N., D'Esposito, M., & Hickok, G. (2011). Conduction aphasia, sensory-motor integration, and phonological short-term memory—an aggregate analysis of lesion and fMRI data. *Brain and Language, 119*(3), 119–128.

Butterworth, B., & Hadar, U. (1989). Gesture, speech, and computational stages: a reply to McNeilll. *Psychological Review, 96,* 168–174.

Buxbaum, L. J. (2001). Ideomotor apraxia: a call to action. *Neurocase, 7,* 445–458.

Buxbaum, L. J., & Kalénine, S. (2010). Action knowledge, visuomotor activation, and embodiment in the two action systems. *Annals of the New York Academy of Sciences, 1191,* 201–218.

Buxbaum, L. J., Kyle, K., Grossman, M., & Coslett, H. B. (2007). Left inferior parietal representations for skilled hand-object interactions: evidence from stroke and corticobasal degeneration. *Cortex, 43*(3), 411–423.

Buxbaum, L. J., Kyle, K. M., & Menon, R. (2005). On beyond mirror neurons: internal representations subserving imitation and recognition of skilled object-related actions in humans. *Brain Research Cognitive Brain Research, 25*(1), 226–239.

Buxbaum, L. J., & Saffran, E. M. (2002). The semantics of object manipulation and object function: A double dissociation. *Brain and Language, 82,* 179–199.

Buxbaum, L. J., Vermonti, T., & Schwartz, M. F. (2000). Function and manipulation tool knowledge in apraxia: Knowing 'what for' but not 'how'. *Neurocase, 6,* 83–97.

Calvert, G. A., Campbell, R., & Brammer, M. J. (2000). Evidence from functional magnetic resonance imaging of crossmodal binding in the human heteromodal cortex. *Current Opinion in Biology, 10,* 649–657.

Campbell, R., MacSweeney, M., Surguladze, S., Calvert, G., McGuire, P., Suckling, J., ... David, A. S. (2001). Cortical substrates for the perception of face actions: an fMRI study of the specificity of activation for seen speech and for meaningless lower-face acts (gurning). *Cognitive Brain Research, 12,* 233–243.

Cardinali, L., Frassinetti, F., Brozzoli, C., Urquizar, C., Roy, A. C., & Farnè, A. (2009). Tool-use induces morphological updating of the body schema. *Current Biology, 19*(12), R478–R479.

Carmo, J. C., & Rumiati, R. I. (2009). Imitation of transitive and intransitive actions in healthy individuals. *Brain and Cognition, 69,* 460–464.

Caute, A., Pring, T., Cocks, N., Cruice, M., Best, W., & Marshall, J. (2013). Enhancing communication through gesture and naming therapy. *Journal of Speech, Language, and Hearing Research, 56,* 337–351.

Chao, L.L., & Martin, A. (2000). Representation of manipulable man-made objects in the dorsal stream. *NeuroImage, 12,* 478–484.

Cherney, L., Patterson, J., & Raymer, A. (2011). Intensity of aphasia therapy: evidence and efficacy. *Current Neurology and Neuroscience Reports, 11*(6), 560–569.

Cherney, L. R., Patterson, P., Raymer, A., Frymark, T., & Schooling, T. (2008). Evidence-based systematic review: effects of intensity of treatment and constraint-induced language therapy for individuals with stroke-induced aphasia. *Journal of Speech, Language, and Hearing Research, 51,* 1282–1299.

Cicone, M., Wapner, W., Foldi, N., Zurif, E., & Gardner, H. (1979). The relation between gesture and language in aphasic communication. *Brain and Language, 8,* 324–349.

Clerget, E., Winderickx, A., Fadiga, L., & Olivier, E. (2009). Role of Broca's area in encoding sequential human actions: a virtual lesion study. *Neuroreport, 20,* 1496–1499.

Code, C., & Gaunt, C. (1986). Treating severe speech and limb apraxia in a case of aphasia. *International Journal of Language & Communication Disorders, 21*(1), 11–20.

Coelho, C. (1991). Manual sign acquisition and use in two aphasic subjects. In T. Prescott (Ed.), *Clinical aphasiology* (Vol. 19, pp. 185–194). Texas: Pro-Ed.

Condon, W. S., & Ogston, W. D. (1967). A segmentation of behavior. *Journal of Psychiatric Research, 5,* 221–235.

Conlon, C., & McNeill, M. (1991). The efficacy of treatment for two globally aphasic adults using visual action therapy. In T. Prescott (Ed.), *Clinical aphasiology* (Vol. 19, pp. 185–194). Texas: Pro-Ed.

Corballis, M. C. (2003). From mouth to hand: gesture, speech, and the evolution of right handedness. *Behavioral and Brain Sciences, 26,* 199–208.

Corballis, M. C. (2002). *From hand to mouth: the origins of language.* Princeton, NJ: Princeton University Press.

Creem, S. H., & Proffitt, D. R. (2001). Grasping objects by their handles: a necessary interaction between cognition and action. *Journal of Experimental Psychology: Human Perception and Performance, 27*(1), 218–228.

Crosson, B., Fabrizio, K. S., Singletary, F., Cato, M. A., Wierenga, C. E., Parkinson, R. B., ... Gonzalez Rothi, L. J. (2007). Treatment of naming in nonfluent aphasia through manipulation of intention and attention: a phase 1 comparison of two novel treatments. *Journal of the International Neuropsychological Society, 13,* 582–594.

Crosson, B. (2012). Thalamic mechanisms in language: a reconsideration based on recent findings and concepts. *Brain and Language, 126*(1), 73–88.

Cubelli, R., Marchetti, C., Boscolo, G., & Della Sala, S. (2000). Cognition in action: testing a model of limb apraxia. *Brain and Cognition, 44,* 144–165.

D'Ausillio, A., Pulvermüller, F., Salmas, P., Bufalari, I., Begliomini, C., & Fadiga, L. (2009). The motor somatotopy of speech perception. *Current Biology, 19*(5), 381–385.

Davis, C., Farias, D., & Baynes, K. (2009). Implicit phoneme manipulation for the treatment of apraxia of speech and co-occurring aphasia. *Aphasiology, 23*(4), 503–528.

Davis, G. A., & Wilcox, M. J. (1985). *Adult aphasia rehabilitation: applied pragmatics.* San Diego, CA: Pro-Ed.

De Leon, J., Gottesman, R. F., Kleinman, J. T., Newhart, M., Davis, C., Heidler-Gary, J., … Hillis, A. E. (2007). Neural regions essential for distinct cognitive processes underlying picture naming. *Brain, 130,* 1408–1422.

De Renzi, E. (1989). Apraxia. In F. Boller & J. Grafman (Eds.), *Handbook of neuropsychology,* (Vol. 2, pp. 245–263). Amsterdam: Elsevier.

De Renzi, E. & Luchelli, F. (1988). Ideational apraxia. *Brain, 111,* 1173–1185.

De Renzi, E., Motti, F., & Nichelli, P. (1980). Imitating gestures. A quantitative approach to ideomotor apraxia. *Archives of Neurology, 37*(1), 6–10.

De Renzi, E., Pieczuro, A., & Vignolo, L. A. (1968). Ideational apraxia: a quantitative study. *Neuropsychologia, 6,* 41–55.

de Ruiter, J. (2000). The production of gesture and speech. In D. McNeill (Ed.), *Language and gesture* (pp. 284–311). Cambridge, UK: Cambridge University Press.

Dewey, D., Roy, E. A., Square-Storer, P. A., & Hayden, D. C. (1988). Limb and oral praxic abilities of children with verbal sequencing deficits. *Developmental Medicine & Child Neurology, 30,* 743–751.

Dittman, A. T. (1972). *Interpersonal messages of emotion.* New York: Springer.

Dronkers, N. F. (1996). Frenchay aphasia screening test: validity and comparability. *Disability and Rehabilitation, 18,* 238–240.

Druks, J. (2002). Verbs and nouns: a review of the literature. *Journal of Neurolinguistics, 15,* 289–315.

Duffy, R. J., & Duffy, J. R. (1981). Three studies of deficits in pantomimic expressions and pantomimic recognition in aphasia. *Journal of Speech and Hearing Research, 46,* 70–84.

Fadiga, L., Fogassi, L., Pavesi, G., & Rizzolatti, G. (1995). Motor facilitation during action observation: a magnetic stimulation study. *Journal of Neurophysiology, 73,* 2608–2611.

Farias, D., Davis, C., & Harrington, G. (2006). Drawing: Its contribution to naming in aphasia. *Brain and Language, 97*(1), 53–63.

Faroqui-Shah, Y., & Virion, C. (2009). Constraint-induced language therapy for agrammatism. Role of grammaticality constraints. *Aphasiology, 23,* 977–988.

Fazio, P., Cantagallo, A., Craighero, L., D'Ausilio, A., Roy, A.C., Pozzo, T., … Fadiga, L. (2009). Encoding of human action in Broca's area. *Brain, 132,* 1980–1988.

Feyereisen, P., & Seron, X. (1982). Nonverbal communication and aphasia, a review: II. Expression. *Brain and Language, 16,* 213–236.

Feyereisen, P. (1997). The competition between gesture and speech production in dual-task paradigms. *Journal of Memory and Language, 36,* 13–33.

Fiebach, C. J., & Friederici, A. D. (2004). Processing concrete words: fMRI evidence against a specific right-hemisphere involvement. *Neuropsychologia, 42*(1), 62–70.

Fiebach, C. J., & Schubotz, R. I. (2006). Dynamic anticipatory processing of hierarchical sequential events: a common role for Broca's area and ventral premotor cortex across domains? *Cortex, 42,* 499–502.

Fischer, M. H. (2003). Spatial representation in number processing—evidence from a pointing task. *Visual Cognition, 10*(4), 493–508.

Fogassi, L., & Luppino, G. (2005). Motor functions of the parietal lobe. *Current Opinion in Neurobiology, 15,* 626–631.

Fogassi, L., & Ferrari, P. F. (2007). Mirror neurons and the evolution of embodied language. *Current Directions in Psychological Science, 16*(3), 136–141.

Fogassi, L., Ferrari, P. F., Gesierich, B., Rozzi, S., Chersi, F., & Rizzolatti, G. (2005). Parietal lobe: from action organization to intention understanding. *Science, 308*(5722), 662–667.

Foundas, A. L., Macauley, B. L., Raymer, A. M., Maher, L. M., Heilman, K. M., & Gonzalez Rothi, L. J. (1995). Gesture laterality in aphasic and apraxic stroke patients. *Brain and Cognition, 29*(2), 204–213.

Fowler, C. A. (1986). An event approach to the study of speech perception from a direct-realist perspective. *Journal of Phonetics, 14*, 3–28.

Frey, S. H. (2007). What puts the how in where? Tool use and the divided visual streams hypothesis. *Cortex, 43*, 368–375.

Frey, S. H. (2008). Tool use, communicative gesture and cerebral asymmetries in the modern human brain. *Philosophical Transactions of the Royal Society B, 363*, 1951–1957.

Frick-Horbury, D., & Guttentag, R. E. (1998). The effects of restricting hand gesture production on lexical retrieval and free recall. *American Journal of Psychology, 111*(1), 43–62.

Fridriksson, J., Moss, J., Davis, B., Baylis, G. C., Bonilha, L., & Rorden, C. (2008). Motor speech perception modulates the cortical language areas. *NeuroImage, 41*, 605–613.

Fridriksson, J., Kjartansson, O., Morgan, P. S., Hjaltason, H., Magnusdottir, S., Bonilha, L., & Rorden, C. (2010). Impaired speech repetition and left parietal lobe damage. *Journal of Neuroscience, 30*(33), 11057–11061.

Friederici, A. D. (2006). Broca's area and the ventral premotor cortex in language: functional differentiation and specificity. *Cortex, 42*(4), 472–475.

Gainotti, G., & Lemmo, M. (1976). Comprehenion of symbolic gestures in aphasia. *Brain and Language, 3*, 451–460.

Gallese V., Fadiga, L., Fogassi, L., & Rizzolatti, G. (1996). Action representation and the inferior parietal lobule. In W. Prinz & B. Hommel (Eds.), *Attention and performance: XIX. Common mechanisms in perception and action.* Oxford, UK: Oxford University Press.

Garrod, S., & Pickering, M. J. (2004). Why is conversation so easy? *Trends in Cognitive Science, 8*, 8–11.

Gentilucci, M., Benuzzi, F., Bertolani, L., Daprati, E., & Gangitano, M. (2000) Language and motor control. *Experimental Brain Research, 133*, 468–490.

Gentilucci, M., & Corballis, M. C. (2006). From manual gesture to speech: a gradual transition. *Neuroscience and Biobehavioral Reviews, 30*, 949–960.

Gentilucci, M., & Dalla Volta, R. (2008). Spoken language and arm gestures are controlled by the same motor control system. *The Quarterly Journal of Experimental Psychology, 61*(6), 944–957.

Geschwind, N. (1965). Disconnexion syndromes in animals and man. I. *Brain, 88*, 237–294.

Geschwind, N., Quadfasel, F. A., & Sagarra, J. M. (1968). Isolation of the speech area. *Neuropsychologia, 6*(4), 327–40.

Gibson, K. R, & Ingold, T. (1993). *Tools, language and cognition in human evolution.* Cambridge, UK: Cambridge University Press.

Glenberg, A. M., & Kaschak, M. P. (2002). Grounding language in action. *Psychonomic Bulletin & Review, 9*, 558–565.

Glover, S., Rosenbaum, D. A., Graham, J., & Dixon, P. (2004). Grasping the meaning of words. *Experimental Brain Research, 154*, 103–108.

Goldenberg, G., & Hagmann, S. (1997). The meaning of meaningless gestures: a study of visuo-imitative apraxia. *Neuropsychologia, 35*, 333–341.

Goldenberg, G., & Hagmann, S. (1998). Tool use and mechanical problem solving in apraxia. *Neuropsychologia, 36*, 581–589.

Goldenberg, G., Hermsdörfer, J., Glindemann, R., Rorden, C., & Karnath, H. O. (2007). Pantomime of tool use depends on integrity of left inferior frontal cortex. *Cerebral Cortex, 17*, 2769–2776.

Goldenberg, G. (2009). Apraxia and the parietal lobes. *Neuropsychologia, 47*, 1449–1459.

Goldenberg, G., & Spatt, J. (2009). The neural basis of tool use. *Brain, 132*, 1645–1655.

Goodglass, H., & Kaplan, E. (1963). Disturbance of gesture and pantomime in aphasia. *Brain, 86*, 703–720.

Goral, M., & Kempler, D. (2009). Training verb production in communicative context: evidence from a person with chronic non-fluent aphasia. *Aphasiology, 23*(12), 1383–1397.

Greenfield, P. M. (1991). Language, tools and brain: the ontogeny and phylogeny of hierarchically organized sequential behavior. *Behavioral and Brain Sciences, 14*, 531–595.

Hadar, U., Burstein, A., Krauss, R. M., & Soroker, N. (1998a). Ideational gestures and speech: a neurolinguistic investigation. *Language and Cognitive Processes, 13*, 59–76.

Hadar, U., Wenkert-Olenik, D., Krauss, R. M., & Soroker, N. (1998b). Gesture and the processing of speech: neuropsychological evidence. *Brain and Language, 62*, 107–126.

Hall, D. A., Fussell, C., & Summerfield, A. Q. (2005). Reading fluent speech from talking faces: typical brain networks and individual differences. *Journal of Cognitive Neuroscience, 17*, 939–953.

Hanlon, R. E., Brown, J. W., & Gerstman, L. J. (1990). Enhancement of naming in nonfluent aphasia through gesture. *Brain and Language, 30*, 298–314.

Hauk, O., Johnsrude, I., & Pulvermüller, F. (2004). Somatotopic representation of action words in the motor and premotor cortex. *Neuron, 41*, 301–307.

Heath, M., Roy, E. A., Westwood, D., & Black, S. E. (2001). Patterns of apraxia associated with the production of intransitive limb gestures following left and right hemisphere stroke. *Brain and Cognition, 46*, 165–169.

Hebb, D. O. (1949). *The organization of behavior*. Hoboken, NJ: Wiley.

Heilman, K. M., & Rothi, L. J. (1997). Limb apraxia: a look back. In L. J. Rothi & K. M. Heilman (Eds), *Apraxia: the neuropsychology of action* (pp. 7–18). Hove, UK: Psychology Press.

Heilman, K. M., & Rothi, L. J. (2003). Apraxia. In K. M. Heilman & E. E. Valenstein (Eds.), *Clinical neuropsychology*, 4th ed. (pp. 215–236). New York: Oxford University Press.

Heilman, K.M., Rothi, L.J., & Valenstein, E. (1982). Two forms of ideomotor apraxia. *Neurology, 32*, 342–346.

Helm-Estabrooks, N., Albert, M.L., & Nicholas, M. (2014). *Manual of aphasia and aphasia therapy*. Austin, TX: Pro-Ed.

Hermsdörfer, J., Terlinden, G., Mühlau, M., Goldenberg, G., & Wohlschläger, A. M. (2007). Neural representations of pantomimed and actual tool use: evidence from an event-related fMRI study. *Neuroimage, 36*, T109–T118.

Herrmann, M., Reichle, T., Lucius-Hoene, G., Wallesch, C. W., & Johannsen-Horbach, H. (1988). Nonverbal communication as a compensatory strategy for severely nonfluent aphasics? A quantitative approach. *Brain and Language, 33*, 41–54.

Hewes, G. W. (1973) Primate communication and the gestural origin of language. *Current Anthropology, 14*(1–2), 5–24.

Hickok, G. (2009). Eight problems for the mirror neuron theory of action understanding in monkeys and humans. *Journal of Cognitive Neuroscience, 21*(7), 1229–1243.

Hickok, G. (2010). The role of mirror neurons in speech perception and action word semantics. *Language and Cognitive Processes, 25*(6), 749–776.

Hickok, G., & Peoppel, D. (2007). The cortical organization of speech processing. *Nature Reviews Neuroscience, 8*(5), 393–402.

Hickok, G., & Poeppel, D. (2000). Towards a functional neuroanatomy of speech perception. *Trends in Cognitive Sciences, 4*, 131–138.

Hillis, A. E. (2007). Aphasia: progress in the last quarter of a century. *Neurology, 69*, 200–213.

Hillis, A. E., Barker, P. B., Wityk, R. J., Aldrich, E. M., Restrepo, L. & Breese, E. L., & Work, M. (2004). Variability in subcortical aphasia is due to variable sites of cortical hypoperfusion. *Brain and Language, 89*(3), 524–530.

Hillis, A. E., Tuffiash, E., Wityk, R. J., & Barker, P. B. (2002). Regions of neural dysfunction associated with impaired naming of actions and objects in acute stroke. *Cognitive Neuropsychology, 19*, 523–524.

Hodges, J. R., Bozeat, S., Lambon Ralph, M. A., Patterson, K., & Spatt, J. (2000). The role of conceptual knowledge in object use evidence from semantic dementia. *Brain, 123*, 1913–1925.

Hoodin, R., & Thompson, C. (1983). Facilitaion of verbal labeling in adult aphasia by gesture, verbal or verbal plus gesture training. In R. H. Brookshire (Ed.), *Clinical aphasiology* (pp. 62–64). Minneapolis, MN: BRK Publishers.

Iacoboni, M., & Wilson, S. M. (2006). Beyond a single area: motor control and language within a neural architecture encompassing Broca's area. *Cortex, 42*, 503–506.

Iriki, A., Tanaka, M., & Iwamura, Y. (1996). Coding of modified body schema during tool use by macaque postcentral neurones. *Neuroreport, 7*, 2325–2330.

Jacobs, S., Danielmeier, C., & Frey, S. H. (2010). Human anterior intraparietal and ventral premotor cortices support representations of grasping with the hand or a novel tool. *Journal of Cognitive Neuroscience, 22*, 2594–2608.

Jirak, D., Menz, M. M., Buccino, G., Borghi, A. M., & Binkofski, F. (2010). Grasping language—a short story on embodiment. *Consciousness and Cognition, 19*, 711–720.

Johns, D. F., & Darley, F. L. (1970). Phonemic variability in apraxia of speech. *Journal of Speech and Hearing Research, 13*, 556–583.

Johnson-Frey, S. H. (2003). What's so special about human tool use? *Neuron, 39*(2), 201–204.

Johnson-Frey, S. H. (2004).The neural bases of complex tool use in humans. *Trends in Cognitive Science, 8*, 71–78.

Johnson-Frey, S. H., Funnell, M. G., Gerry, V. E., & Gazzaniga, M. S. (2005). A dissociation between tool use skills and hand dominance: insights from left and right-handed callosotomy patients. *Journal of Cognitive Neuroscience, 17*, 262–272.

Kellenbach, M. L., Brett, M., & Patterson, K. (2003). Actions speak louder than functions: the importance of manipulability and action in tool representation. *Journal of Cognitive Neuroscience, 15*(1), 30–46.

Kemmerer, D., & Tranel, D. (2003). A double dissociation between the meanings of action verbs and locative prepositions. *NeuroCase, 9*, 421–435.

Kendon, A. (1980). Gesticulation and speech: two aspects of the process of utterance. In M. Key (Ed.), *The relationship of verbal and nonverbal communication* (pp. 207–227). The Hague: Mouton.

Kertesz, A., & Ferro, J. M. (1984). Lesion size and location in ideomotor apraxia. *Brain, 107,* 921–933.

Kertesz, A., Ferro, J. M., & Shewan, C. M. (1984). Apraxia and aphasia: the functional-anatomical basis of their dissociation. *Neurology, 34,* 40–47.

Kertesz, A., & Hooper, P. (1982). Praxis and language: the extent and variety of apraxia in aphasia. *Neuropsychologia, 20,* 275–286.

Kimura, D. (1977). Acquisition of a motor skill after left-hemisphere damage. *Brain, 100,* 527–542.

Kimura, D., & Archibald, Y. (1974). Motor functions of the left hemisphere. *Brain, 97,* 337–350.

Kiran, S. (2008). Typicality of inanimate category exemplars in aphasia treatment: further evidence for semantic complexity. *Journal of Speech, Language, and Hearing Research, 51*(6), 1550–1568.

Kita, S., & Davies, T. S. (2009). Competing conceptual representations trigger co-speech representational gestures. *Language and Cognitive Processes, 24*(5), 761–775.

Kita, S., Özyürek, A., Allen, S., Brown, A., Furman, R., & Ishizuka, T. (2007). Relations between syntactic encoding and co-speech gestures: implications for a model of speech and gesture production. *Language and Cognitive Processes, 22*(8), 1212–1236.

Kleim, J. A., & Jones, T. A. (2008). Principles of experience-dependent neural plasticity: implications for rehabilitation after brain damage. *Journal of Speech, Language and Hearing Research, 51*(1), S225–S239.

Knecht, S., Deppe, M., Dräger, B., Bobe, L., Lohmann, H., Ringelstein, E., & Henningsen, H. (2000). Language lateralization in healthy right-handers. *Brain, 123*(Pt 1), 74–81.

Kobayashi, S., & Ugawa, Y. (2013). Relationships between aphasia and apraxia. *Journal of Neurology and Translational Neuroscience, 2*(1), 1028.

Koskia, L., Iacoboni, M., & Mazziotta, J. C. (2002). Deconstructing apraxia: understanding disorders of intentional movement after stroke. *Current Opinion in Neurology, 15,* 71–77.

Krauss, R. M., Chen, Y., & Gottesman, R. F. (2000). Lexical gestures and lexical access: a process model. In D. McNeill (Ed.), *Language and gesture* (pp. 261–283). New York: Cambridge University Press.

Krauss, R. M., & Hadar, U. (1999). Iconic gestures: the grammatical categories of lexical affiliates. *Journal of Neurolinguistics, 12*(1), 1–12.

Kurland, J., Baldwin, K., & Tauer, C. (2010). Treatment-induced neuroplasticity following intensive naming therapy in a case of chronic Wernicke's aphasia. *Aphasiology, 24*(6–8), 737–751.

Kurland, J., Pulvermüller, F., Silva, N., Burke, K., & Adrianopoulous, M. (2012). Constrained versus unconstrained intensive language therapy in two individuals with chronic, moderate-to-severe aphasia and apraxia of speech: behavioral and fMRI outcomes. *American Journal of Speech-Language Pathology, 21*(2), S65–S87.

Lanyon, L., & Rose, M. (2009). Do the hands have it? The facilitation effects of arm and hand gestures in word retrieval in aphasia. *Aphasiology, 23*(7–8), 809–822.

Le May, A., David, R., & Thomas, P. (1988). The use of spontaneous gesture by aphasic patients. *Aphasiology, 2,* 137–145.

Levelt, W. J., Richardson, G., & La Heij, W. (1985). Pointing and voicing deictic expressions. *Journal of Memory and Language, 24*, 133–164.

Lewis, J. W. (2006) Cortical networks related to human use of tools. *Neuroscientist, 12*, 211–231.

Liberman, A. M., Cooper, F. S., Shankweiler, D. P., & Studdert-Kennedy, M. (1967). Perception of the speech code. *Psychological Review, 74*(6), 431–461.

Liberman, A. M., & Mattingly, I. G. (1985). The motor theory of speech perception revised. *Cognition, 21*, 1–36.

Liepmann, H. (1908). *Drei aufs "Atze aus dem Apraxiegebiet."* Berlin: Karger.

Liepmann, H. (1920). Apraxie. *Ergebnisse der Gesamten Medzin, 1*, 516–543.

Lott, P. (1999). *Gesture and aphasia*. Berlin: Lang.

Lotto, A. J., Hickok, G. S., & Holt, L. L. (2008). Reflections on mirror neurons and speech perception. *Trends in Cognitive Sciences, 13*(3), 110–114.

Luria, A. (1972). *Traumatic aphasia*. The Hague: Mouton.

Maher, L. M., Kendall, D., Swearengin, J., Rodriguez, A., Leon, S., Pingel, K., … Rothi, G. (2006). A pilot study of use-dependent learning in the context of constraint induced language therapy. *Journal of the International Neuropsychological Society, 12*, 843–852.

Mahon, B. Z., & Caramazza, A. (2008). A critical look at the embodied cognition hypothesis and a new proposal for grounding conceptual content. *Journal of Physiology—Paris, 102*, 59–70.

Marshall, J., Best, W., Cocks, N., Cruice, M., Pring, T., Bulcock, G., … Caute, A. (2012). Gesture and naming therapy for people with severe aphasia: a group study. *Journal of Speech, Language, and Hearing Research, 55*(3), 726–738.

Martin, P. I., Treglia, E., Naeser, M. A., Ho, M. D., Baker, E. H., Martin, E. G., Bashir, S., & Pascual-Leone A. (2014). Language improvements after TMS plus modified CILT: pilot, open-protocol study with two, chronic nonfluent aphasia cases. *Restorative Neurology and Neuroscience (RNN), 32*(4), 483–505.

McNeill, D. (1985). So you think gestures are nonverbal. *Psychological Review*, 92 (3), 350–371.

McNeill, D. (2005). *Gesture and Thought*. Chicago: University of Chicago Press.

McNeill, M. R., Robin, D. A., & Schmidt, R. A. (2009). Apraxia of speech: definition and differentiational diagnosis. In M. R. McNeill (Ed.), *Clinical management of sensorimotor speech disorders* (2nd ed., pp. 249–268). New York: Thieme.

McNeill, D. (1992). *Hand and mind: what gestures reveal about thought*. Chicago: University of Chicago Press.

Meinzer, M., Djundja, D., Barthel, G., Elbert, T., & Rockstroh, B. (2005). Long-term stability of improved language functions in chronic aphasia after constraint-induced aphasia therapy. *Stroke, 36*, 1462–1466.

Meinzer, M., Elbert, T., Weinbruch, C., Djundja, D., Barthel, G., & Rockstroh, B. (2004). Intensive language training enhances brain plasticity in chronic aphasia. *BioMed Central Biology, 2*(20), 1–9.

Meinzer, M., Flaisch, T., Breitenstein, C., Weinbruch, C., Elbert, T., & Rockstroh, B. (2008). Functional re-recruitment of dysfunctional brain areas predicts language recovery in chronic aphasia. *NeuroImage, 39*, 2038–2046.

Meinzer, M., Mohammadi, S., Kugel, H., Schiffbauer, H., Floel, A., Albers, J., … Deppe, M. (2010). Integrity of the hippocampus and surrounding white matter is correlated with language training success in aphasia. *NeuoImage, 53*, 283–290.

Melinger, A., & Levelt, W. (2004). Gesture and the communication intention of the speaker. *Gesture, 4*, 119–141.

Menke, R., Meinzer, M., Kugel, H., Deppe, M., Baumgartner, A., Schiffbauer, H., ... Breitenstein, C. (2009). Imaging short- and long-term training success in chronic aphasia. *BioMed Central Neuroscience, 10*, 118.

Maeshima, S., Toshiro, H., Sekiguchi, E., Okita, R., Yamaga, H., Ozaki, F., ... Roger, P. (2002). Transcortical mixed aphasia due to cerebral infarction in left inferior frontal lobe and temporo-parietal lobe. *Neuroradiology, 44*(2), 133–137.

Morgan, A., & Helm-Estabrooks, N. (1987). Back to the drawing board: a treatment program for nonverbal aphasic patients. In R. H. Brookshire (Ed.), *Clinical aphasiology proceedings* (pp. 34–39). Minneapolis, MN: BRK Publishers.

Morrel-Samuels, P., & Krauss, R. M. (1992). Word familiarity predicts the temporal asynchrony of hand gestures and speech. *Journal of Experimental Psychology: Learning, Memory and Cognition, 18*, 615–623.

Morin, O., & Grezes, J. (2008). What is "mirror" in the premotor cortex? A review. *Clinical Neurophysiology, 38*(3), 189–195.

Morsella, E., & Krauss, R. (2004). The role of gestures in spatial working memory and speech. *American Journal of Psychology, 111*(3), 411–424.

Mosely, R., Carota, F., Hauk, O., Mohr, B., & Pulvermüller, F. (2012). A role for the motor system in binding abstract emotional meaning. *Cerebral Cortex, 22*, 1634–1647.

Motomura, N. (1994). Motor performance in aphasia and ideomotor apraxia. *Perceptual and Motor Skills, 79*, 719–722.

Mozaz, M., Rothi, L. J., Anderson, J.M., Crucian, G. P., & Heilman, K. M. (2002). Postural knowledge of transitive pantomimes and intransitive gestures. *Journal of the International Neuropsychological Society, 8*, 958–962.

Myung, J., Blumstein, S.E., & Sedivy, J. C. (2006). Playing on the typewriter, typing on the piano: manipulation knowledge of objects. *Cognition, 98*, 223–243.

Myung, J., Blumstein, S. E., Yee, E. Sedivy, J. C., Thompson-Schill, S. L., & Buxbaum, L. J. (2010). Impaired access to manipulation features in apraxia: evidence from eyetracking and semantic judgment tasks. *Brain and Language, 112*(2), 101–112.

Neininger, B., & Pulvermüller, F. (2003). Word-category specific deficits after lesions in the right hemisphere. *Neuropsychologia, 41*(1), 53–70.

Nelissen, N., Pazzaglia, M., Vandenbulcke, M., Sunaert, S., Fannes, K., Dupont, P., ... Vandenberghe, R. (2010). Gesture discrimination in primary progressive aphasia: the intersection between gesture and language processing pathways. *Journal of Neuroscience, 30*, 6334–6341.

Obayashi, S., Suhara, T., Kawabe, K., Okauchi, T., Maeda, J., Akine, Y., ... Iriki, A. (2001), Functional brain mapping of monkey tool use. *Neuroimage, 14*, 853–861.

Ochipa, C., Rothi, L. J., & Heilman, K. M. (1994). Conduction apraxia. *Journal of Neurology, Neurosurgery and Psychiatry, 57*, 1241–1244.

Ogar, J., Slama, H., Dronkers, N., Amici, S., & Gorno-Tempini, M. L. (2005). Apraxia of speech: an overview. *Neurocase, 11*, 427–432.

Papagno, C., Della Sala, S., & Basso, A. (1993). Ideomotor apraxia without aphasia and aphasia without apraxia: the anatomical support for a double dissociation. *Journal of Neurology, Neurosurgery & Psychiatry, 56*(3), 286–289.

Pashek, G. V. (1997). A case study of gesturally cued naming in aphasia: dominant versus nondominant hand training. *Journal of Communication Disorders, 30*, 349–366.

Pazzaglia, M., Smania, N., Corato, E., & Aglioti, S. M. (2008). Neural underpinnings of gesture discrimination in patients with limb apraxia. *Journal of Neuroscience, 28*, 3030–3041.

Pedelty, L. (1987). Gesture in aphasia (unpublished doctoral dissertation). Chicago: University of Chicago.

Pickering, M. J., & Garrod, S. (2007). Do people use language production to make predictions during comprehension? *Trends in Cognitive Sciences, 11*(3), 105–10.

Pulvermüller, F., & Berthier, M. L. (2008). Aphasia therapy on a neuroscience basis. *Aphasiology, 22*(6), 563–599.

Pulvermüller, F., & Fadiga, L. (2010). Active perception: sensorimotor circuits as a cortical basis for language. *Nature Reviews Neuroscience, 11*, 351–360.

Pulvermüller, F., Hauk, O., Nikulin, V. V., & Ilmoniemi, R. J. (2005). Functional links between motor and language systems. *European Journal of Neuroscience, 21*, 793–797.

Pulvermüller, F., Neininger, B., Elbert, T., Mohr, B., Rockstroh, B., Koebbel, P., & Taub, E. (2001). Constraint-induced therapy of chronic aphasia after stroke. *Stroke, 32*, 1621–1626.

Pyers, J., Grossmith, S., Magid, R., Dikanovic, M., Gollan, T., & Emmorey, K. (2010). Individual differences in the role of gesture in lexical retrieval. Poster presented at the 22nd annual meeting of the Association for Psycholoical Science, Boston.

Ramsberger, G., & Helm-Estabrooks, N. (1989). Visual action therapy for bucco-facial apraxia. In T. Prescott (Ed.), *Clinical aphasiology* (pp. 395–406). Cambridge, MA: College-Hill.

Randerath, J., Li, Y., Goldenberg, G., & Hermsdörfer, J. (2009). Grasping tools, effects of task and apraxia. *Neuropsychologia, 47*, 497–505.

Rao, P. (1994). Use of amer-ind code by persons with aphasia. In Chapey, R. (Ed.), *Language intervention strategies in adult aphasia* (3rd ed., pp.395–406). Cambridge, MA: College-Hill.

Rapcsak, S., Ochipa, C., Beeson, P.M., & Rubens, A.B. (1993). Praxis and the right hemisphere. *Brain and Cognition, 23*, 181–202.

Rauscher, F.H., Krauss, R.M., & Chen, Y. (1996). Gesture, speech, and lexical access: The role of lexical movements in speech production. *Psychological Science, 7*(4), 226–231.

Raymer, A. M., & Thompson, C. K. (1991). Effects of verbal plus gestural treatment in a person with aphasia and severe apraxia of speech. In T. Prescott (Ed.), *Clinical Aphasiology* (pp. 285–298). Austin, TX: Pro-Ed.

Raymer, S., McHose, B., Smith, K., Iman, L., Ambrose, A., & Casselton, C. (2012). Contrasting effects of errorless naming treatment and gestural facilitation for word retrieval in aphasia. *Neuropsychological Rehabilitation, 22*(2), 235–266.

Richter, M., Miltner, W., & Straube, T. (2008). Association between therapy outcome and right-hemisphere activation in chronic aphasia. *Brain, 131*, 1391–1401.

Rizzolatti, G., & Arbib, M. A. (1998). Language within our grasp. *Trends in Neuroscience, 21*(5), 188–194.

Rizzolatti, G., & Craighero, L. (2004). The mirror-neuron system. *Annual Review of Neuroscience, 27*, 169–192.

Rizzolatti, G., Fadiga, L., Gallese, V., & Fogassi, L. (1996). Premotor cortex and the recognition of motor actions. *Cognitive Brain Research, 3*, 131–141.

Rizzolatti, G., Fogassi, L., & Gallese, V. (2001). Neuropsychological mechanisms underlying the understanding and imitation of action. *Nature Reviews Neuroscience, 2*(9), 661–670.

Rizzolatti, G., & Luppino, G. (2001). The cortical motor system. *Neuron, 31*(6), 889–901.

Roby-Brami, A., Hermsdörfer, J., Roy, A. C., & Jacobs, S. (2012). A neuropsychological perspective on the link between language and praxis in modern humans. *Philosophical Transactions of the Royal Society B: Biological Sciences, 367,* 144–160.

Rochon, E., Caplan, D., & Waters, G. S. (1991). Short-term memory processes in patients with apraxia of speech: implications for the nature and structure of the auditory verbal short-term memory system. *Journal of Neurolinguistics, 5,* 237–264.

Rodriguez, A. D., Raymer, A. M., & Rothi, L. J. (2006). Effects of gesture plus verbal and semantic-phonologic treatments for verb retrieval in aphasia. Presented at the 35th Clinical Aphasiology Conference, Sanibel Island, FL.

Rogalsky, C., Love, T., Driscoll, D., Anderson, S. W., & Hickok, G. (2011). Are mirror neurons the basis of speech perception? Evidence from five cases with damage to the purported human mirror system. *Neurocase, 17*(2), 178–187.

Rose, M. (2006). The utility of gesture treatments in aphasia. *International Journal of Speech Language Pathology, 8*(2), 92–109.

Rose, M., & Attard, M. (2011). *Multi-Modality aphasia therapy (M-MAT): A procedural manual.* Melbourne, Australia: La Trobe University.

Rose, M., & Douglas, J. (2001). The differential faciliatory effects of gesture and visualization processes on object naming in aphasia. *Aphasiology, 15*(10), 977–990.

Rose, M., Douglas, J., & Matyas, T. (2002). The comparative effectiveness of gesture and verbal treatments for a specific phonologic naming impairment. *Aphasiology, 16,* 1001–1030.

Rose, M. L. (2013). Releasing the constraints on aphasia therapy: the positive impact of gesture and multimodality treatments. *American Journal of Speech-Language Pathology, 22*(2), S227–S239.

Rothi, L.J.G. (1995). Behavioral compensation in the case of treatment of acquired language disorders resulting from brain damage. In R. A. Dixon & L. Mackman (Eds.), *Compensating for psychological deficits and declines: managing losses and promoting gains* (pp. 219–230). Mahwah, NJ: Earlbaum.

Rousseaux, M., Daveluy, W., & Kozlowski, O. (2010). Communication in conversation in stroke patients. *Journal of Neurology, 257,* 1099–1107.

Roy, A. C., & Arbib, M. A. (2005). The syntactic motor system. *Gesture, 1,* 7–37.

Roy, E. A., & Square, P. (1985). Common considerations in the studies on limb, verbal and oral apraxia. In E. Roy (Ed.), *Neuropsychological studies of apraxia and related disorders* (pp. 111–162). Amsterdam: Elsevier.

Rozzi, S., Ferrari, P. F., Bonini, L., Rizzolatti, G., & Fogassi, L. (2008). Functional organization of inferior parietal lobule convexity in the macaque monkey: electrophysiological characterization of motor, sensory and mirror responses and their correlation with cytoarchitectonic areas. *European Journal of Neuroscience, 28,* 1569–1588.

Saygin, A. P., Wilson, S. M., Dronkers, N. F., & Bates, E. (2004). Action comprehension in aphasia: linguistic and non-linguistic deficits and their lesion correlates. *Neuropsychologia, 42*(13), 1788–1804.

Schmid, G., & Ziegler, W. (2006). Audio-visual matching of speech and non-speech oral gestures in patients with aphasia and apraxia of speech. *Neuropsychologia, 44*(4), 546–555.

Schnider, A., Hanlon, R. E., Alexander, D. N., & Benson, D. F. (1997). Ideomotor apraxia: behavioral dimensions and neuroanatomical basis. *Brain and Language, 58,* 125–136.

Schoppe, K. J. (1974). Das MLS-Gerat: ein neuer Testapparat zur Messung feinmotorischer Leistungen. *Diagnostica, 20*, 43–47.

Schwartz, M. F., Kimberg, D. Y., Walker, G. M., Faseyitan, O., Breecher, A., Dell, G. S., & Coslett, H. B. (2009). Anterior temporal involvement in semantic word retrieval: voxel-based lesion-symptom mapping evidence from aphasia. *Brain, 132*, 3411–3427.

Scott, S. K. (1998). The point of P-centres. *Psychological Research, 61*, 4–11.

Scott, S.K., McGettigan, C., & Eisner, F. (2009). A little more conversation, a little less action—candidate roles for the motor cortex in speech perception. *Nature Reviews Neuroscience, 10*, 295–302.

Sekine, K., & Rose, M. (2013). The relationship between aphasia type and severity to gesture production in people with aphasia. *American Journal of Speech-Language Pathology, 22*, 622–672.

Skelly, M., Schinsky, L., Smith, R., & Fust, R. (1974). American Indian sign (Amer-Ind) as a facilitator of verbalization for the oral verbal apraxic. *Journal of Speech and Hearing Disorders, 34*, 445–455.

Stamenova, V., Roy, E. A., & Black, S. E. (2010). Associations and dissociations of transitive and intransitive gestures in left and right hemisphere stroke patients. *Brain and Cognition 72*(3), 483–490.

Steele, J., & Uomini, N. (2009). Can the archaeology of manual specialization tell us anything about language evolution? A survey of the state of play. Steps to a (neuro-) archaeology of mind. *Cambridge Archeological Journal, 19*(1), 97–110.

Steele, J., Ferrari, P. F., & Fogassi, L. (2012). From action to language: comparative perspectives on primate tool use, gesture and the evolution of human language. *Philosophical Transactions of the Royal Society B: Biological Sciences, 367*, 4–9.

Steinthal, H. (1871). Einleitung in die Psychologie und Sprachwissenschaft. *Abriss der sprachwissenschaft*. Berlin: Dümmlers.

Szaflarski, J., Ball, A., Grether, S., Al-Fwaress, F., Griffith, N., Strunjas, J., ... Reichhardt, R. (2008). Constraint induced aphasia therapy stimulates language recovery in patients with chronic aphasia after ischaemic stroke. *Medical Science Monitor, 14*, 243–250.

Taub, E. (2004). Harnessing brain plasticity through behavioral techniques to produce new treatments in neurorehabilitation. *American Psychologist, 59*(8), 692–704.

Taub, E., Uswatte, G., Mark, V., & Morris, D. (2006). The learned non-use phenomenon: implications for rehabilitation. *Europa Medicophysica, 42*(3), 241–255.

Tettamanti, M., Buccino, G., Saccuman, M. C., Gallese, V., Danna, M., Scifo, P., ... Perani, D. (2005). Listening to action-related sentences activates fronto-parietal motor circuits. *Journal of Cognitive Neuroscience, 17*, 273–281.

Thompson, C. K., Shapiro, L. P., Kiran, S., & Sobecks, J. (2003). The role of syntactic complexity in treatment of sentence deficits in agrammatic aphasia: the complexity account of treatment efficacy (CATE). *Journal of Speech, Language, and Hearing Research, 46*(3), 591–607.

Toni, I., de Lange, F. P., Noordzij, M. L., & Hagoort, P. (2008) Language beyond action. *Journal of Physiology—Paris, 102*, 71–79.

Tranel, D., Adolphs, R., Damasio, H., & Damasio, A. R. (2001). A neural basis for the retrieval of words for actions. *Cognitive Neuropsychology, 18*(7), 655–674.

Tranel, D., Kemmerer, D., Adolphs, R., Damasio, H., & Damasio, A. R. (2003). Neural correlates of conceptual knowledge for actions. *Cognitive Neuropsychology, 20*, 409–432.

Umilta, M. A., Escola, L., Intskirveli, I., Grammont, F., Rochat, M., Caruana, F., ... Rizzolatti, G. (2008). When pliers become fingers in the monkey motor system. *Proceedings of the National Academy of Sciences of the United States of America, 105*, 2209–2213.

Van Heugten, C. M., Dekker, J., Deelman, B. G., Stehmann-Saris, J. C., & Kinebanian, A. (1999). A diagnostic test for apraxia in stroke patients: internal consistency and diagnostic value. *Clinical Neuropsychologist, 13*(2), 182–192.

Vicario, C. M., & Newman, A. (2013). Emotions affect the recognition of hand gestures. *Fronteirs in Human Neuroscience, 7*, 906.

Wang, L., & Goodglass, H. (1992). Pantomime, praxis, and aphasia. *Brain and Language, 42*, 402–418.

Warren, J. E., Sauter, D. A., Eisner, F., Wiland, J., Dresner, M. A., Wise, R. J., ... Scott, S. K. (2006). Positive emotions preferentially engage an auditory–motor "mirror" system. *The Journal of Neuroscience, 26*(50), 13067–13075.

Waters, G. S., Rochon, E., & Caplan, D. (1992). The role of high-level speech planning in rehearsal: evidence from patients with apraxia of speech. *Journal of Memory and Language, 31*, 54–73.

Wertz, R. T. (1985). Neuropathologies of speech and language: an introduction to patient management. In D. R. Johns (Ed.), *Clinical management of neurogenic communicative disorders* (2nd ed.). Boston: Little Brown.

Wertz, R. T., LaPointe, L. L., & Rosenbek, J. C. (1984). *Apraxia of speech in adults: the disorder and its management.* New York: Grune & Stratton.

Wise, R. J., Howard, D., Mummery, C. J., Fletcher, P., Leff, A., Büchel, C., & Scott, S. K. (2000). Noun imageability and the temporal lobes. *Neuropsychologia, 38*(7), 985–994.

Zwaan, R. A., & Taylor, L. J. (2006). Seeing, acting, understanding: motor resonance in language comprehension. *Journal of Experimental Psychology: General, 135*, 1–11.

Zwinkels, A., Geusgens, C., van de Sande, P. & van Heugten, C. (2004). Assessment of apraxia: inter-rater reliability of a new apraxia test, association between apraxia and other cognitive deficits and prevalence of apraxia in a rehabilitation setting. *Clinical Rehabilitation, 18*, 819–827.

8

Visual Processing in Recovery from Aphasia

Introduction

This chapter takes us one step further along the nonlinguistic path toward recovery from aphasia by addressing the neural bases underlying the interaction between visual and language processing in aphasia. For many years, processing of visual and linguistic information was assumed to be neuroanatomically distinguishable, largely based on early lesion studies associating deficits in visual recognition (agnosia) with the right hemisphere and impaired language use (aphasia) with the left hemisphere (e.g., Geschwind, 1965). Within this system, links between visual and linguistic information were established through the transmittal of information via interhemispheric commissural fibers—the corpus callosum. Confirmatory evidence for this hemispheric specialization was found in studies of split-brain patients, whose commissural fibers were surgically removed, a procedure that, for some, resulted in a reduction in the ability to process linguistic material presented to them in their right visual field (reviewed in Gazzaniga, 2005).

Additional support for this right/left hemispheric division came from studies of optic aphasia, a language impairment that selectively affects a person's ability to name an object but leaves intact his or her object recognition (e.g., Caramazza & Hillis, 1990; Freund, 1889; Hillis & Caramazza, 1995; Margolin, Friedrich, & Carlson, 1985; Plaut & Schallice, 1993; Riddoch & Humphreys, 1987). This failure is vision system-specific, as the same object can be named when it is presented in auditory, tactile, olfactory, or gustatory modalities as well as from verbal definitions of it (e.g., Gainotti, 2004; Girkin &

Miller, 2001; Manning, 2000). The brain damage underlying these behavioral patterns involves both a left occipital lesion, which presumably blocks visual object processing in the left hemisphere, and a lesion in the corpus callosum, which prevents the transfer of visual information about the object from the right to the left hemisphere, where it would be named.

Against this background emerged a flurry of studies of category-specific deficits in aphasia (reviewed in De Bleser, 2009), which aimed to explain how perceptual information, vision included, contributes to the creation of semantic concepts in the brain. These works were inspired by Wernicke's (1874) and Freud's (1891/1953) neuroanatomy of "concept fields" and gave rise to Damasio's (1989) influential notion of supramodal processing in high-level convergence zones, situated amid modal sensorimotor systems (restated in more recent terms in Binder & Desai, 2011).

Our focus in this chapter, however, is not on the hotly debated questions concerning the neural bases of the semantic system in aphasia as related to the visual modality but rather on the somewhat more overlooked topic of how persons with aphasia process visual cues—inherent in naturalistic speech situations and clinical settings—as a means of augmenting linguistic performance. Specifically we present evidence, to the extent that the literature allows, that speaks to (1) the effects of visual cues encoded in images (pictures and scenes) and faces (mouth movements) on aphasic language performance, (2) the brain activation patterns associated with the use of these visual cues, (3) the benefits associated with the inclusion of these cues in aphasia treatment protocols, and (4) the neural underpinnings of these cues and their contribution to reshaping the neural pathways mediating the recovery of language functions in aphasia.

We open with a discussion of how the healthy brain supports visual perception and recognition, harnessing visual information to support language performance. We first show that the healthy brain distinguishes the processing of naming to picture as compared with naming to definitions (Hamberger et al., 2013). We then review studies demonstrating that healthy adults engage in visual scanning of the scene in which the speech situation is embedded in order to determine the veracity of linguistic input they hear vis-à-vis the available visual information they analyze (Goolkasian, 1996; Reichle, Carpenter, & Just, 2000; Singer, 2006; Underwood, Jebbett, & Roberts, 2004). We also discuss neurophysiological findings indicating several time points during which visual context affects neural activation in response to online picture-based sentence comprehension (Knoeferle et al., 2011).

In addition, we introduce evidence demonstrating that healthy adults visually track the articulatory movements produced by others so as to improve identification of speech sounds (and by extension lexical processing) by matching bits of visual and acoustic information against one another (Campbell, 1996; Dodd, 1977; Erber, 1969; Grant & Seitz, 2000; Green, 1996; Reisberg, McLean, & Goldfield, 1987; Schwartz et al., 2004; Stein & Meredith, 1993; Sumby & Pollack, 1954; Summerfield, 1979). We briefly summarize the neural correlates of these behavioral patterns, which suggest maximal brain activation primarily in the superior temporal gyrus for incongruent audiovisual stimuli (van Atteveldt et al., 2010; Stevenson et al., 2010).

We then discuss findings from aphasia studies that speak to these visual behaviors. Specifically we review evidence which suggests that persons with aphasia have more facility processing pictorial versus verbal materials (Stead & colleagues, 2012). We describe studies indicating that high-context images are particularly informative for persons with aphasia (e.g., Hux et al., 2010; McKelvey, Hux, Dietz, & Beukelman, 2010; Wallace et al., 2014). In addition, we present neuroimaging studies of picture naming in aphasia that have identified the neural substrates associated with nonverbal visual functions—substrates that contribute to lexical selection and retrieval (e.g., Baldo, Arevalo, Pattereson, & Dronkers, 2013). Some of these findings demonstrate a putative convergence of neural substrates subserving visual, linguistic, and higher-order cognitive functions during language performance (Baldo, Bunge, Wilson, & Dronkers, 2010), much in the spirit of the neural multifucntionality approach espoused throughout this book.

We then turn to findings concerning audiovisual effects in aphasia, which portray a mixed picture of patterns of impairments (Schmid & Ziegler, 2006) and sparing (Baum, Martin, Hamilton, & Beauchamp, 2012), calling into question the extent to which persons with aphasia can derive benefits from information encoded in visual cues. Where available, we discuss the neural underpinnings of these patterns (Baum et al., 2012) and the implications they might have for our view of neural multifunctionality in the course of recovery of aphasia.

We conclude with a review of aphasia treatment protocols incorporating visual components, which demonstrate the clinical utility of using visual cues in therapeutic settings (e.g., Harnish et al., 2014). We focus on the behavioral and neural underpinnings of exposure to pictorial stimuli (e.g., Abel et al., 2014; Szalfarski et al., 2011) and audiovisual cues (e.g., Fridriksson et al., 2009; Sarasson et al., 2014) and discuss the extent to which they support the idea that neural activation induced by visual information in right hemisphere and perilesional areas assists in lexical processing/retrieval.

The Use of Visual Information During Language Performance

In most speech situations, language users utilize visual information from their surroundings in order to enhance their language processing. Just picture yourself in a crowded restaurant trying to hear your server listing today's specials. Most likely you will look to see if there is mention of these items in the written menu, or you will look at him intently in the hope that watching his face will clue you in to what he is saying. However, incorporation of visual information into speech processing is not a prerequisite for successful language performance. We can clearly express and/or understand the content of a spoken word or sentence when blindfolded. And, of course, persons who are blind can understand and express language. By the same token, we usually understand the content of the verbal exchange during a phone conversation even in the absence of eye contact with the conversational partner. If optional, what is it that visual processing contributes to language processing? We turn to a discussion of this question below.

EFFECTS OF PICTURES AND VISUAL SCENES ON LANGUAGE PROCESSING

Studies exploring the extent to which the processing of pictorial representations affects language performance in healthy adults are limited in number, and the neurocognitive mechanisms underlying these effects remain underspecified. Sparse neuroimaging evidence suggests that naming to pictures (visual naming) relies on some shared but also distinct neural pathways from those associated with naming to definitions (responsive naming) (Hamberger et al., 2013; Tomaszewski-Farias et al., 2005).

Specifically, Hamberger et al. (2013) found that visual naming activated anterior and posterior portions of the left superior, middle, and inferior temporal gyri, the right superior and middle temporal gyri, and the fusiform gyrus, while responsive naming appeared to activate the left posterior, middle, and inferior temporal gyri. An ordinal trend analysis of the data revealed additional task-related differences, where responsive naming induced increased expression in the left middle temporal gyrus, fusiform gyrus, precentral gyrus, and middle and inferior frontal gyri for, whereas visual naming increased expression in the left middle temporal and fusiform gyrus, and in the left inferior temporal gyrus, post central gyrus, parahippocampal gyrus, the right postcentral, middle temporal, and inferior temporal gyri. These patterns are shown in Figure 8.1. Visual naming did not invoke frontal activation. The authors speculate that the differences between these activation patterns might lie in the possibility that visual materials induce less linguistic competition than verbal definitions and that the resolution of this presumed competition is reflected by unique frontal activation in the responsive naming condition.

Results from Hamberger et al.'s (2013) study clearly indicate that naming to pictorial stimuli engages distinct neural processes, but conclusions cannot be made about whether or not such neural activity aids in lexical retrieval. Moreover, their results need to be evaluated against recent neural accounts of visual naming, based on neural stimulation mapping in awake participants, which propose that picture-induced language performance implicates parallel, segregated, large-scale corticosubcortical subnetworks, which directly interact with executive functions (Duffau et al., 2014), not inconsistent with our own view of neural multifunctionality of language.

More direct evidence for the ameliorating effects that visual cues have on language performance comes from eye-tracking studies monitoring eye gaze during act-out or passive listening comprehension tasks, which have shown that visual scenes help to resolve linguistic/referential ambiguities (e.g., Altmann, 2004; Chambers et al., 2004; Knoeferle et al., 2005; Knoeferle & Crocker, 2007; Sedivy et al., 1999; Spivey et al., 2002). Specifically, the matching of linguistic and visual inputs facilitates sentence-verification against pictorial information, as measured by decreased verification times.

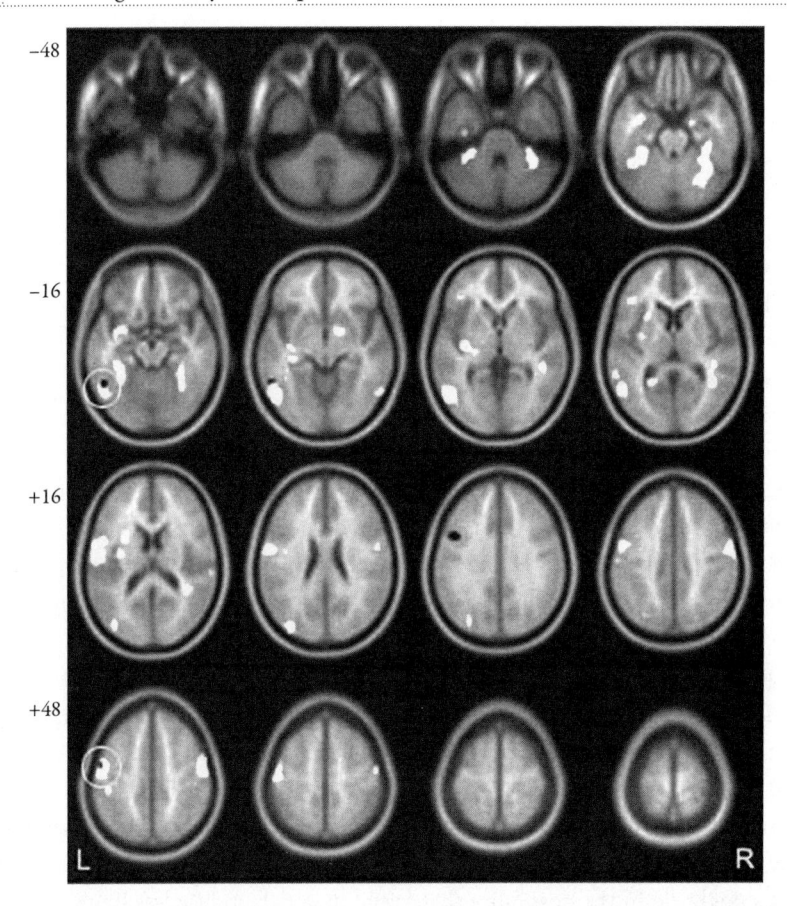

FIGURE 8.1 Neural correlates of visual and responsive naming in Hamberger's et al.'s (2013) study (See color insert.)

GLM results for visual and description naming. There was visual naming activation (yellow, VN > VC) in the bilateral parahippocampal gyrus and fusiform gyrus (row 1, fourth panel), temporooccipital cortex (row 2, bottom clusters), and bilateral pre/postcentral and inferior frontal gyrus (row 3 and 4). There was description naming activation (red, DN > DC) in left temporo-occipital cortex (row 2, left two panels), left inferior frontal gyrus (row 3, third panel), and left precentral gyrus (row 4, first panel). Regions of overlap for description and visual naming are indicated with circles (temporo-occipital cortex, second row, and pre/post central gyrus, fourth row).

Source: From Hamberger, M.J., Habeck, C.G., Pantazatos, S.P., Williams, A.C., & Hirsch, J. (2013). Shared space, separate processes: Neural activation patterns for auditory description and visual object naming in healthy adults. *Human Brain Mapping 35*(6), 2507–2520, figure 1. Reprinted by permission from John Wiley and Sons [Human Brain Mapping], copyright 2013.

Visual sentence-verification has been argued to reflect a temporally coordinated reciprocal relationship between processing of a linguistic input, which directs attention to objects/actions, and rapid feedback from scene-based visual representations (Knoeferle & Crocker, 2007; Mayberry, Crocker, & Knoeferle, 2009). Indeed, the extraction of information from visual images interacts with mechanisms of visual attention, resulting in distinguishable visual fixation times (e.g., Rayner, 2009). These include two main eye fixation patterns: (1) rapid and preferential fixation on human figures (Judd et al., 2009), regardless of size and position of the figure within the scene (Wilkinson & Light, 2011), and (2) fixation on objects with which one or more human are engaged (Fletcher-Watson et al., 2008).

However, some have argued that scene-sentence matching through sentence verification is an offline process that does not capture the visual effects of online incremental language processing (e.g., Kounios & Holocomb, 1992; Tanenhaus, Carroll, & Bever, 1976). To address this problem, researchers combined sentence verification response time with online event-related brain potential (ERP) measures (Knoeferle et al., 2011; Szücs et al., 2007; Vissers et al., 2008; Wassenaar & Hagoort, 2007). The important findings pertain to picture-sentence-congruence manipulations, which elicit a negativity effect (N400) (as in Szücs et al., 2007 and Wassenaar & Hagoort, 2007) independently associated with language comprehension tasks (e.g., Holcomb & Neville, 1991).

Knoeferle et al. (2011) measured sentence-verification response times and ERP responses among participants who were asked to match syntactically simple subject-verb-object sentences with a previous pictorial presentation of an action. They found differential patterns for congruent and noncongruent materials, which speak to multiple points in which visual context affects sentence comprehension. For noncongruent materials, verification response times were longer, and negativity N400 effects were found in the centroparietal areas for verbs and more anteriorly for objects. For congruent materials, sentence-verification response times showed a negative correlation with the verb N400 and a positive correlation with the object negativity effect. Interestingly, sentence-verification response times were predicted by both negativity effects and by measures of verbal working memory rather than by negativity effects alone, indicating a complex interaction between visual, memory, and language processes in the course of picture-based sentence comprehension—thus, it seems, presenting more evidence for neural multifunctionality.

LOOKING THE OTHER PERSON IN THE MOUTH: AUDIOVISUAL LANGUAGE PROCESSING

Studied somewhat more extensively are visual effects associated with audiovisual speech, during which participants listen for the acoustic properties of the sounds they hear and at the same time visually scan mouth movements of the speaker with whom they are interacting (Campbell, 1990). Unlike the acoustic speech signal, which provides the full array of distinctive features of the sound, speech information encoded in the visual signal is by definition incomplete; it specifies only a subset of the sound's distinctive features, typically place of articulation (Campbell, 1990). This partial specification generates visually noncontrastive sounds, known as *visemes* (e.g., /m/, /b/, /p/, all of which are bilabial and thus visually indistinguishable) (Fisher, 1968; Owens & Blazek, 1985).

Despite the poverty of its phonological properties, the visual stimulus has been found to play an important role in successful speech perception, especially in noisy conditions (e.g., Campbell, 1996; Dodd, 1977; Erber, 1969; Grant & Seitz, 2000; Green, 1996;

Reisberg, McLean, & Goldfield, 1987; Schwartz et al., 2004; Stein & Meredith, 1993; Sumby & Pollack, 1954; Summerfield, 1979). Studies have revealed improved language performance in response to simultaneous presentation of visual and auditory material as compared with unimodal auditory presentation (Callan et al., 2003; Helfer, 1997; MacLeod & Summerfield, 1990; Ross et al., 2007; Sumby & Pollack, 1954; Zion Golumbic et al., 2013). When the auditory and visual speech information conflicts, the visual presentation of the speech sound can modify the auditory speech percept, resulting in what is known as the McGurk effect (McGurk & MacDonald, 1976). Specifically, when auditory presentation of a syllable, "ba," is coupled with visual presentation of a mismatching syllable, "ga," the resulting percept is a fused syllable, "da" (see also Schmid, Thielmann, & Ziegler, 2009).

The contribution of audiovisual information to speech processing, especially in challenging listening conditions, has been argued to go beyond facilitation of sound detection, involving extraction of useful articulatory information that enhances speech intelligibility and hence speech comprehension (Schwartz et al., 2004). For example, in a study investigating the effects of lip reading on speech processing in noisy environments, participants showed improved discrimination of voicing cues when presented with audiovisual versus auditory-only input. This gain disappeared when the visual lip gestures were replaced by nonspeech visual input, suggesting a speech-specificity component to articulatory movement as visual cues. It is interesting to note in this regard that visual cues— even in the absence of acoustic information (lip reading)—encoded in articulatory movements appear to allow access to phonological representations that promote speech comprehension (Erber, 1969; Summerfield, 1987), although performance is less accurate and subject to more individual variability than that observed for bimodal stimuli (Auer, 2002; Campbell, 1990).

The nature of the neurocognitive mechanism mediating audiovisual processing, however, remains an open-ended question. For example, based on findings from electrophysiological studies reporting visually induced neural activation in the auditory cortex at time points as early as 50 to 100 ms, some have proposed a system in which audiovisual processing proceeds in an analysis-by-synthesis fashion, where the visual information imposes early constraints on speech processing before explicit auditory input is registered (e.g., Lebib, Papo, de Bode, & Baudonnière, 2003; Skipper et al., 2007; van Wassenhove, Grant, & Poeppel, 2005). The incoming auditory representations are evaluated in the context of the visually initiated predictions, during which redundancies between the phonetic features of visual prediction and those of the auditory input are decorrelated. The rate of decorrelation is determined on the basis of the strength of the visual prediction, which is derived from the salience of its features (e.g., bilabial /p/ is more salient than velar /k/). The stronger the prediction, the faster the decorrelation proceeds (van Wassenhove, Grant, & Poeppel, 2005). However, the precise temporal window during which this audiovisual integration occurs remains elusive (e.g., van Wassenhove, Grant, & Poeppel, 2007).

In a related electrophysiological study, Hessler et al. (2013) proposed that audiovisual processing reflects not merely an additive process but rather a synergistic effect whereby processing of visual information promotes language comprehension. The authors examined brain activity induced by auditory, visual, and audiovisual stimuli. Analyses comparing the audiovisual with the auditory materials (which adjusted for visual brain activity) revealed distinct evoked brain responses to the audiovisual stimuli compared with the auditory stimuli, with smaller amplitudes (P3) and shorter latencies (N2) associated with the audiovisual items. These findings were interpreted as indicative of the facilitating role multisensory integration has in correct phoneme identification (see also Möttönen, Krause, Tiippana, & Sams, 2002).

Note that the benefits of simultaneous presentation of visual and speech information interact in important ways with selective attention to facilitate speech processing, especially in multitalker environments (Zion Golumbic et al., 2013). Using magnetoenceohalographic measures, Zion Golumbic and colleagues (2013) demonstrated that visual input from an attended speaker improved the selectivity of auditory tracking of the auditory cortex, which helps parse continuous linguistic input into smaller units (also known as temporal tracking of the speech envelope). Because this attention modulation was not found in the absence of visual input, the authors proposed that visual enhancement aids in directing attentional resources to those future time points during which the auditory input will engage the language processing system.

Interaction among visual, attentional, and speech processes is exactly what we would expect in a brain that is neurally multifunctional in nature. Mesulam's (1998) early work elucidating the neural foundation underlying the transformation of sensation into cognition clearly indicates that sensory information necessarily undergoes attentional modulation, following a synaptic hierarchy comprising primary sensory, upstream unimodal, downstream unimodal, heteromodal, paralimbic, and limbic brain structures. Within this system, the midtemporal cortex, Wernicke's area, the hippocampal formation, and posterior parietal cortices partake in the conversion of sensation into recognition, engaging analogous computational epicenters that give rise to resultant cognitive processes.

It should come as no surprise, then, that from a neuroanatomical perspective, the neural imprint of audiovisual speech processing has been found in early sensory cortices as well as in higher-order speech areas (Besle, Fort, Delpuech, & Giard, 2004; Davis et al., 2008; McGettigan et al., 2012). These include primary sensory regions and posterior inferior frontal gyrus and ventral premotor cortex, supramarginal gyrus, posterior superior temporal gyrus, planum temporale, and posterior superior temporal sulcus (e.g., Bernstein, Lu, & Jiang, 2008; Callan et al., 2004; Calvert & Campbell, 2003; Miller & D'Esposito, 2005; Skipper et al., 2007; Skipper, Nusbaum & Small, 2005).

Indeed, Musacchia and Schroeder (2009) described a web of subcortical-cortical networks that feed forward and backward and connect laterally to accomplish multisensory integration during audiovisual processing. They argue that this integration is observed even at the lowest levels of the auditory system and acts to coordinate new sensory input with ongoing cortical processes. A good example of such lower-level audiovisual integration is the reduction in neural activation of Heschl's gyrus found in response to stimuli that share acoustic and visual features compared with those that are acoustically identical but visually distinct (Hasson et al., 2007).

Many neuroimaging studies of audiovisual effects have focused on the role of the left superior temporal sulcus (STS) in multimodal processing (Beauchamp, 2005; Miller & D'Esposito, 2005; Nath & Beauchamp, 2011, 2012; Scott & Johnsrude, 2003; Stevenson & James, 2009). For example, neuroimaging studies comparing neural responses to uni- and multisensory stimuli have shown greater blood oxygen level dependent (BOLD) activation in the left STS for the latter (Beauchamp et al., 2004; Calvert, Campbell, & Brammer, 2000; Stevenson & James, 2009). Other studies have shown that the degree of McGurk effect is associated with amplitude of activity in the STS (Nath & Beauchamp, 2012) or that the McGurk effect can be reduced if transcranial magnetic stimulation is temporarily applied to the left STS (Beauchamp et al., 2010). Based on these and similar findings, some have proposed that unimodal information is integrated in multisensory cortices, such as the STS, and feed back onto primary sensory structures, leading to enhanced activation of auditory cortices (e.g., van Wassenhove, Grant, & Poeppel, 2005).

Audiovisual effects have also been found to activate Broca's area (Callan et al., 2003; Campbell et al., 2001; Nishitani & Hari, 2002; Ojanen et al., 2005; Paulesu et al., 2003; Sekiyama et al., 2003). For example, Ojanen et al. (2005) found that processing of congruent and incongruent audiovisual stimuli induced activation in Broca's area and Brodmann's area 6 but that incongruent materials led to greater BOLD responses. Figure 8.2 depicts these brain activation patterns.

These and similar findings have led some to propose that motor systems are foundational for audiovisual processing. Paulesu et al. (2003), for example, proposed that phonological processing during audiovisual speech involves matching of articulatory motor plans between speaker and viewer. Similarly, Callan et al. (2003) suggested that audiovisual speech is supported by internal simulation of the intended speech act of the observed speaker, feeding into what has been termed a supramodal phonological unit (Campbell, 1990; De Gelder, Bertelson, & Vroomen, 1996; Kim et al., 2004).

Activation of frontal circuits during audiovisual processing has been argued to reflect encoding of abstract representations at a sublexical level, independent of the properties of the sensory cues from which they are assumed to derive (e.g., Hasson et al., 2007). For example, in a neuroimaging study, Hasson et al. (2007) compared brain activation during passive observation of four types of audiovisual stimuli presented prior to the target stimulus /pk/: (1) /pa/, which involved auditory overlap with /pk/; (2) /ka/, which involved visual overlap with /pk/; (3) /ta/ which involved perceptual but no sensory overlap with /pk/; and (4) /pk/, which involved both perceptual and sensory overlap. They found a reduction in neural activation in the left hemisphere (pars opercularis and planum polare) when the target /pk/ was preceded by /ta/, which is perceptually

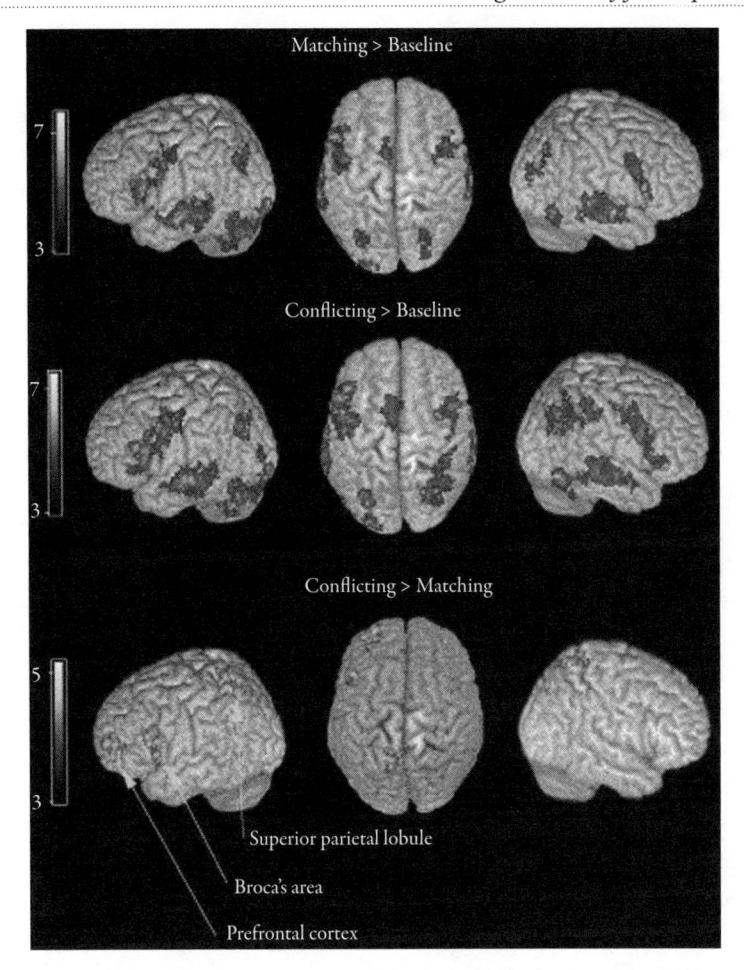

8. *Visual Processing in Recovery from Aphasia* 233

FIGURE 8.2 Brain activation in response to audiovisual processing (See color insert.)
Across-subjects (N = 10) z statistical maps overlaid on an anatomical template. Matching audiovisual speech activated the auditory and visual cortical areas as well as the inferior frontal, premotor, and the visual-parietal areas bilaterally (upper panel). Conflicting audiovisual speech caused a similar but more extensive pattern of brain activity (middle panel). The difference in the contrast conflicting N matching AV-stimulation reached significance in three left-hemisphere areas: Broca's area (BA44/45), the superior parietal lobule (BA7), and the prefrontal cortex (BA10) (lower panel). In the contrast matching N conflicting no statistically significant voxels were detected. Activation maps were thresholded using clusters determined by voxelwise Z N 3.0 and a cluster significance threshold of P b.05, corrected for multiple comparisons.

Source: From Ojanen, V., Möttönen, R., Pekkola, J., Jääskeläinen, I.P., Joensuu, R., Autti, T., & Sams, M. (2005). Processing of audiovisual speech in Broca's area, *Neuroimage, 25,* 333–338, figure 2. Reprinted by permission from Elsevier Limited [NeuroImage], copyright, 2005.

comparable to the target, but shared none of its visual and auditory features. The authors concluded that processing of the percept /ta/ cannot simply be attributed to the joint activation of visual and auditory inputs in unisensory brain structures and suggested considering an abstract level of speech representation at the level of the speech percept.

Some researchers have explicitly linked the activation of frontal brain structures during audiovisual processing to a visuomotor mirror neuron system (e.g., Ojanen et al.,

2005), on the assumption that these neurons allow for the convergence of phonetic and visual features in a motor representational space and thus serve as the basis for categorization (e.g., Fadiga, Fogassi, Gallese, & Rizzolatti, 2000). In this context, Skipper and colleagues (2006, 2007) proposed that during audiovisual processing, frontal brain structures actively generate hypotheses about the communicated speech category, which is then reconciled with input from auditory and somatosensory structures. However, it is difficult to rule out the possibility that patterns of frontoparietal activation result from increased task demands, as in the incongruent audiovisual stimuli in Ojanen et al.'s (2005) study, which, they themselves argue, engage additional neural mechanisms of conflict resolution and divided attention (as in Badre & Wagner, 2004; Durston et al., 2003; Loose et al., 2003; Mazoyer et al., 2002).

Nonetheless, the grounding of audiovisual processing in neural systems of motor function is strongly supported by studies attesting to visual effects on other types of movement, including head movements and cospeech gestures, implicating the superior temporal cortex posterior to primary auditory cortex, the supramarginal gyrus of the inferior parietal lobule, and ventral and dorsal premotor and primary motor cortices (e.g., Dick et al., 2009; Munhall et al., 2004; Skipper et al., 2009). For example, in Skipper et al.'s (2009) neuroimaging study, visual processing of face movements was associated with neural activation (as measured by strength of BOLD signal) in brain circuits mediating motor planning and production as well as in posterior regions subserving phonological processing, suggesting that visual processing of oral gestures supports phonological disambiguation. For visual processing of cospeech manual gestures, they found activation of motor and production areas alongside anterior brain structures associated with semantic processing, indicating that manual gestures contribute to semantic interpretation of communicative goals. Relatedly, Dick et al. (2009) found that manual gestures activate a distributed bilateral cortical network comprising the posterior temporal and inferior parietal structures, along with the inferior frontal gyrus (IFG), where the right IFG is activated more strongly in response to audiovisual presentation of meaningless gestures.

However, the extent to which motor systems play a central role in predicting audiovisual effects remains a matter of debate. Hickok (2012), for example, has rejected the idea that motor systems are foundational to audiovisual processing and more generally to speech perception (as reviewed in Chapter 7). His objection is rooted in the mixed empirical picture regarding the neural underpinnings of additive and supraadditive effects of audiovisual speech, which are not always mediated by frontal brain structures (e.g., Calvert, Campbell, & Brammer, 2000; Miller & D'Esposito, 2005). He also notes developmental studies demonstrating audiovisual effects in infants, who clearly lack the motor-speech experience that supposedly underlies speech processing. Instead, he proposes that the ventral rather than the dorsal stream generates forward predictions that guide speech perception.

Hickok and colleagues do not completely rule out involvement of motor systems in speech perception but instead suggest a modulatory role within a sensory feedback control model of speech production (for a detailed review, see Hickok, Houde, & Rong, 2011). The frontal networks in this system do not engage in phonemic analysis in service of speech perception but rather activate sensory-to-motor feedback circuits aimed at correcting motor speech patterns based on speech input from self or others. In this system, motor-based forward predictions generate a sensory expectation, which focuses attention on relevant sensory properties and allows the detection of deviations from the expected target. Thus motor systems function as an internal feedback control mechanism through top-down attention modulation of sensory systems. The attentional focus is assumed to enhance the detection of the expected features but also increase detection of deviations.

From a neural perspective, Hickok et al. (2011) proposed that target neurons mediate coarse sensory discrimination whereas flanking neurons, which are tuned slightly away from the target neurons (e.g., Jazayeri & Movshon, 2006, 2007), subserve fine discrimination. Their suggestion is based on the observation that flanking neurons have been shown to adapt to slight changes in stimulus features and are presumably good candidates for this type of neural processing. Our discussion here is not meant to endorse this particular proposal as an account for audiovisual or other speech perception effects. Rather, it is intended to highlight the model's direct incorporation of selective attention into its mechanism, which expands the discussion of neural integration beyond the scope of sensorimotor systems much in the spirit of our notion of neural multifunctionality in recovery from aphasia.

Visual Processing of Pictures/Visual Scenes in Aphasia: Behavioral and Neural Correlates

The use of pictorial stimuli in studies of aphasia rests on the assumption that the ability to process pictorial information requires functionality of the visual system and that this system is spared among persons with aphasia (e.g., Radanovic & Mansur, 2011). However, studies exploring the neurobehavioral underpinnings of picture and/or visual scene processing in aphasia are scant (Baldo et al., 2010; 2013; Gardner et al., 2012; Stead, Savage, & Buckingham, 2012). This gap is somewhat surprising given that the characterization of aphasic language impairments frequently relies on the use of pictorial materials. One would be hard pressed to find someone in the aphasia world who is not familiar with the "cookie theft" picture from the Boston Diagnostic Aphasia Examination (Goodglass & Kaplan, 1983). In fact, we performed a google search using the phrase "cookie theft picture in aphasia" and received over a million hits! Even granting that some of these links were not relevant to our current discussion, they clearly speak to the popularity of this test. Google searches aside, it is well known that the Boston Naming Test, a test based on the visual processing of pictures, is the most widely used test in neuropsychological testing (Rabin, Barr, & Burton, 2005).

Although early work on visual processing in aphasia has shown that deficits in the visual processing of nonverbal symbols are dissociable from language impairments (e.g., Farah, 1990; Geschwind, 1965), researchers at the time disagreed about whether or not persons with aphasia in fact retain the ability to process such symbols visually. Some demonstrated compromised symbol naming (e.g., Duffy, Duffy, & Pearson, 1975; Gardner, 1974), while others showed preservation of symbol use (Goodglass & Kaplan, 1983; Luria, 1970).

Evidence emerging from more recent behavioral work endorses the claim that persons with aphasia have more facility while processing pictorial than verbal materials. For example, Stead and colleagues (2012) compared pictorial and graphemic processing in which three participants with fluent aphasia were asked to determine whether or not the final stimulus in a sequence of four was congruent with the three preceding stimuli. Pictorial materials consisted of pictures of objects and of action scenes. The corresponding graphemic stimuli comprised word categories. Participants performed better on all pictorial stimuli, as measured by accuracy and reaction time, but only the participant with conduction aphasia showed a significant advantage in pictorial over graphemic processing. The authors leave open the interpretation regarding the source of variation in performance, but suggest that the use of nonverbal pictorial materials might be beneficial as an alternative mode of communication at least for some persons with fluent aphasia.

High-context images, which portray people or objects relating to one another in a naturalistic setting in reference to a central action in a scene, have been found to be particularly informative for persons with aphasia (Blackstone, 2004; Dietz, McKelvey, & Beukelman, 2006; Dietz, Hux, McKelvey, Beukelman, & Weissling, 2009; Hux et al., 2010; McKelevy et al., 2010; Weissling & Beukelman, 2006). For example, in a recent eye-tracking study, Thiessen and colleagues (2014) demonstrated that persons with aphasia are much like neurologically intact participants in processing visually rich images in that they quickly and repeatedly fixate on human figures in a visual image as well as on the object with which such figures are engaged.

In addition, a comparison of aphasic performance on word-image matching tasks among high-, low-, and no-context images revealed better object, person, and action naming in response to the high-context images (McKelvey et al., 2010). Relatedly, the use of information encoded in high-context images among persons with aphasia has been found to result in a greater amount of content and level of cognitive complexity expressed during communicative interaction (Hux et al., 2010). Wallace et al. (2014), however, caution that high-context images laden with information may pose a visual, inferential, and cognitive burden that may exceed the processing capacities of persons with aphasia. Indeed, persons with aphasia are slower and less accurate than healthy adults in matching sentences conveying background and inferential information to high-context images as compared with those relaying action-based information (Wallace et al., 2014).

To the best of our knowledge, neuroimaging studies directly contrasting naming to verbal cues with naming to visual cues have yet to be conducted. Nonetheless, evidence for the neural correlates of visual naming in aphasia can be derived indirectly from neuroimaging studies of picture naming, which delineate the discrete contributions of nonverbal visual and motor functions from those associated with lexical selection and retrieval. For example, using a voxel-based lesion analysis of the performance of 96 aphasic participants on the Boston Naming Test (Kaplan et al., 2001), Baldo et al. (2013) revealed that picture naming implicates a large network in the left peri-Sylvian cortex comprising the middle temporal gyrus (MTG), the superior temporal gyrus (STG) and underlying white matter, and the left inferior parietal cortex. After they adjusted for impairments in visual recognition and motor speech, the areas that remained significant in their analysis involved the left midposterior MTG and underlying white matter. They interpret their findings as an indication that the left MTG is a core brain structure subserving naming, in line with findings from many other studies of naming deficits in aphasia, including studies comparing picture- to definitional naming (e.g., Corina et al., 2005; Damasio et al., 1996; Edwards et al., 2010; Hamberger, Goodgman, Perrine, & Tamny, 2001; Hillis et al., 2006; Indefrey & Levelt, 2004; Martin, 2007; Tomaszewski-Farias et al., 2005).

Although Baldo and colleagues (2013) did not set out to characterize visual effects on picture naming, their results clearly suggest that this process is based on a multimodal interaction between visual and language processing. They, in fact, note that the MTG is positioned in the brain to function as a "supramodal" processing center, where object recognition, mediated by the inferior temporal cortex, visual perception, subserved by visual association cortex, and language functions, supported by MTG/STG all converge (see also Turken & Dronkers, 2011). This claim is consistent with the proposal that an occipitotemporal tract underlies visual recognition in picture naming (Mandonnet, Gatignol, & Duffau, 2009).

Interestingly, these findings are consistent with results from a recent neuroimaging study by Sandberg & Kiran (2014) of concreteness effects among persons with and without aphasia. They used word judgment and synonym judgment tasks to compare neural activation patterns associated with the processing of concrete and abstract words, which differ semantically in terms of the visual features they encode. Aphasic and nonaphasic participants alike showed brain activation patterns for both word classes in the left inferior frontal and middle temporal gyrus, where semantic processing is assumed to occur (Lau, Phillips, & Poeppel, 2008; Vigneau et al., 2006). The aphasic participants showed strong perilesional activation even where brain damage was extensive as well as right homologous activation, suggesting left-sided restoration of function coupled with right-sided reorganization or ancillary processing. For the concrete words, both groups showed additional activation in multimodal brain regions, with stronger activation observed in the aphasic group. Although the authors do not note this possibility, this stronger multimodal activation may reflect overreliance on perceptual information to aid in lexical processing.

INTERACTIONS WITH OTHER COGNITIVE DOMAINS

Gardner et al. (2012) found that persons with aphasia with lesions to the left prefrontal cortex (PFC) but not to the left temporoparietal cortex showed an interaction among visual, nonverbal auditory, verbal, and semantic control abilities. The authors compared (1) spoken word-picture matching to picture-picture matching, (2) spoken word-picture matching to sound-picture matching—pairing an environmental sound with a thematically related picture (e.g., the sound of a horn with a picture of a horn), and (3) associative matching in verbal and visual modalities. They found that repeated and rapid presentations of semantically related stimuli across all conditions led to declines in the participants' word-picture matching abilities. This effect, also known as refractory effect, was found only among the PFC participants; the authors took this to reflect impaired control of multimodal semantic retrieval, likely linked to deficiency in executive function systems, as discussed in Chapter 3.

Relatedly, in another voxel-based lesion/symptom-mapping study, Baldo and colleagues (2010) considered the interaction among visual pattern matching, relational reasoning, and language functions among aphasic persons and nonaphasic persons with left hemisphere brain damage. They used Raven's colored progressive matrices (RCPMs), where participants are required to complete a visual pattern by choosing one of six possible options (see also Chapter 3). For some of these items, the solution can be derived by simple visual matching, whereas for others complex relational reasoning is needed (DeShon, Chan, & Wessbein, 1995; Villardita, 1985). The investigators found worse performance on the RCPMs among persons with aphasia versus the other patient group. These participants, especially those with more severe aphasia, showed greater difficulty on the relational than on the visual-matching items. The deficient relational reasoning was associated with damage to brain structures central for language processing, including the left middle and superior temporal gyri, whereas visual-matching performance was linked to damage to occipital inferotemporal regions, which mediate visual processing. Thus, while certain aspects of visual processing and executive functions might be neuroanatomically distinguishable, their integration is called upon in the service of language functions, in line with the neural multifunctionality approach espoused throughout this book.

AUDIOVISUAL PROCESSING IN APHASIA:
BEHAVIORAL AND NEURAL CORRELATES

As discussed earlier in this chapter, audiovisual processing in the neurologically unimpaired brain relies heavily on neural activation in the left hemisphere. While articulatory movements undoubtedly also engage visuospatial face recognition functions of the right hemisphere (Moskovitch, Scullion, & Christie, 1976), evidence from lesion studies suggests that audiovisual and visuospatial face processing are dissociable (Campbell, 1990; Campbell et al., 1986). Campbell et al. (1986), for example, showed that a right hemisphere participant with prosopagnosia maintained the capacity to speech read and that a left hemisphere participant with impaired audiovisual performance retained face recognition functions.

Very few studies have explored audiovisual effects in aphasia (e.g., Baum et al., 2012; Schmid & Ziegler, 2006). In a small number of studies of participants with word deafness, benefits from visual input have been reported (Morris et al., 1996; Shindo et al., 1991). However, the extent to which persons with aphasia can derive benefits from information encoded in visual cues remains unclear. In a study comparing audiovisual performance between persons with and without aphasia and/or apraxia of speech, Schmid and Ziegler (2006) found significant impairment in the aphasic/apraxic compared with the healthy control group. They used a discrimination task comprised of speech (sounds that differed in manner of articulation and in lip rounding) and nonspeech stimuli (lip gestures such as "kiss" and "whistle"), which were presented in four conditions: auditory only, visual only, a simultaneous bimodal audiovisual presentation, and a sequential cross-modal presentation of auditory followed by visual.

Results indicated that persons with aphasia and/or apraxia erred more than healthy controls on speech and nonspeech stimuli in all four conditions. Healthy controls produced very few errors but showed great interindividual variability in their cross-modal matching for nonspeech materials. The patients' impairments in cross-modal matching were differentially predicted by their nonspeech and speech abilities, with poor cross-modal matching of nonspeech stimuli being associated with low facial apraxia scores and impaired cross-modal matching of speech stimuli being related to deficits in verbal repetition. Based on these findings, Schmid and Ziegler (2006) concluded that there exists a distinction between audiovisual processing for speech and nonspeech oral gestures and that impaired speech perception among aphasic/apraxic participants reflects disrupted phonological access at the supramodal level, where visual and auditory data are integrated.

However, brain damage to the left hemisphere does not always result in a reduction in audiovisual processing in aphasia. In a recent neuroimaging study, Baum et al. (2012) showed, at 5 years poststroke, preserved multisensory integration in a participant with anomic aphasia due to a lesion to the left middle and posterior superior temporal sulcus (STS) and surrounding temporal and parietal structures. The participant demonstrated greater BOLD responses in the right STS, induced by the McGurk effect, which in age-matched controls was observed bilaterally. The authors took these findings to reflect a role for the right STS in the reorganization of language networks in recovery from aphasia, at least in terms of multisensory integration of speech.

Baum et al. (2012) noted that unlike neurologically intact participants, in whom maximal brain activation is observed for incongruent audiovisual stimuli (Stevenson et al., 2010; van Atteveldt et al., 2010), their participant showed enhanced and uniform activation in response to all speech stimuli. They attributed this pattern to attention modulation, which presumably supports the participant's effortful speech. Such an interpretation is consistent with our view of neural multifunctionality during the course of recovery of aphasia, where the neural constellation of cognitive, emotional, motor, and sensory functions dynamically reshapes aphasic language performance.

Aphasia Assessment/Treatment Studies Incorporating Visual Components

The observation that the processing of pictorial/visual scene information and of articulatory movement facilitates aphasic language performance speaks to the clinical utility of incorporation of visual components into therapeutic settings. For example, a recent study by Harnish et al. (2014) has shown that a high dosage of intensive training in picture naming for persons with anomia results in rapid and significant naming gains for trained items. Cued picture naming was administered over 2 weeks, with eight presentations of pictures per session. Six of the participants increased performance over 400 presentations, which is the equivalent of a 1-hour training session, and the other two improved over 1,200, which translated into 3 hours. Thus the understanding the contribution of visual processing to aphasic language performance is central to determining the type, amount, and frequency of cueing provided during the assessment and treatment of aphasia (for a related comment, see Stead, Savage, & Buckingham, 2012).

USE OF PICTORIAL STIMULI

It is well established that persons with aphasia have the capacity to use visual symbols, such as photographs or drawings, as a means for alternative communication (e.g., Beck & Fritz, 1998; Cress & King, 1999; Dietz et al., 2009; Fox & Fried-Oken, 1996; Hux et al., 2010; Jacobs et al., 2004; Johanssen-Horbach et al., 1985; Kagan, 1998; Koul & Lloyd, 1998; Levin et al., 2007; McKelvey et al., 2010; Simmons-Mackie et al., 2014; van de Sandt-Koenderman, 2004; Wallace et al., 2012; see also Chapter 3). These are particularly popular among persons with severe aphasia, who often resort to using photographic visual images, iconic drawings, communication books and boards, as well as low-, and high-tech mobile devices in lieu of speech (Garrett & Lasker, 2013; King, 2013; Lasker, Garrett, & Fox, 2007).

The use of pictorial stimuli requires extensive reliance on the visual system to locate, identify, and recognize the pictured images (Wilkinson et al., 2012; Wilkinson & Jagaroo, 2004). However, little is known about the nature of information processing in which persons with aphasia engage as they attempt to analyze visual images, nor is much known about the degree to which they rely on visual strategies during treatment.

Nonetheless, neurobehavioral evidence is now emerging that speaks to the involvement of brain structures mediating visual processing during the assessment and treatment of aphasia. For example, in the course of lexical processing, picture-identification tasks have been found to activate recovered perilesional brain structures of the left hemisphere among persons with chronic aphasia (Szaflarski et al., 2011). Using functional neuroimaging, Szalfarski and colleagues (2011) examined patterns of brain activation among participants with and without aphasia induced by picture-word matching versus picture-shape matching tasks over a 10-week period. Both groups performed similarly in the picture-shape matching condition, but the healthy controls showed an advantage in the picture-word matching condition. Brain activation patterns differed between the groups, with healthy control showing left-to-right positive BOLD activation in frontotemporal networks and in retrosplenial posterior cingulate areas along with negative BOLD in bilateral frontotemporal areas. Aphasic participants, on the other hand, demonstrated positive BOLD activations in perilesional areas and negative BOLD activations in the right hemisphere. The authors interpreted these findings as indicating that visual lexical processing is required in order to engage recovered perilesional brain structures in the left hemisphere. However, their sample size was too small (four aphasic participants) to determine whether changes in performance are related to greater recruitment of language networks, as the investigators themselves note.

In a recent model-oriented word-production aphasia therapy study, Abel et al. (2014) documented brain activation of regions mediating visual processing as related to naming, although the goal of the treatment protocol was not to assess the effects of visual cues on aphasic performance. They administered increasingly complex phonological and semantic cues to participants with phonologically and semantically based naming deficits, defined by Dell's spreading activation model (mentioned in Chapter 5) over a 4-week period with the aim of identifying general treatment effects, potential differences between trained and untrained items, differential effects of treatment methods, and analysis of error patterns in terms of Dell's model. The interesting finding in the current context is that brain areas mediating visual processing, especially the precuneus and thalamus, were activated only for trained items, which overall showed better treatment gains versus untrained items. Because the left precuneus has been associated with visual imagery (Price, 2012) and cognitive strategy (Calvert, Campbell, & Brammer, 2000), the authors interpreted their findings as suggesting strategic use of visual imagery to assist in lexical retrieval.

AUDIOVISUAL CUEING

A long-standing method to boost word-finding difficulties among participants with aphasia is phonological cueing (Best, Herbert, Hickin, Osborne, & Howard, 2002; Bruce & Howard, 1988; Herbert, Best, Hickin, Howard, & Osborne, 2001; Hickin, Best, Herbert, Howard, & Osborne, 2002; Howard & Harding, 1998; Lorenz &

Nickels, 2007; Lorenz & Ziegler, 2009; Marshall, Freed, & Karow, 2001; Myers-Pease & Goodglass, 1978; Nickels, 2002). Phonological cueing is particularly common among persons with anomic aphasia, in whom a disruption of the mapping between preserved phonological and semantic systems is observed (e.g., Lambon Ralph et al., 2000). There is some controversy regarding the precise mechanism by which phonological facilitation occurs, specifically whether it involves lexical or sublexical processes (an association between phonological cueing and nonwords would distinguish these views) (e.g., Best et al., 2002).

Phonological information encoded in the phonological cue is typically bimodal—auditory and visual—although selective use of either modality in treatment is possible (e.g., mouthing speech sounds without generating acoustic output). For most persons with anomia, bimodal cues have been found to be efficacious in improving word production (e.g., Best et al., 2002; Howard & Harding, 1998; Li & Williams, 1990; Podraza & Darley, 1977; Stimley & Noll, 1991), which is somewhat surprising given the mixed picture regarding audiovisual abilities among persons with aphasia discussed earlier.

In a recent study, Wunderlich and Ziegler (2011) considered the utility of visual phonological information as compared with auditory cueing in promoting word retrieval among persons with anomia. They used picture-naming tasks in which the first segment of the target served as a cue. For visual cues, mouth shapes were presented; for auditory ones, the first phoneme was given. Both cue types enhanced naming among participants as a group as measured by reductions in reaction times. However, case-by-case analyses demonstrated that participants were differentially affected by cue type, with some deriving benefits from auditory input while others benefitted from a visual one. The results were taken to indicate that the phonologic information encoded in visual input—place of articulation—even though incomplete, is sufficiently informative to activate its associated phonemes and serves as an effective aid in word retrieval difficulties among persons with anomia.

Support for this claim comes from a computerized aphasia treatment study by Choe and Stanton (2011) in which two aphasic participants underwent a naming treatment program consisting of audiovisual and auditory-only cues. One participant benefited from the combined presentation significantly more than the one involving auditory cues only while the other gained from both types of cues. Gains were measured by word counts of items that the participant produced spontaneously without prompting. These findings point to the clinical promise of incorporating visual cues into naming treatment protocols.

Some treatment studies exploring the contribution of visual speech perception to language performance in aphasia have focused on the potential gains of targeting visual speech for persons with nonfluent aphasia (e.g., Fridriksson et al., 2009). The underlying logic rests on the observation that the brain structures compromised in nonfluent aphasia (Broca's area and the left anterior insula—e.g., Dronkers, 1996; Hillis et al., 2004) are the very areas that are activated during speech perception and audiovisual speech, as reviewed earlier in the chapter. Thus targeting audiovisual speech perception during treatment of nonfluent aphasia could presumably stimulate residual frontal networks without requiring patients to engage in effortful production. Evidence supporting this idea comes from Fridriksson et al.'s (2009) visual aphasia treatment study; it compared two types of aphasia interventions, one involving auditory presentation of target words with matching pictures and the other comprising auditory word presentations and a video of a speaker mouthing the heard words. Findings showed improvements in picture naming of trained and untrained items following the audiovisual but not the auditory-picture treatment protocols, in spite of far less than perfect audiovisual performance. The authors thus argued that the incorporation of a motor speech perception component in the therapy program could result in gains among nonfluent aphasic participants even in the face of a deficit in audiovisual processing. Note, however, that because the study was behavioral, it is difficult to determine whether these treatment-based changes were a function of neural activation of perilesional brain structures or right hemisphere homologues of traditional language areas, as the authors themselves note. Also, recovery patterns were highly variable and were not related to the presence of apraxia, suggesting that speech production in and of itself is not a predictor of the success of this visual therapy.

More direct evidence for brain changes induced by aphasia treatment incorporating observation of mouth movements has been reported by Sarasson et al. (2014). They explored changes in EEG sleep slow-wave activity (SWA) in response to an intensive mouth-imitation aphasia protocol designed to stimulate bilateral links between the inferior parietal lobule and ventral premotor areas. A single administration of the treatment protocol results in posttreatment increases in SWA activity in these cortical structures, especially in the undamaged right hemisphere, as well as in left precentral cortices. The latter were found to be predictive of participants' repetition scores, emphasizing the role of perilesional brain activation in the restoration of language function in aphasia. As the authors note, these patterns clearly reflect short-term treatment-induced plastic changes in the aphasic brain but do not provide information of long-term therapy-based neural changes.

References

Abel, S., Weiller, C., Huber, W., & Willmes, K. (2014). Neural underpinnings for model-oriented therapy of aphasic word production. *Neuropsychologia, 57*, 154–165.

Altmann, G. T. (2004). Language-mediated eye movements in the absence of a visual world: the 'blank screen paradigm'. *Cognition, 93*(2), B79–B87.

Auer, E. T. (2002). Spoken word recognition by eye. *Scandinavian Journal of Psychology, 50*(5), 419–425.

Badre, D., & Wagner, A. D. (2004) Selection, integration, and conflict monitoring; assessing the nature and generality of prefrontal cognitive control mechanisms, *Neuron, 41*(3), 473–487.

Baldo, J. V., Arevalo, A., Patterson, J. P., & Dronkers, N. F. (2013). Grey and white matter correlates of picture naming: evidence from a voxel-based lesion analysis of the Boston Naming Test. *Cortex, 49*(3), 658–667.

Baldo, J. V., Bunge, S. A., Wilson, S. M., & Dronkers, N. F. (2010). Is relational reasoning dependent on language? *Brain and Language, 113*(2), 59–64.

Baum, S. H., Martin, R. C., Hamilton, A. C., & Beauchamp, M. S. (2012). Multisensory speech perception without the left temporal sulcus. *Neuroimage, 62*(3), 1825–1832.

Beauchamp, M. S. (2005). See me, hear me, touch me: multisensory integration in lateral occipital-temporal cortex. *Current Opinion in Neurobiology, 15*(2), 145–145.

Beauchamp, M. S., Argall, B. D., Bodurka, J., Duyn, J. H., & Martin, A. (2004). Unraveling multisensory integration: patchy organization within human STS multisensory cortex. *Nature Neuroscience, 7*, 1190–1192.

Beauchamp, M. S., Nath, A. R., & Pasalar, S. (2010). fMRI-guided transcranial magnetic stimulation reveals that the superior temporal sulcus is a cortical locus of the McGurk Effect. *The Journal of Neuroscience, 30*, 2414–2417.

Beck, A., & Fritz, H. (1998). Can people who have aphasia learn iconic codes? *Augmentative and Alternative Communication, 14*(3), 184–196.

Besle, J., Fort, A., Delpuech, C., & Giard, M. H., (2004). Bimodal speech: early suppressive visual effects in human auditory cortex. *The European Journal of Neuroscience, 20*(8), 2225–2234.

Best, W., Herbert, R., Hickin, J., Osborne, F., & Howard, D. (2002). Phonological and orthographic facilitation of word-retrieval in aphasia: immediate and delayed effects. *Aphasiology, 16*, 151–168.

Bernstein, L. E., Lu, Z.-L., & Jiang, J. (2008). Quantified acoustic-optical speech signal incongruity identifies cortical sites of audiovisual speech processing. *Brain Research, 1242*, 172–184.

Binder, J. R., & Desai, R. H. (2011). The neurobiology of semantic memory, *Trends in Cognitive Sciences, 15*(11), 527–536.

Blackstone, S. (2004). Visual scene displays. *Augmentative Communication News, 16*(2), 1–8.

Bruce, C., & Howard, D. (1988). Why don't Broca's aphasics cue themselves? An investigation of phonemic cueing and tip of the tongue information. *Neuropsychologia, 26*(2), 253–264.

Callan, D. E., Jones, J. A., Munhall, K., Callan, A. M, Kroos, C., & Vatikiotis-Bateson, E. (2003). Neural processes underlying perceptual enhancement by visual speech gestures. *Neuroreport, 14*(17), 2213–2218.

Callan, D. E., Jones, J.A., Munhall, K., Kroos, C., Callan, A. M., & Vatikiotis-Bateson, E. (2004). Multisensory integration sites identified by perception of spatial wavelet filtered visual speech gesture information. *Journal of Cognitive Neuroscience, 16*(5), 805–816.

Calvert, G. A., & Campbell, R. (2003). Reading speech from still and moving faces: the neural substrates of visible speech. *Journal of Cognitive Neuroscience, 15*(1), 57–70.

Calvert, G. A., Campbell, R., & Brammer, M. J. (2000). Evidence from functional magnetic resonance imaging of crossmodal binding in the human heteromodal cortex. *Current Biology, 10*(11), 649–657.

Campbell, R. (1990). Lipreading, neuropsychology, and immediate memory. In G. Vallar & T. Shallice (Eds.), *Neuropsychological impairments of short-term memory* (pp. 268–286). Cambridge, UK: Cambridge University Press.

Campbell, R. (1996). Seeing brain reading speech: a review and speculations. In D. G. Stork & M. E. Hennecke (Eds.), *Speechreading by humans and machines* (pp. 115–133). Berlin: Springer.

Campbell, R., Landis T., & Regard M. (1986). Face recognition and lipreading. A neurological dissociation. *Brain, 109*(Pt 3), 509–521.

Campbell, R., MacSweeney, M., Surguladze, S., Calvert, G., McGuire, P., Suckling, J., ... David, A. S. (2001). Cortical substrates for the perception of face actions: an fMRI study of the specificity of activation for seen speech and for meaningless lower-face acts (gurning). *Brain Research. Cognitive Brain Research, 12*(2), 233–243.

Caramazza, A., & Hillis, A. E. (1990). Where do semantic errors come from? *Cortex, 26*(1), 95–122.

Chambers, C. G., Tanenhaus, M. K., & Magnuson, J. S. (2004). Actions and affordances in syntactic ambiguity resolution. *Journal of Experimental Psychology: Learning, Memory, and Cognition, 30*(3), 687–696.

Choe, Y., & Stanton, K., (2011). The effects of visual cues provided by computerized aphasia treatment. *Aphasiology, 25*(9), 983–997.

Corina, D. P., Gibson, E. K., Martin, R., Poliakov, A., Brinkley, J., & Ojemann, G. A. (2005). Dissociation of action and object naming: evidence from cortical stimulation mapping. *Human Brain Mapping, 24*(1), 1–10.

Cress, C., & King, J. (1999). AAC strategies for people with primary progressive aphasia without dementia: two case studies. *Augmentative and Alternative Communication, 15*(4), 248–259.

Damasio, A. R. (1989). Time-locked multiregional retroactivation: a systems-level proposal for the neural substrates of recall and recognition. *Cognition, 33*(1–2), 25–62.

Damasio, H., Grabowski, T. J., Tranel, D., Hichwa, R., & Damasio, A. R. (1996). A neural basis for lexical retrieval. *Nature, 380*, 499–505.

Davis, C., Kleinman, J. T., Newhart, M., Gingis, L., Pawlak, M., & Hillis, A. E. (2008). Speech and language functions that require a functioning Broca's area. *Brain and Language, 105*(1), 50–58.

De Bleser, R. (2009). History of Aphasia: Negative optic aphasia: How much semantics does a name need? Wolff's re-examination of Voit. *Aphasiology, 23*(12), 1427–1437.

De Gelder, B., Bertelson, B., & Vroomen, J. (1996). Aspects of modality in audio-visual processes. In D. G. Stork & M. E. Hennecke (Eds.), *Speechreading by humans and machines* (pp. 179–191). Berlin: Springer Verlag.

DeShon, R., Chan, D., & Weissbein, D. (1995). Verbal overshadowing effects on Raven's advanced progressive matrices: evidence for multidimensional performance determinants. *Intelligence, 21*, 135–155.

Dick, A. S., Goldin-Meadow, S., Hasson, U., Skipper, J. I., & Small, S. L. (2009). Co-speech gestures influence neural activity in brain regions associated with processing semantic information. *Human Brain Mapping, 30*, 3509–3526.

Dietz, A., Hux, K., McKelvey, M. L., Beukelman, D. R., & Weissling, K. (2009). Reading comprehension by people with chronic aphasia: a comparison of three levels of visuographic contextual support. *Aphasiology, 23*(7–8), 1053–1064.

Dietz, A., McKelvey, M., & Beukelman, D. R. (2006). Visual scene display (VSD): new AAC interfaces for persons with aphasia. *Perspectives on Augmentative and Alternative Communication, 15*(1), 13–17.

Dodd, B. (1977). The role of vision in the perception of speech. *Perception*, *6*(1), 31–40.

Dronkers, N. F. (1996). A new brain region for coordinating speech articulation. *Nature*, *384*(6605), 159–161.

Duffau, H., Moritz-Gasser, S., & Mandonnet, E. (2014). A re-examination of neural basis of language processing: proposal of a dynamic hodotopical model from data provided by brain stimulation mapping during picture naming. *Brain and Language*, *131*, 1–10.

Duffy, R. J., Duffy, J. R., & Pearson, K. (1975). Pantomime recognition in aphasics. *Journal of Speech and Hearing Disorders*, *44*, 156–168.

Durston, S., Davidson, M. C., Thomas, K. M., Worden, M. S., Tottenham, N., Martinez, A., . . . Casey, B. J. (2003). Parametric manipulation of conflict and response competition using rapid mixed-trial event-related fMRI. *Neuroimage*, *20*(4), 2135–2141.

Edwards, E., Nagarajan, S. S., Dalal, S. S., Canolty, R. T., Kirsch, H. E., Barbaro, N. M., & Knight, R. T. (2010). Spatiotemporal imaging of cortical activation during verb generation and picture naming. *Neuroimage*, *50*(1), 291–301.

Erber, N. P. (1969) Interaction of audition and vision in the recognition of oral speech stimuli. *Journal of Speech and Hearing Research*, *12*(2), 423–425.

Fadiga, L., Fogassi, L., Gallese, V., & Rizzolatti, G. (2000). Visuomotor neurons: ambiguity of the discharge or 'motor' perception? *International Journal of Psychophysiology*, *35*, 165–177.

Farah, M. J. (1990). *Visual agnosia: disorders of object recognition and what they tell us about normal vision*. Cambridge, MA: MIT Press.

Fisher, C. G. (1968). Confusions among visually perceived consonants. *Journal of Speech and Hearing Research*, *11*(4), 796–804.

Fletcher-Watson, S., Findlay, J. M., Leekman, S. R., & Benson, V. (2008). Rapid detection of person information in a naturalistic scene. *Perception*, *37*, 571–583.

Fox, L. E., & Fried-Oken, M. (1996). AAC aphasiology: partnership for future research. *Augmentative and Alternative Communication*, *12*, 257–271.

Freud, S. (1953). On aphasia: A critical study. In E. Stengel (Ed.), *Freud on aphasia*. New York: International Universities Press. (Original work published 1891)

Freund, D. C. (1889). Über optische Aphasie und Seelenblindheit. *Archiv für Psychiatrie und Nervenkrankheinten*, *20*, 371–416.

Fridriksson, J., Baker, J. M., Whiteside, J., Eoute, D. Jr., Moser, D., Vesselinov, R., & Rorden, C. (2009). Treating visual speech perception to improve speech production in nonfluent aphasia. *Stroke*, *40*(3), 853–858.

Gardner, H. (1974). The naming and recognition of written symbols in aphasic and alexic patients. *The Journal of Communication Disorders*, *7*(2), 141–153.

Gardner, H. E., Lambon Ralph, M. A., Dodds, N., Jones, T., Ehsan, S., & Jefferies, E. (2012). The differential contributions of the pFC and temporo-parietal cortex to multimodal semantic control: exploring refractory effects in semantic aphasia. *Journal of Cognitive Neuroscience*, *24*(4), 778–793.

Garrett, K., & Lasker, J. P. (2013). Adults with severe aphasia and apraxia of speech. In D. Beukelman & P. Mirenda (Eds.), *Augmentative and alternative communication: supporting children and adults with complex communication needs* (4th ed., pp. 405–445). Baltimore: Brookes.

Gazzaniga, M. S. (2005). Forty-five years of split-brain research and still going strong. *Nature Reviews Neuroscience*, *6*(8), 653–659.

Geschwind, N. (1965). Disconnexion syndromes in animals and man. *Brain*, *88*, 237–294.

Gainotti, G. (2004). A metanalysis of impaired and spared naming for different categories of knowledge in patients with a visuo-verbal disconnection. *Neuropsychologia*, *42*(3), 299–319.

Girkin, C. A., & Miller, N. R. (2001). Central disorders of vision in humans. *Survey of Ophthalmology*, *45*(5), 379–405.

Goodglass, H., & Kaplan, E. (1983). *Boston diagnostic aphasia examination*. Lea & Febiger.

Goolkasian, P. (1996). Picture-word differences in a sentence verification task. *Memory and Cognition*, *24*(5), 584–594.

Grant, K. W., & Seitz, P. F. (2000). The use of visible speech cues for improving auditory detection of spoken sentences. *Journal of the Acoustical Society of America*, *108*(3 Pt 1), 1197–208.

Green, K. P. (1996). The use of auditory and visual information in phonetic perception. In D. G. Stork & M. E. Hennecke (Eds.), *Speechreading by humans and machines: models, systems, and applications* (Vol. 150, pp. 55–77). Berlin: Springer Verlag.

Hasson, U., Skipper, J. I., Nusbaum, H. C., & Small, S. L. (2007). Abstract coding of audiovisual speech: beyond sensory representation. *Neuron*, *56*, 1116–1126.

Hamberger, M. J., Goodgman, R. R., Perrine, K., & Tamny, T. (2001). Anatomic dissociation of auditory and visual naming in the lateral temporal cortex. *Neurology*, *56*(1), 56–61.

Hamberger, M. J., Habeck, C.G., Pantazatos, S. P., Williams, A. C., & Hirsch, J. (2013). Shared space, separate processes: neural activation patterns for auditory description and visual object naming in healthy adults. *Human Brain Mapping 35*(6), 2507–2520.

Harnish, S. M., Lundine, J. P., Bauer A., Singletary, F., Benjamin, M. L., & Crosson, B. (2014). Dosing of a cued picture-naming treatment for anomia, *American Journal of Speech-Language Pathology*, *23*, 285–299.

Helfer, K. S., (1997). Auditory and auditory-visual perception of clear and conversational speech, *Journal of Speech and Hearing Research*, *40*(2), 432–443.

Herbert, R., Best, W., Hickin, J., Howard, D., & Osborne, F. (2001). Phonological and orthographic approaches to the treatment of word retrieval in aphasia. *International Journal of Language & Communication Disorders*, *36*(1), 7–12.

Hessler, D., Jonkers, R., Stowe, L., & Bastiaanse, R. (2013). The whole is more than the sum of its parts—audiovisual processing of phonemes investigated with ERPs. *Brain & Language*, *124*, 213–224.

Hickok, G. (2012). The cortical organization of speech procession: feedback control and predictive coding the context of a dual-stream model. *Journal of Communication Disorders*, *45*(6), 393–402.

Hickin, J., Best, W., Herbert, R., Howard, D., & Osborne, F. (2002). Phonological therapy for word-finding difficulties: a re-evaluation. *Aphasiology*, *16*(10–11), 981–999.

Hickok, G., Houde, J., & Rong, F. (2011). Sensorimotor integration in speech processing: computational basis and neural organization. *Neuron*, *69*, 407–419.

Hillis, A. E., & Caramazza, A. (1995). Cognitive and neural mechanisms underlying visual and semantic processing: implications from "optic aphasia". *Journal of Cognitive Neuroscience*, *7*(4), 457–478.

Hillis, A. E., Barker, P. B., Wityk, R. J., Aldrich, E. M., Restrepo, L., Breese, E. L., & Work, M. (2004). Variability in subcortical aphasia is due to variable sites of cortical hypoperfusion. *Brain and language*, *89*(3), 524–530.

Hillis, A. E., Kleinman, J. T., Newhart, M., Heidler-Gary, J., Gottesman, R., Barker, P. B., ... Chaudhry, P. (2006). Restoring cerebral blood flow reveals neural regions critical for naming. *The Journal of Neuroscience, 26*(31), 8069–8073.

Holcomb, P. J., & Neville, H. J. (1991). Natural speech processing: an analysis using event-related brain potentials. *Psychobiology, 19*(4), 286–300.

Howard, D., & Harding, D. (1998). Self-cueing of word retrieval by a woman with aphasia: why a letter board works. *Aphasiology, 12*(4–5), 399–420.

Hux, K., Buechter, M., Wallace, S., & Weissling, K. (2010). Using visual scene displays to create a shared communication space for a person with aphasia. *Aphasiology, 24*(5), 643–660.

Indefrey, P., & Levelt, W. J. (2004). The spatial and temporal signatures of word production components. *Cognition, 92*(1), 101–144.

Jacobs, B., Drew, R., Ogletree, B. T., & Pierce, K. (2004). Augmentative and alternative communication (AAC) for adults with severe aphasia: where we stand and how we can go further. *Disability & Rehabilitation, 26*(21–22), 1231–1240.

Jazayeri, M., & Movshon, J. A. (2006). Optimal representation of sensory information by neural populations, *Natural Neuroscience, 9*(5), 690–696.

Jazayeri, M., & Movshon, J. A. (2007). A new perceptual illusion reveals mechanisms of sensory decoding, *Nature, 446*(7138), 912–915.

Johanssen-Horbach, H., Cegla, B., Mager, U., Schemmp, B., & Wallesch, C. W. (1985). Treatment of chronic global aphasia with a nonverbal communication system. *Brain and Language, 24*(1), 74–82.

Judd, T., Ehinger, K., Durand, F., & Torralba, A. (2009). Learning to predict where humans look. Presented at the 2009 IEEE 12th international conference on Computer Vision, Kyoto, Japan.

Kagan, A. (1998). Supported conversation for adults with aphasia: methods and resources for training conversation partners. *Aphasiology, 12*(9), 816–830.

Kaplan, E., Goodglass, H., & Weintraub, S. (2001). *The Boston naming test*. Philadelphia: Lippincott Williams & Wilkins.

Kim, J., Davis, C., & Krins, P. (2004). A modal processing of visual speech as revealed by priming. *Cognition, 92*, 67–99.

King, J. (2013). Communication support. In Simmons-Mackie, J., King, J., & Beukelman, D. (Eds.), *Supporting communication for adults with acute and chronic aphasia* (pp. 54–73). Baltimore: Brookes.

Knoeferle, P., & Crocker, M. W. (2007). The influence of recent scene events on spoken comprehension: evidence from eye movements. *Journal of Memory and Language, 57*(4), 519–543.

Knoeferle, P., Crocker, M. W., Scheepers, C., & Pickering, M. J. (2005). The influence of the immediate visual context on incremental thematic role-assignment: evidence from eye-movements in depicted events. *Cognition, 95*(1), 95–127.

Knoeferle, P., Urbach, T. P., & Kutas, M. (2011). Comprehending how visual context influences incremental sentence processing: insights from ERPs and picture-sentence verification. *Psychophysiology, 48*, 495–506.

Koul, R. K., & Lloyd, L. L. (1998), Comparison of graphic symbol learning in individuals with aphasia and right hemisphere brain damage., *Brain and Language, 62*(3), 398–421.

Kounios, J., & Holocomb, P. J. (1992). Structure and process in semantic memory: evidence from event-related brain potentials and reaction times. *Journal of Experimental Psychology, General 121*(4), 459–479.

Lambon Ralph, M. A., Sage, K., & Roberts, J. (2000). Classical anomia: a neuropsychological perspective on speech production. *Neuropsychologia, 38*, 186–202.

Lau, E. F., Phillips, C., & Poeppel, D. (2008). A cortical network for semantics: (de)constructing the N400. *Nature Reviews Neuroscience, 9*(12), 920–933.

Lasker, J. P., Garrett, K. L., & Fox, L. E. (2007). Severe aphasia. In D. R. Beukelman, K. L. Garrett & K. M. Yorkston (Eds.), *Augmentative communication strategies for adults with acute or chronic medical conditions*. Baltimore: Brookes.

Lebib, R., Papo, D., de Bode, S., & Baudonnière, P. M. (2003). Evidence of a visual-to-auditory cross-modal sensory gating phenomenon as reflected by the human P50 event-related brain potential modulation. *Neuroscience Letters, 341*(3), 185–188.

Levin, T., Scott, B. M., Borders, B., Hart, K., Lee, J., & Decanini, A. (2007). Aphasia talks: photography as a means of communication, self-expression, and empowerment in persons with aphasia. *Topics in Stroke Rehabilitation, 14*(1), 72–84.

Li, E. C., & Williams, S. E. (1990). The effects of grammatic class and cue type on cueing responsiveness in aphasia. *Brain and Language, 38*(1), 48–60.

Loose, R., Kaufmann, C., Auer, D. P., & Lange, K. W. (2003). Human prefrontal and sensory cortical activity during divided attention tasks. *Human Brain Mapping, 18*(4), 249–259.

Lorenz, A., & Nickels, L. (2007). Orthographic cueing in anomic aphasia: how does it work? *Aphasiology, 21*(6–8), 670–686.

Lorenz, A., & Ziegler, W. (2009). Semantic vs. word-form specific techniques in anomia treatment: a multiple single-case study. *Journal of Neurolinguistics, 22*(6), 515–537.

Luria, A. R. (1970). *Traumatic aphasia: its syndromes, psychology and treatment* (Vol. 5). The Hague, The Netherlands: Walter De Gruyter.

MacLeod, A., & Summerfield, Q. (1990). A procedure for measuring auditory and audio-visual speech-reception thresholds for sentences in noise: rationale, evaluation, and recommendations for use. *Brain Journal of Audiology, 24*(1), 29–43.

Mandonnet, E., Gatignol, P., & Duffau, H. (2009). Evidence for an occipito-temporal tract underlying visual recognition in picture naming. *Clinical Neurology and Neurosurgery, 111*(7), 601–605.

Manning, L. (2000). Loss of visual imagery and defective recognition of parts of wholes in optic aphasia. *Neurocase, 6*(2), 111–128.

Margolin, D. I., Friedrich, F. J., & Carlson, N. R. (1985). Visual agnosia—optic aphasia: Continuum or dichotomy? Presented at the annual meeting of the International Neuropsychological Society, San Diego, CA.

Marshall, R. C., Freed, D. B., & Karow, C. M. (2001). Learning of subordinate category names by aphasic subjects: a comparison of deep and surface-level training methods. *Aphasiology, 15*(6), 585–598.

Martin, A. (2007). The representation of object concepts in the brain. *Annual Review of Psychology, 58*, 25–45.

Mayberry, M. R., Crocker, M. W., & Knoeferle, P. (2009). Learning to attend: a connectionist model of situated language comprehension. *Cognitive Sciences, 33*(3), 449–496.

Mazoyer, P., Wicker, B., & Fonlupt, P. (2002). A neural network elicited by parametric manipulation of the attention load. *NeuroReport, 13*, 2331–2334.

McGettigan, C., Faulkner, A., Altarelli, I., Oblesser, J., Baverstock, H., & Scott, S. K. (2012). Speech comprehension aided by multiple modalities: behavioural and neural interactions. *Neuropsychologia, 50*(5), 762–776.

McGurk, H., & MacDonald, J. (1976). Hearing lips and seeing voices. *Nature, 264*(5588), 746–748.

McKelvey, M. L., Hux, K., Dietz, A., & Beukelman, D. R. (2010). Impact of personal relevance and contextualization on word-picture matching by people with aphasia. *American Journal of Speech-Language Pathology, 19*(1), 22–33.

Mesulam, M. M. (1998). From sensation to cognition. *Brain, 121*, 1013–1052.

Miller, B. D., & D'Esposito, M. (2005). Searching for "the top" in top-down control. *Neuron, 48*(4), 535–538.

Morris, J., Franklin, S., Ellis, A. W., Turner, J. E., & Bailey, P. J. (1996). Remediating a speech perception deficit in an aphasic patient. *Aphasiology, 10*(2), 137–158.

Moskovitch, M., Scullion, D., & Christie, D. (1976). Early versus late stages of processing and their relation to functional hemispheric asymmetries in face recognition. *Journal of Experimental Psychology, 2*(3), 401–416.

Möttönen, R., Krause, C. M., Tiippana, K., & Sams, M. (2002). Processing of changes in visual speech in the human auditory cortex. *Cognitive Brain Research, 13*(3), 417–425.

Munhall, K.G., Jones, J. A., Callan, D. E., Kuratate, T., & Vatikiotis-Bateson, E. (2004). Visual prosody and speech intelligibility: head movement improves auditory speech perception. *Psychological Science, 15*(2), 133–137.

Musacchia, G., & Shroeder, C. E. (2009). Neuronal mechanisms, response dynamics and perceptual functions of multisensory interactions in auditory cortex. *Hearing Research, 258*, 72–79.

Myers-Pease, D. M., & Goodglass, H. (1978). The effects of cuing on picture naming in aphasia. *Neuron, 14*(2), 178–189.

Nath, A. R., & Beauchamp, M. S. (2011). Dynamic changes in superior temporal sulcus connectivity during perception of noisy audiovisual speech. *Journal of Neuroscience, 31*(5), 1704–1714.

Nath, A. R., & Beauchamp, M. S. (2012). A neural basis for interindividual differences in the McGurk effect, a multisensory speech illusion. *Neuroimage, 59*(1), 781–787.

Nishitani, N., & Hari, R. (2002). Viewing lip forms: cortical dynamics. *Neuron, 36*(6), 1211–1220.

Nickels, L. (2002). Improving word finding: practice makes (closer to) perfect? *Aphasiology, 16*(10–11), 1047–1060.

Ojanen, V., Möttönen, R., Pekkola, J., Jääskeläinen, I. P., Joensuu, R., Autti, T., & Sams, M. (2005). Processing of audiovisual speech in Broca's area, *Neuroimage, 25*, 333–338.

Owens, E., & Blazek, B. (1985). Visemes observed by hearing-impaired and normal-hearing adult viewers. *Journal of Speech and Hearing Research, 28*(3), 381–393.

Paulesu, E., Perani, D., Blasi, V., Silani, G., Borghese, N. A., De Giovanni, U., ... Fazio, F. (2003). A functional-anatomical model for lipreading. *Journal of Neurophysiology, 90*(3), 2005–2013.

Plaut, D. C., & Shallice, T. (1993). Perseverative and semantic influences on visual object naming errors in optic aphasia: a connectionist account. *Journal of Cognitive Neuroscience, 5*(1), 89–117.

Podraza, B. L., & Darley, F. L. (1977). Effect of auditory prestimulation on naming in aphasia, *Journal of Speech and Hearing Research, 20*(4), 669–683.

Price, C. J. (2012). A review and synthesis of the first 20 years of PET and fMRI studies of heard speech, spoken language and reading. *Neuroimage, 62,* 816–847.

Rabin, L. A., Barr, W. B., & Burton, L. A. (2005). Assessment practices of clinical neuropsychologists in the United States and Canada: a survey of INS, NAN, and APA Division 40 members. *Archives of Clinical Neuropsychology, 20*(1), 33–65.

Radanovic, M., & Mansur, L. L. (2011). *Language disturbances in adulthood: New advances from the neurolinguistics perspective.* Sharjah, UAE: Bentham Science.

Rayner, K. (2009). Eye movements and landing positions in reading: a retrospective. *Perception, 38*(6), 895–899.

Reichle, E. D., Carpenter, P. A., & Just, M. A. (2000). The neural basis of strategy and skill in sentence-picture verification. *Cognitive Psychology, 40,* 261–295.

Reisberg, D., McLean, J., & Goldfield, A. (1987). Easy to hear but hard to understand: A lip-reading advantage with intact auditory stimuli. In B. Dodd & R. Campbell (Eds.), *Hearing by eye: the psychology of lip-reading* (pp. 97–114). Hillsdale, NJ: Erlbaum.

Riddoch, M. J., & Humphreys, G. W. (1987). A case of integrative visual agnosia, *Brain, 110*(6), 1431–1462.

Ross, L. A., Saint-Amour, D., Leavitt, V. M., Molholm, S., Javitt, D. C., & Foxe, J. J. (2007). Impaired multisensory processing in schizophrenia: deficits in the visual enhancement of speech comprehension under noisy environmental conditions. *Schizophrenia Research, 97*(1), 173–183.

Sandberg, C., & Kiran, S. (2014). Analysis of abstract and concrete word processing in persons with aphasia and age-match neurologically healthy adults using fMRI. *Neurocase, 20*(4), 361–388.

van de Sandt-Koenderman, M. (2004). High-tech AAC and aphasia: widening horizons? *Aphasiology, 18*(3), 245–263.

Sarasson, S., Määttä S., Ferrarelli, F., Poryazova, R., Tononi, G., & Small, S. L. (2014). Plastic changes following imitation-based speech and language therapy for aphasia: a high-density sleep EEG study. *Neurorehabilitation and Neural Repair, 28*(2), 129–138.

Schmid, G., Thielmann, A., & Ziegler, W. (2009). The influence of visual and auditory information on the perception of speech and non-speech oral movements in patients with left hemisphere lesions. *Clinical Linguistics and Phonetics, 23*(3), 208–221.

Schmid, G., & Ziegler, W. (2006). Audio-visual matching of speech and non-speech oral gestures in patients with aphasia and apraxia of speech. *Neuropsychologia, 44,* 546–555.

Schwartz, J., Berthommier, F., & Savariaux, C. (2004). Seeing to hear better: evidence for early audio-visual interactions in speech identification. *Cognition, 93,* B69–B78.

Scott, S. K., & Johnsrude, I. S. (2003). The neuroanatomical and functional organization of speech perception. *Trends in Neurosciences, 26*(2), 100–107.

Sedivy, J. C., Tanenhaus, M. K., Chambers, C. G., & Carlson, G. N. (1999). Achieving incremental semantic interpretation through contextual representation. *Cognition, 71*(2), 109–147.

Sekiyama, K., Kanno, I., Miura, S., & Sugita, Y. (2003). Auditory-visual speech perception examined by fMRI and PET. *Neuroscience Research, 47,* 277–287.

Shindo, M., Kaga, K., & Tanaka, Y. (1991). Speech discrimination and lip reading in patients with words deafness or auditory agnosia. *Brain and Language, 40*, 153–161.

Simmons-Mackie, N., Savage, M. C., & Worrall, L. (2014). Conversation therapy for aphasia: a qualitative review of the literature. *International Journal of Language & Communication Disorders*. doi: 10.1111/1460-6984.12097

Singer, M. (2006). Verification of text ideas during reading. *Journal of Memory and Language, 54*, 574–591.

Skipper, J. I., Goldin-Meadow, S., Nusbaum, H. C., & Small, S. L. (2007). Speech-associated gestures, Broca's area, and the human mirror system. *Brain and Language, 101*(3), 260–277.

Skipper, J. I., Goldin-Meadow, S., Nusbaum, H. C., & Small, S. L. (2009). Gestures orchestrate brain networks for language understanding. *Current Biology, 19*, 661–667.

Skipper, J. I., Nusbaum, H. C., & Small, S. L. (2005). Listening to talking faces: motor cortical activation during speech perception. *Neuroimage, 25*(1), 76–89.

Spivey, M. J., Tanenhaus, M. K., Eberhard, K. M., & Sedivy, J. C. (2002). Eye movements and spoken language comprehension: effects of visual context on syntactic ambiguity resolution. *Cognitive Psychology, 45*(4), 447–481.

Stead, A., Savage, M. C., & Buckingham, H. W. (2012). Pictorial and graphemic processing in fluent aphasia. *Imagination, Cognition and Personality, 31*(4), 279-295.

Stein, B. E., & Meredith, M. A. (1993). *The merging of the senses*. Cambridge, MA: MIT Press.

Stevenson, R. A., Altieri, N. A., Kim, S., Pisoni, D. B., & James, T. W. (2010). Neural processing of asynchronous audiovisual speech perception. *Neuroimage, 49*(4), 3308–3318.

Stevenson, R.A., & James, T.W. (2009). Audiovisual integration in human superior temporal sulcus: Inverse effectiveness and the neural processing of speech and object recognition. *Neuroimage, 44*(3), 1210–1223.

Stimley, M. A., & Noll, J. D. (1991). The effects of semantic and phonemic prestimulation cues on picture naming in aphasia. *Brain and Language, 41*(4), 496–509.

Sumby, W. H., & Pollack, I. (1954). Visual contribution to speech intelligibility in noise. *The Journal of the Acoustical Society of America, 26*(2), 212–215.

Summerfield, Q. (1979). Use of visual information for phonetic perception. *Phonetica, 36*(4–5), 314–331.

Szaflarski, J. P., Eaton, K., Ball, A. L., Banks, C., Vannest, J., Allendorfer, J. B., ... Holland, S. K. (2011). Post-stroke aphasia recovery assessed with fMRI and a picture identification task. *Journal of Stroke and Cerebrovascular Diseases, 20*(4), 336–345.

Szűcs, D., Soltész, F., Czigler, I., & Csépe, V. (2007). Electroencephalography effects to semantic and non-semantic mismatch in properties of visually presented single-characters: the N2b and the N400. *Neuroscience Letters, 412*, 18–23.

Tanenhaus, M. K., Carroll, J. M., & Bever, T. G. (1976). Sentence-picture verification models as theories of sentence comprehension: a critique of Carpenter and Just. *Psychological Review, 83*(4), 310–317.

Thiessen, A., Beukelman, D., Ullman, C., & Longenecker, M., (2014). Measurement of the visual attention patterns of people with aphasia: a preliminary investigation of two types of human engagement in photographic images, *Augmentative and Alternative Communication, 30*(2), 120–129.

Tomaszewski-Farias, S., Harrington, G., Broomand, C., & Seyal, M. (2005). Differences in functional MR imaging activation patterns associated with confrontation naming and responsive naming. *American Journal of Neuroscience, 26*(10), 2492–2499.

Turken, A. U., & Dronkers, N. F. (2011). The neural architecture of the language comprehension network: converging evidence from lesion and connectivity analyses. *Frontiers in Systems Neuroscience, 5*, 1.

Underwood, G., Jebbett, L., & Roberts, K. (2004). Inspecting pictures for information to verify a sentence: eye movements in general encoding and in focused search. *The Quarterly Journal of Experimental Psychology, 57*(1), 165–182.

Van Atteveldt, N. M., Blau, V. C., Blomert, L., & Goebel, R. (2010). fMR-adaptation indicates selectivity to audiovisual content congruency in distributed clusters in human superior temporal cortex. *BMC Neuroscience, 11*(1).

Villardita, C. (1985). Raven's colored progressive matrices and intellectual impairment in patients with focal brain damage. *Cortex, 21*(4), 627–634.

Vigneau, M., Beaucousin, V., Hervé, P. Y., Duffau, H., Crivello, F., Houdé, O., & Tzourio-Mazoyer, N. (2006). Meta-analyzing left hemisphere language areas: phonology, semantics, and sentence processing. *Neuroimage, 30*(4), 1414–1432.

Vissers, C., Kolk, H., Van de Meerendonk, N., & Chwilla, D. (2008). Monitoring in language perception: evidence from ERPs in a picture-sentence matching task. *Neuropsychologia, 46*, 967–982.

Wallace, S. E., Dietz, A., Hux, K., & Weissling, K. (2012). Augmented input: the effect of visuographic supports on the auditory comprehension of people with chronic aphasia. *Aphasiology, 26*(2), 162–176.

Wallace, S. E., Hux, K., Brown, J., & Knollman-Porter, K. (2014). High-context images: Comprehension of main, background, and inferential information by people with aphasia, *Aphasiology, 28*(6), 713–730.

van Wassenhove, V., Grant, K.W., & Poeppel, D. (2005). Visual speech speeds up the neural procession of auditory speech. *Proceedings of the National Academy of Sciences of the United States of America, 102*(4), 1181–1186.

van Wassenhove, V., Grant, K. W., & Poeppel, D. (2007). Temporal window of integration in auditory-visual speech perception. *Neuropsychologia, 45*, 598–607.

Wassenaar, M., & Hagoort, P. (2007). Thematic role assignment in patients with Broca's aphasia: sentence–picture matching electrified. *Neuropsychologia, 45*(4), 716–740.

Weissling, K.S.E., & Beukelman, D. R. (2006) Visual scenes displays: low-tech options. *Augmentative and Alternative Communication, 17*, 15–17.

Wernicke, C. (1874). *Der aphasische Symptomenkomplex.* Breslau: Teschen.

Wilkinson, K. M., & Jagaroo, V. (2004). Contributions of principles of visual cognitive science to AAC system display design. *Augmentative and Alternative Communication, 20*(3), 123–136.

Wilkinson, K. M., & Light, J. (2011). Preliminary investigation of visual attention to human figures in photographs: potential considerations for the design of aided AAC visual scene displays. *Journal of Speech, Language and Hearing Research, 54*(6), 1644–1657.

Wilkinson, K. M., Light, J., & Drager, K. (2012). Considerations for the composition of visual scene displays: potential contributions of information from visual and cognitive sciences. *Augmentative and Alternative Communication, 28*, 137–147.

Wunderlich, A., & Ziegler, W. (2011). Facilitation of picture-naming in anomic subjects: sound vs mouth shape. *Aphasiology*, 25(2), 202–220.

Zion Golumbic, E. M., Ding, N., Bickel, S., Lakatos, P., Schevon, C. A., McKhann, G. M., ... Schroeder, C. E. (2013). Mechanisms underlying selective neuronal tracking of attended speech at a "cocktail party." *Neuron*, 77(5), 980–991.

9

Redefining Recovery from Aphasia

What Have We Learned?

By this point in the book, the reader will surely have understood that we have been addressing two fundamental aspects of brain-language relations: one, theoretical, regarding the neural organization of nonlinguistic-linguistic interconnections in the healthy brain; the other, clinical, regarding the use of such knowledge to characterize functional recovery from aphasia more precisely and to enhance the understanding of treatment-based neural changes that lead to this recovery. This chapter summarizes our thoughts on these two issues and relates to our conceptualization of language as a constant and dynamic neurally multifunctional system.

Before we address our own hypotheses, we wish to acknowledge those whose research and analyses, prior to ours, influenced the directions of own thinking—in particular, Antonio Damasio, David Poeppel, Gregory Hickok, Angela Friederici, and Sheila Blumstein. Each of these scientists powerfully contributed to what has clearly come to be recognized as a paradigm shift in the understanding of brain-language relations within the contemporary field of cognitive neuroscience.

In the late 1980s Damasio propounded a theory that came to have considerable influence on subsequent ideas regarding memory, consciousness, and the binding problem (Damasio, 1989a,b). In two key papers, he introduced his theory of convergence zones and time-locked, multiregional retroactivation. He proposed that the experience of reality occurs when widely dispersed clusters of neuronal assemblies (responsible for recall and recognition of features, entities, and events) are activated in a time-locked fashion, directed by information transmitted to (and from) convergence zones in a reciprocal, feedforward, feedback system, the convergence zones representing higher order clusters of neuronal assemblies that serve as control systems. Much of the research evidence provided in this book is consistent with Damasio's theory of convergence zones.

This call to conceive of language from a theory-driven integrative perspective was later expressed in the works of Gregory Hickok and David Poeppel, who, together and separately, have taken a leading role in carrying the study of neurolinguistics and its relation to cognitive neuroscience out of the 19th-century classical mold of strict, lesion-based clinicoanatomical correlations into the contemporary world of science. Despite their sometimes hyperbolic statements (e.g., "worth pointing out explicitly, the era of the classical model is over"; Poeppel et al., 2012, p. 14125), they have more often than not been right. In particular, and especially for our purposes in this book, they have repeatedly emphasized the necessity of understanding brain-language relations not only within a contemporary analysis of neuroanatomy and neurobiology, based in large part on the newest technologies for representing the spatial and temporal aspects of brain activity, but also with a seriously sophisticated analysis of language, without which no theory of brain-language relations can be meaningful. In papers with titles like "Towards a New Functional Anatomy of Language" (Poeppel and Hickok, 2004) and "Towards an Integrated Psycholinguistic, Neurolinguistic, Sensorimotor Framework for Speech Production" (Hickok, 2014), they have braved the single-discipline tradition (neuroscientists speak only to neuroscientists, linguists speak only to linguists) and asserted that "integrating across fields requires us to tear down some of what we have built, re-think long-held assumptions and submit to the fact that the early stages of an integrated research agenda will lack some of the theoretical crispness of the separate areas alone" (Hickok, 2014, p. 52). As the reader will no doubt see, when we offer our own speculations regarding how the brain creates language, we will be taking up the challenge of rethinking long-held assumptions.

One of the most reliable sources of neural evidence that was brought to bear on these ideas comes from studies led by Angela Friederici, who is among the most respected specialists in the field of cognitive neuroscience of language of the past quarter century. Her scientific contributions, especially her neuroimaging studies of brain-language relations, have certainly influenced our own thinking. Of the more than 350 publications from her research in collaboration with other scholars in this domain, in which she has used sophisticated, theory-based psycholinguistic analyses and contemporary neuroimaging techniques, we note three studies that have had particular relevance for our own theses. In one, she reviews the brain basis of language processing from structure to function and summarizes evidence supporting the conclusion that language functions are organized throughout the entire brain—with local, regional, and wide area connections depending on the specific language function being studied (Friederici, 2011). The anatomical connectivity of this widely dispersed network has been dubbed "the language connectome" (Dick et al., 2013). In two other papers she discusses the relation of Broca's area to syntactic integration, syntactic processing, and working memory (Fiebach et al, 2005; Makuuchi & Friederici, 2013). While dissecting mechanisms of syntax into subcomponents (syntactic integration versus syntactic working memory) and demonstrating the role of Broca's area in syntactic working memory, she also provided evidence to support the following assertion: "Language processing inevitably involves working memory (WM) operations" (p. 2416). Her findings and assertions, of course, fit neatly into our concept of neural multifunctionality.

Our own evolving perspective on the neural multifunctional organization of language has been most eloquently expressed by Sheila Blumstein, who has made immeasurable contributions to the understanding of the cognitive neuroscience of language. As we were approaching the final chapter of this book, she and her colleague Dima Amso published a paper titled, in part, "Dynamic Functional Organization of Language," which brilliantly reviews and reconceptualizes much of the research we have been referring to in this chapter and serves as the jumping-off point for our own view of how the brain creates language. One of the key points of this article, in their own words, is that "there is a dynamic functional architecture, rather than a fixed neural architecture, that emerges across the lifespan, pursuant to injury and in response to language experience" (Blumstein & Amso, 2013, p. 44). This statement and the evidence supporting it lie at the heart of the concept of neural multifunctionality.

Indeed, increasingly more and more models are emerging that explore the interplay among the neural networks mediating language and those that underlie other nonlinguistic functions. Most such models do not present interactions with neural substrates of emotion, but Duffau et al. (2014) note the importance of incorporating such a component into the picture, with an emphasis on characterizing interconnections with right hemisphere networks, which appear to support certain aspects of emotional language (Beaucousin et al., 2007; Vigneau et al., 2011; Willems et al., 2011). It would appear, then, that the theoretical climate within which the neural underpinnings of language are currently discussed is ripe for considering the nonlinguistic components that help create language in the healthy and the compromised brain.

An Argument for the Neural Multifunctionality of Language: Converging Evidence

The key themes discussed in the preceding chapters strongly support the postulate that the neural basis of language can best be understood by the concept of *neural multifunctionality* (Cahana-Amitay & Albert, 2014). Findings from lesion, neuroimaging, and electrophysiological studies provide information instrumental to the claim that nonlinguistic functions need to be incorporated into language models of the intact brain, reflecting a multifunctional perspective whereby there exists a constant and dynamic interaction among neural networks subserving cognitive, emotional, and sensorimotor functions and neural networks specialized for lexical retrieval, sentence comprehension, and discourse processing, giving rise to language as we know it (Cahana-Amitay & Albert, 2014). Such an approach relates to the influence of neural plasticity in the intact brain, to interindividual variability, to the realm of language recovery from aphasia following brain damage, and to the role of nonlinguistic factors in reshaping neural circuitry for aphasia rehabilitation, be this behavioral therapy (e.g., speech/language therapy), high-tech biological interventions (e.g., transcranial magnetic stimulation), or neurochemical manipulations (e.g., pharmacotherapy).

We demonstrated, for example, that impaired *executive functions* among persons with aphasia interact with aspects of lexical retrieval so as to negatively affect performance, in line with current neural models of semantic control in the healthy brain. We showed that in aphasia, damage to the prefrontal cortex results in deficits on lexical selection tasks involving strong semantic competition and/or open-ended task demands, reducing cognitive control of task-appropriate responses that activate semantic information within the semantic store. We then presented evidence that these problems are also apparent in people with aphasia, with lesions in white matter tracts connecting frontal, temporal, and parietal regions, as well as with damaged subcortical circuits. We concluded by discussing aphasia treatment studies, which show that targeting specific executive support systems improves naming in aphasic people with stroke-induced cortical lesions by stimulating right hemisphere activation.

Similarly, we showed that *attention* deficits among persons with aphasia impair multiple language functions and lead to increased error rates and prolonged reaction times that further worsen language performance. We reviewed studies identifying attention problems across domains of attention with complex attention functions—assessed primarily using dual-task paradigms—being identified as the most devastating for language performance. We also discussed how these attention effects on aphasic language performance are best understood as a deficit in accessing linguistic knowledge, which can account for much of the interindividual variability found in almost all aphasia (and non-aphasia) language studies. We noted that attention deficits in aphasia typically appear in persons with brain damage in the left frontal lobe and subcortical structures, including the thalamus, anterior cingulate gyrus, and caudate nucleus.

With respect to attention-based interventions, we cited evidence that speaks to the benefits of directing attention to stimuli in the left hemispace, which harnesses preserved right hemisphere attention abilities to naming, especially among aphasic persons with parietal brain damage. We further noted the proposal of pharmacotherapeutic treatment aimed at reducing effects of attention deficits on aphasic language using dopaminergic and noradrenergic systems, which presumably act on damaged prefrontal, motor, and association areas that enhance impaired linguistic functions subserved by these areas. We also mentioned recent findings that indicate that intensive naming treatment results in improved connectivity of the default mode network, which presumably mediates attention functions.

In our discussion of *memory*, we related the theoretical distinctions among working memory (WM), short-term memory (STM), and long-term memory to findings from aphasia studies which indicate that STM/WM tasks, typically measured in terms of digit span, challenge persons with aphasia and can adversely affect their language performance. We also suggested that neuroimaging findings converge to indicate that STM/WM and language functions share certain neural substrates, including the left inferior frontal, left posterior temporal, and left posterior temporoparietal cortex.

In addition, we pointed out that many of these observations of the relationship between memory and language have guided the selection of therapy targets for anomia treatment studies. The neural picture that emerges from these studies is one of treatment-based activations in bilateral temporal regions or left perilesional brain structures. We also discussed neuroimaging studies that expand the neuroanatomical maps of recovery of language functions in aphasia to neural structures traditionally associated with learning and memory, such as the hippocampus, where short- and long-term effects of naming training were associated with differential brain activation patterns. Here short-term therapy gains implicated bilateral activation of the hippocampus and fusiform gyrus and right precuneus and cingulate gyrus while long-term effects emerged in well-established language regions.

Our review of altered *emotional states* in aphasia, specifically of depression and anxiety, clearly demonstrated that such emotional changes can adversely affect aphasic language performance. For psychophysiological stress responses, which are typically associated with anxiety, we presented findings documenting involvement of biomarkers of the autonomic nervous system (ANS) (blood pressure, heart rate) and hypothalamic-pituitary-adrenal axis (salivary cortisol). In addition, we introduced findings from aphasia pharmacotherapy studies, which speak to the benefits of targeting biomarkers of the ANS with the beta blocker propranolol as a means of ameliorating language performance. We related these findings to results from studies of healthy adults, in whom poorer physiologic regulation of an ANS biomarker (heart-rate variability) in a high-threat condition was associated with greater decrements in cognitive and neural functioning. We offered the speculation that the inferior frontal gyrus might be implicated in this treatment effect, based on neuroimaging findings from healthy adults, which suggested that administration of propranolol induces a compensatory brain response in the inferior frontal region without impairing cognitive performance.

Regarding the interactions of *motor* and language functions in the aphasic brain, we portrayed links among action recognition, repetition, imitation, gestural communication, and vocalizations, which propelled the development of models that speak to the integration of systems of motor control and language in the brain. In this context, we discussed the controversy surrounding the notion that mirror neurons serve as the neural foundation upon which action and language are integrated in the brain. We then reviewed theoretical accounts that have equated apraxic deficits (pantomiming, gesture imitation and recognition) with aphasic language difficulties (repetition), where the presumed parallels reflect damage to a shared left-lateralized neural system. We demonstrated that contemporary accounts of impaired voluntary control of movement indicate that the neural foundation of praxis and aphasia implicates activation of dynamic brain networks, in which complex motor and linguistic processes interact, both drawing on semantic and conceptual knowledge.

We then discussed how insights about motor-linguistic integration have informed current clinical practices in aphasia treatment. We described multimodal interventions that incorporate gesture in aphasia treatment, on the assumption that preserved gesturing can serve as crossmodal adjunct method to reestablish language use, through activation of all available neural networks that support language function. We also presented the opposite view, that is, variants of constraint-induced language protocols, which exclude gesture use in aphasia treatment, on the assumption that deficient language use can be reshaped through strategic, repetitive, intensive, learning, where the coupling of gesture nonuse and intensive use of residual language leads to neuronal activation in perilesional brain areas. We reviewed neuroimaging and neurophysiological findings showing that improvement posttreatment involves neural changes both perilesionally and bilaterally, with long-term effects being left-lateralized, leading to the proposal that the left hemisphere takes on a primary role in recovery of language functions in aphasia, and the right hemisphere provides ancillary support.

The final strand of experimental evidence we covered in the book concerns the effects of *visual processing* on aphasic language performance. We examined evidence indicating that persons with aphasia process pictorial cues with greater ease than they do verbal ones and that they derive particular benefit from high-context images. In addition, we reviewed neuroimaging studies of picture naming in aphasia where neural correlates of the visual contribution to lexical retrieval were identified, with some findings pointing to the potential convergence of neural substrates subserving vision, language, and higher-order cognitive functions during picture naming. We then considered evidence of audiovisual effects on language processing in aphasia, where both impairment and sparing have been documented, questioning the utility of bimodal cues for persons with aphasia. We described the neural underpinnings of these patterns, which indicate increased brain activation in the superior temporal sulcus regardless of whether or not auditory and visual stimuli were congruent, whereas in the healthy brain such activation occurs only in response to incongruent audiovisual stimuli. We concluded with a discussion of aphasia treatment programs demonstrating the efficacy of incorporating visual cues into clinical assessments and interventions, highlighting the degree to which they support the idea that visually based neural activation in the right hemisphere and perilesional areas supports lexical processing and lexical retrieval.

Rethinking the Neural Organization of Language: What Is New?

The scope of the evidence presented here clearly suggests that we need to reevaluate the way we think about the neurocognitive imprint of language in the brain and develop a neural multifunctional characterization. What would such a description require? Consider, for example, the multiple processes underlying word retrieval. They engage a web of brain structures that extend well beyond the traditional language region, including (1) heteromodal structures (Brodmann's area 37 and 39) to mediate phonological and lexical processing; (2) temporal structures to support concept and word retrieval; (3) sensorimotor connections to subserve action perception; (4) hippocampal, fusiform gyrus, and inferior parietal lobe structures to activate memory systems; and (5) pre- and supplementary motor cortices and subcortical structures (basal ganglia, insula, putamen) that partake in executive functions (Kurland et al., 2012; see also Chapter 7).

How might such an interconnected system work? As we note in Cahana-Amitay and Albert (2014), one possibility is to follow Cabeza and Moscovitch (2013) in proposing a view of language in the brain in terms of a *component process framework*, where region-specific neural bundles subserve multiple cognitive tasks simultaneously. The component interactions in this framework are conceived as "process-specific alliances," which comprise small brain regions that are temporarily recruited to perform a particular cognitive task with specific task demands. Each component in the alliance has a specific function, and they converge to yield a complex operation. These neural bundles dissipate once task demands are met and are thus distinct from larger-scale stable networks, which remain connected at rest. The connections within the stable larger-scale networks can affect which alliances are shaped, but they do not drive their selection. Thus operations within our neural multifunctionality model would manifest as interactions of "neural cohorts" that mediate multiple functions in cognitive, emotional, motor, and perceptual domains.

One question that remains unanswered, however, is what happens at the neuronal level. Here, we leave behind a book filled with scientific evidence supporting the concept of *neural multifunctionality* and gingerly enter the realm of speculation—testable speculation, it is true, but speculation nonetheless. In this section we shall assert that the concept of *neural multifunctionality* lends itself to the support of a basic understanding of brain function in the service of brain-language relations.

As we have shown, expert scientists have made prodigious strides, empirically based and theory-driven, towards the understanding of brain-language relations. What pieces, if any, are missing from the emerging puzzle? How close are we to revealing how the brain creates language? It would, of course, be outrageously presumptuous for anyone to claim to have a definitive answer to that question, but it would not be unfair to say that one could reasonably speculate on the possibilities of such an answer. To provide the steps that might eventually lead to an answer, we should first answer the question of what is missing from the other theories. Two things are missing, we believe: *multifunctionality* and *timing*.

With regard to *multifunctionality*, we would argue that none of the other theories insists, as we do, that language does not exist independently of its interactions with nonlinguistic aspects of cognition, emotion, and sensorimotor functions. The evidence, it seems to us, is clear that language is created constantly, as it is being used, only insofar as it is intimately entwined with executive system function, attention, memory, emotion, and sensorimotor functions. Whereas the basic building blocks of language may well be organized in a neural language network that is local or regional, the full flower of language itself—in conversation, self-reflection, dreaming—is the instantaneous, constantly changing, product of the dynamic interaction of language networks with networks underlying other aspects of the individual's entire personhood. It is our belief that language cannot be understood as being supported by neurally based language networks alone. In other words, language is a *whole-brain phenomenon*.

But, how does this whole-brain phenomenon come together to produce a single, well-chosen word at just the right moment, or a poem or a book? We think the answer to that as yet unanswered question lies in the concept of *timing*. With regard to the issue of timing, we have observed throughout this book that there is a "constant and dynamic interaction" of language networks with other, nonlanguage, networks creating language as we know it. The question then arises as to how the brain manages to maintain the constancy of this dynamic interaction.

We address this question with reference to the laws of physics and, in particular, to the notion of space-time. Space-time is a phenomenon in physics that combines space and time into a single interwoven continuum (Einstein, 1920). The space-time continuum serves to explain physical phenomena at the level of the universe and throughout every layer of quantification down to subatomic levels (Isaacson, 2007). According to Einstein's general theory of relativity, (1) the wave-like fabric of space-time is influenced by the objects within it (planets, for example, if one is talking about the universe), especially by the relative movement of these objects; (2) mass and energy are interconvertible and interactive; (3) it is not the charges or the particles but the field in the space between the charges and the particles that is essential for the description of physical phenomena.

We are proposing that the brain itself follows the same laws of physics as does the universe. By analogy with the laws of physics within the universe, the following image represents what is, or may be, happening in the brain to explain the immediate, constant, and dynamic interaction of elements. The particles—such as, for example, packets of neurotransmitters that travel from one nerve fiber to another crossing synaptic clefts in local, regional, and widely distributed networks—and the electric charges that travel throughout these networks represent only part of the neural support for language. It is the *neuronal space-time field*, we suggest, that allows the constancy, the continuousness, of the dynamic interaction that creates language. Stated another way, the creation of language is determined by physical neurochemical reactions taking place at all times but also, simultaneously, the creation of language determines the activity of the brain's neurochemistry. Consequently the creation of language and the brain's neurochemistry influence each other dynamically. To understand this dynamic process, both must be considered. According to this proposal, language is not sitting in the brain waiting to be pulled out but is created as we use it by the constant, dynamic interaction of language and nonlanguage networks. We further propose that the neural support for language and therefore language itself are in a constant state of flux (development, improvement, adaptation, decrement) throughout life, influenced by aging, health, experience, and life's multitudinous contingencies.

Redefining Recovery from Aphasia

The challenge remains in determining how the concept of *neural multifunctionality* can provide a basis for theory-driven descriptions of aphasia, which can inform clinical practices that would optimize treatment-induced neural activation.

Clearly a person with aphasia caused by a stroke is left with a greater portion of healthy brain than damaged brain. With this simple, straightforward truth came an intense exploration of the degree to which spared brain tissue in the right hemisphere participates in language recovery from aphasia. The question was whether the presumably intact right hemisphere can take over left hemisphere language functions via a mechanism of cerebral plasticity (Kolb et al., 2010).

Initially, the answer to this question was yes. Behavioral studies in which experimental manipulations of right hemisphere behaviors were performed showed negative impact of these manipulations on language performance among persons with aphasia; relatedly, neuroimaging studies of persons with aphasia documented right-sided or bilateral brain activation induced by different language tasks (reviewed in Anglade et al., 2014). These results pointed to a positive role for the right hemisphere in the reorganization of language functions in the course of recovery from aphasia. Some have argued that this right-sided neural support is particularly beneficial to persons with Broca's aphasia, who appeared to activate a right hemispheric homologue of Broca's area (e.g., Naeser et al., 2005) and show a gradual shift from bilateral to left-lateralized language-based brain activation (e.g., Thomas et al., 1997).

In contrast, others have proposed that involvement of right hemisphere structures in the recovery of language functions in aphasia constitutes a maladaptive process (Postman-Caucheteux et al., 2010; Price et al., 1999). In this context, some researchers have claimed that following stroke, the right hemisphere is less able to exert its inhibitory influence on the left hemisphere, which under normal circumstance ensures efficient left-lateralized language processing; in the aphasic brain, however, it reduces processing efficiency. Confirmatory evidence for this claim comes from Naeser and colleagues (2005), who showed that applying repeated transcranial magnetic stimulation to the right homologue of Broca's area, thereby inhibiting the function of the right hemisphere, results in improved naming performance among persons with nonfluent aphasia. However, as counterevidence has also been found, the utility of inhibiting activation of the right hemisphere in the treatment of aphasia remains undetermined (reviewed in Anglade et al., 2014).

It appears, then, that although neuroimaging studies exploring neural changes in aphasia recovery have made considerable progress toward identifying specific networks implicated in this process (e.g., Meizner et al., 2011; Price & Crinion, 2005; Saur et al., 2006; 2010; Warren et al., 2009), findings taken in their entirety and, thus, models of aphasia recovery have yet to converge on a unified coherent account (Hamilton et al., 2011). Some have focused on characterizing the shifts in lateralization of language functions from left to right (e.g., Leff et al., 2002; Raboyeau et al., 2008; Saur et al., 2006; Thompson et al., 2000; Weiller et al., 1995) and others have highlighted the independent contributions of the right hemisphere to aphasic language processing, whether beneficial or counterproductive (e.g., Blank et al., 2003; Naeser et al., 2005; Rosen et al., 2000; Thiel et al., 2001; Winhusien et al., 2007). Yet others have noted the essential role of preserved left hemisphere brain tissue (e.g., Heiss et al., 1999; Rosen et al., 2000; Warburton et al., 1999).

In a recent review of the role of the right hemisphere in recovery from aphasia (spanning studies from 1946 through 2012), Anglade et al. (2014) identified three patterns of language-related activation of the right hemisphere in aphasia, as shown in Figure 9.1. The first is linked to time postonset, where early-stage recovery involves increased right-sided activation, which decreases at later stages. The second concerns preservation of key language areas in the left hemisphere, which predicts limited right-sided contributions along with considerable and even full language recovery. The third is associated with obliteration of core language areas, which is accompanied by constant recruitment of the right hemisphere, which supports mostly automated aspects of speech.

The principal thrust of our argument, then, is that although the language-centric focus on uncovering aphasic impairments and treating them is crucially important, such an approach should be reinforced in every instance by exploration of amodal nonlinguistic functions and right hemispheric functions simultaneously. There is an abundance of evidence that persons with aphasia can be stimulated to perform correctly when a variable set of nonlinguistic factors is manipulated, including, for example, visual properties of the stimulus, stimulus loudness, or duration of interstimulus intervals (e.g., Kurland, 2011). These observations have been taken to suggest that response selection in aphasia is malleable and can be shaped into acquired compensatory strategies (e.g., Hula & McNeil, 2008).

Scientists and clinicians over the years have, in fact, taken advantage of this knowledge to a limited extent. We know, for example, that some patients with language production problems and who therefore cannot speak can nevertheless sing. This clinical fact must necessarily mean that these patients have at least two neuroanatomically

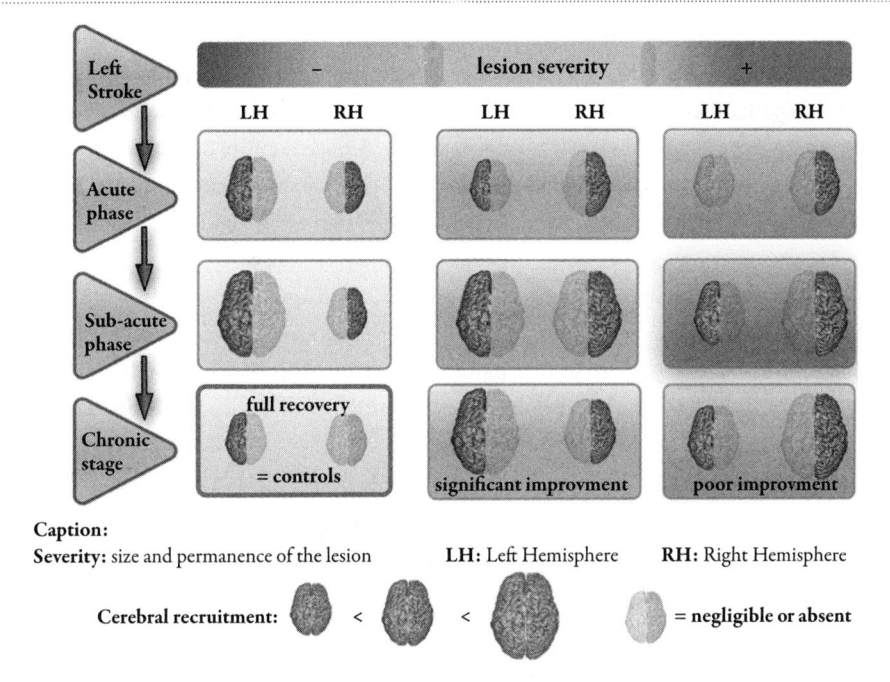

FIGURE 9.1 The role of the right hemisphere in recovery from aphasia. A possible interpretation of the controversial results about the role of the right hemisphere during recovery from aphasia: recruitment depending of lesion severity and time poststroke (See color insert.)
Source: From Anglade, C., Thiel, A., & Ansaldo, A. I. (2014). The complementary role of the cerebral hemispheres in recovery from aphasia after stroke: a critical review of the literature. *Brain Injury, 28(2)*, 138–145. Reprinted by permission from Informa Healthcare [Brain Injury], copyright 2014.

distinct language production systems, one for speaking and the other for singing. The well-known aphasia treatment program known as melodic intonation therapy capitalizes on this knowledge (Albert et al., 1973). We also know that neural mechanisms for attention are intimately interconnected with neural mechanisms that support language and that aphasia treatment programs focusing on the stimulation of attentional systems can facilitate language output (Murray, 2002). We know further that neural mechanisms for motor system function are interlinked with neural mechanisms for language, and that aphasia treatment programs focusing on the activation of motor systems can facilitate the recovery of speech (Goldstein, 1948; Luria, 1970).

The story is the same for each of the nonlinguistic domains touched on in this book. Within each of these domains examples can be found of aphasia therapy programs that have relied on the nonlinguistic aspect of what we are calling neural multifunctionality. Intention treatment, for example, targets mechanisms responsible for action initiation and so necessarily implicates, at the very least, language, executive functions, and motor control. Similarly, motor-related treatment protocols, such as constraint-based interventions, require the active suppression of voluntary motor movement. Treatments incorporating gesture strongly implicate sensory components, especially in imitation protocols where the participants are instructed to view facial gestures produced by others. Interventions focused on visual cueing strongly rely on attention skills, which guide the participant in the visual analysis of the visual cue. By the same token, treatments of attention directly interact with visual abilities, as placement of stimuli in the visual field ipsilateral to the lesion enhances language performance. Engagement of attention mechanisms during treatment can be strongly affected by emotional state, where anxious anticipation of language breakdown reinforces increased psychophysiological stress responses that consume some of the attention resources which would otherwise support the language task at hand. Changes in emotional state, which implicate hypothalamic-pituitary-adrenal axis biomarkers, affect the integrity of limbic structures and so can lead to memory-based or learning-related difficulties on language performance.

As laid out in detail, chapter by chapter, in this book, the evidence is overwhelming that language in the brains of healthy people, in persons with aphasia, and during recovery from aphasia is at all times constantly and dynamically interacting with other, nonlanguage neurobiological elements of the individual's personhood: cognition, emotion, and sensorimotor functions. The evidence is equally abundant that these interconnections comprise local, regional, and wide-area networks within broad swaths of the brain—cortical to cortical, cortical to subcortical, left hemisphere to right hemisphere, anterior to posterior.

The simple argument being put forth in this book regarding recovery of function from aphasia is that clinicians can and should take advantage of the nonlinguistic contributions to the creation of language in persons with aphasia to help them recover better and faster. The evidence in this book is a testament to the "total push" approach for treatment of aphasia, using multimodal and multicategory treatment programs in the same patient at the same time, systematically, the goal being to use the brain's multifunctionality to facilitate the creation and re-creation of language.

References

Albert, M. L., Sparks, R. W., & Helm, N. (1973). Melodic intonation therapy for aphasia. *Archives of Neurology, 29*, 130–131.

Anglade, C., Thiel, A., & Ansaldo, A. I. (2014). The complementary role of the cerebral hemispheres in recovery from aphasia after stroke: a critical review of the literature. *Brain Injury, 28*(2), 138–145.

Beaucousin, V., Lacheret, A., Turbelin, M. R., Morel, M., Mazoyer, B., & Tzourio-Mazoyer, N. (2007). FMRI study of emotional and speech comprehension. *Cerebral Cortex, 17*, 339–352.

Blank, S. C., Bird, H., Turkheimer, F., & Wise. R. J. (2003). Speech production after stroke: the role of the pars opercularis. *Annals of Neurology, 54*, 310–320.

Blumstein, S., & Amso, D. (2013). Dynamic functional organization of language: insights from Functional Neuroimaging. *Perspectives on Psychological Science, 8*(1), 44–48.

Cabeza, R., & Moscovitch, M. (2013). The porous boundaries between explicit and implicit memory: behavioral and neural evidence. *Perspectives and Psychological Sciences, 8*(1), 49–55.

Cahana-Amitay, D. & Albert, M. L. (2014). Brain and language: evidence for neural multifunctionality. *Behavioural Neurology,* http://dx.doi.org/10.1155/2014/260381

Damasio, A. R. (1989a). The brain binds entities and events by multiregional activation from convergence zones. *Neural Computation, 1,* 123–132,

Damasio, A. R. (1989b). Time-locked multiregional retroactivation: a systems-level proposal for the neural substrates of recall and recognition. *Cognition, 33,* 25–62.

Dick, A., Bernal, B., & Tremblay, P. (2013). The language connectome: new pathways, new concepts. *Neuroscientist,* Dec 15, ePub ahead of print.

Duffau, H., Moritz-Gasser, S., & Mandonnet, E. (2014). A re-examination of neural basis of language processing: proposal of a dynamic hodotopical model from data provided by brain stimulation mapping during picture naming. *Brain and Language, 131,* 1–10.

Einstein, A. (1920). *Relativity: the special and the general theory.* New York: Henry Holt.

Fiebach, C., Schlesewsky, M., Lohmann, G., von Cramon, D. Y., & Friederici, A. D. (2005). Revisiting the role of Broca's area in sentence processing: syntactic integration versus syntactic working memory. *Human Brain Mapping, 24*(2), 79–91.

Friederici, A. D. (2011). The brain basis of language processing: from structure to function. *Physiological Reviews, 91*(4),1357–1392.

Goldstein K. (1948). *Language and language disturbances.* New York: Grune and Stratton.

Hamilton, R. H., Chrysikou, E. G., & Coslett, B. (2011). Mechanisms of recovery after stroke and the role of noninvasive brain stimulation. *Brain and Language, 118,* 40–50.

Heiss, W. D., Kessler, J., Thiel, A., Ghaemi, M., & Karbe, H. (1999). Differential capacity of left and right hemispheric areas for compensation of poststroke aphasia. *Annals of Neurology, 45,* 430–438.

Hickok, G. (2014). Towards an integrated psycholinguistic, neurolinguistic, sensorimotor framework for speech production. *Language, Cognition, and Neuroscience, 29,* 52–59.

Cahana-Amitay, D. & Albert, M. L. (2014). Brain and language: evidence for neural multifunctionality. *Behavioural Neurology,* http://dx.doi.org/10.1155/2014/260381

Isaacson, W. (2007). *Einstein: his life and universe.* New York: Simon and Schuster.

Kolb, B., Teskey, G. C., & Gibb, R. (2010). Factors influencing cerebral plasticity in the normal and injured brain. *Frontiers in Human Neuroscience, 4,* 204.

Kurland, J. (2011). The role that attention plays in language processing. *Perspectives on Neurophysiology and Neurogenic Speech and Language Disorders, 21*(2), 44–77.

Kurland, J., Pulvermüller, F., Sliva, N., Burke, K., & Andrianopoulos, M. (2012). Constrained versus unconstrained intensive language therapy in two individuals with chronic, moderate-to-severe aphasia and apraxia of speech: behavioral and fMRI outcomes. *American Journal of Speech-Language Pathology, 21,* S65–S87.

Leff, A., Crinion, J., Scott, S., Turkheimer, F., Howard, D., & Wise, R. (2002). A physiological change in the homotopic cortex following left posterior temporal lobe infarction. *Annals of Neurology, 51,* 553–558.

Luria, A. (1970). *Traumatic aphasia.* The Hague: Mouton.

Meizner, M., Harnish, S., Conway, T., & Crosson, B. (2011). Recent developments in functional and structural imaging of aphasia recovery after stroke. *Aphasiology, 25,* 271–290.

Makuuchi, M., & Friederici, A. D. (2013). Hierarchical functional connectivity between the core language system and the working memory system. *Cortex, 49*(9), 2416–23. DOI:10.1016/j.cortex.2013.01.007

Murray, L. (2002). Attention deficits in aphasia: presence, nature, assessment, and treatment. *Seminars in Speech and Language, 23*(2), 107–116.

Naeser, M., Martin, P., Nicholas, M., Baker, E., Seekins, H., Kobayashi, ... Pascual-Leone A. (2005). Improved picture-naming after TMS to part of the right Broca's area: an open-protcol study. *Brain and Language, 93*, 95–105.

Poeppel, D., Emmorey, K., Hickok, G., & Pylkkanen, L. (2012). Towards a new neurobiology of language. *Journal of Neuroscience, 32*, 14125–14131.

Poeppel, D., & Hickok, G. (2004). Towards a new functional anatomy of language. *Cognition, 92*, 1–12.

Postman-Caucheteux, W. A., Brin, R. M., Pursley, R. H., Butman J. A., Solomon, J. M., Picchioni, D., ... Braun, A.R. (2010). Single-trial fMRI shows contralesional activity linked to overt naming errors in chronic aphasic patients. *Journal of Cognitive Neuroscience, 22*, 1299–1318.

Price, C., & Crinion, J. (2005). The latest on functional imaging studies of aphasic stroke. *Current Opinion in Neurology, 18*, 429–434.

Price, C. J., Mummery, C. J., Moore C. J., Fraowiak, R. S., & Friston, K. J. (1999). Delineating necessary and sufficient neural systems with functional imaging studies of neuropsycological patients. *Journal of Cognitive Neuroscience, 11*, 371–382.

Raboyeau, G., de Boissezon, X., Marie, N., Balduyck, S., Puel, M., Bezy C., ... Cardebat, D. (2008). Right hemisphere activation in recovery from aphasia: lesion effect or function recruitment? *Neurology, 70*, 290–298.

Rosen, H. J., Petersen, S. E., Lineweber, M. R., Snyder, A. Z., White, D. A., Chapman, L., ... Corbetta, M. (2000). Neural correlates of recovery from aphasia after damage to left inferior cortex. *Neurology, 55*, 1883–1894.

Saur, D., Lange, R., Baumgaertner, A., Schraknepper, V., Willmes, K., Rijntjes, M., & Weiller, C. (2006). Dynamics of language reorganization after stroke. *Brain, 129*(6), 1371–1384.

Saur, D., Ronneberger, O., Kummerer, D., Mader, I., Weiller, C., Kloppel, S. (2010). Early functional magnetic resonance imaging activations predict language outcome after stroke. *Brain, 133*, 1252–1264.

Thiel, A., Herholz, K., Koyuncu, A., Ghaemi, M., Kracht, L. W., Habendank, B., & Heiss, W. D. (2001). Plasticity in language networks in patients with brain tumors: a positron emission tomography activation study. *Annals of Neurology, 50*, 620–629.

Thomas, C., Altenmuller, E., Marckmann, G., Kahrs, J., & Dichgans, J. (1997). Language processing in aphasia: changes in lateralization patterns during recovery reflect cerebral plasticity in adults. *Electroencephalography and Clinical Neurophysiology, 102*, 86–97.

Thompson, C. K., Fix, S., Gitelman, D. G., Parrish, T. B., & Mesulam, M. M. (2000). fMRI studies of agrammatic sentence comprehension before and after treatment. *Brain and Language, 74*, 387–391.

Vigneau, M., Beaucousin, V., Hervé, P. Y., Jobard, G., Petit, L., Crivello, F., ... Tzourio-Mazoyer N. (2011). What is the right hemisphere contribution to phonological, lexico-semantic, and sentence processing? Insights from a meta-analysis. *Neuroimage, 54*, 577–593.

Warburton, E., Price, C., Swinburn, K., & Wise R. J. (1999). Mechanisms of recovery from aphasia: evidence from positron emission tomography studies. *Journal of Neurology, Neurosurgery, and Psychiatry, 66*, 155–161.

Warren, J. E., Crinion, J. T., Lambon Ralph, M. A., & Wise, R.J.S. (2009). Anterior temporal lobe connectivity correlates with functional outcome after aphasic stroke. *Brain, 132*, 3428–3442.

Weiller, C., Isensee, C., Rijntjes, M., Huber, W., Muller, S., Bier, D., ... Diener, H. C. (1995). Recovery from Wernicke's aphasia: a positron emission tomographic study. *Annals of Neurology, 37*, 723–732.

Willems, R. M., Clevis, K., & Hagoort, P. (2011). Add a picture of suspense: neural correlations of the interaction between language and visual information in the perception of fear. *Social Cognitive and Affective Neuroscience, 6*, 404–416.

Winhusien, L., Thiel, A., Schumacher, B., Kessler, J., Rudolf, J., Haupt, W. F., & Heiss, W. D. (2007). The right inferior frontal gyrus and poststroke aphasia: a follow-up investigation. *Stroke, 38*, 1286–1292.

Index

Abel, S., 127, 241
abstract reasoning, prognostic values, 55
access deficit, in apraxia, 203
access inhibitory process, 111
action naming, vs. object naming, 203
action understanding, 195
Activities of Daily Living Profile, 45, 47
aging brain, language in, 25–27
agrammatic aphasia, and reduced working memory abilities, 121
Albert, M.L., 261
alertness attention system, 81
Alexander, M.P., 53
alternating attention, 76, 78
American Speech-Language Hearing Association Functional Assessment of Communication Skills for Adults, 52
Amso, Dima, 256
amydala, 151f
Anglade, C., 264, 265f
anomia, 4, 13, 14t
  best predictors of therapy outcome, 55
  treatment protocols, 125
anomic aphasia, 242
ANS biomarkers, role, and language performance, 164–165

anterior cingulate, 162
anxiety, 259
  after stroke, 153–156
  and cognitive function disruption, 149
  linguistic, 161–162
  and linguistic function, 150–152
  neural correlates on executive function, 152
  reactivity in aphasia, 161–166
anxiety-induced stress dysregulation, 146–147
aphasia
  aging brain and, 26
  and apraxia, 197–198
    behavioral and neural correlates, 196–204
    frontoparietal network role, 201–203, 201f
    gesture role in treatment, 204–209
    neural changes in chronic states, 208
  and processing visual cues, 225
aphasia recovery, ix, 1–6
  defining, 1–4
  prognostic factors in success, 4–5, 4t
  stating problem, 4–6
aphasia therapy, incorporating movement constraint into, 206
Aphasic Depression Rating Scale (ADRS), 157

Index

aphasic syndromes, 13, 14*t*
apraxia, 186, 187
  and aphasia, 197–198
    behavioral and neural correlates, 196–204
      frontoparietal network role, 201–203, 201*f*
    behavioral manifestations, 199
    ideational, 198
    ideomotor, 198–199
    theoretical accounts, 198–201
apraxia of speech, 199
Arbib, M.A., 193
arcuate fasciculus, 199
arousal system, in vigilance, 77
articulatory rehearsal process, 109
asymbolia, 198
Atkinson, R.C., 108
attention, 5, 74–94
  alertness attention system, 81
  behavioral patterns, 86–88
  components, 75–78
  functional neuroanatomy of system, 82*f*
  mechanisms in treatment, 266
  mechanisms of allocation, 88–89
  neural approaches to role of, 92–94
  neural basis, 80–83, 86
  neuroanatomical models, 81
  relationship with language, 79–80
  treatment in aphasia, 89–94
attention control, 111
  executive function, 44*t*
  model, 152, 162
attention deficits, 258
attention-language interlinks, neural underpinnings, 83–95
attention networks, categories, 80
attention orienting system, 110
attention process training (APT), 91
audiovisual cueing, 241–243
audiovisual processing, 229–235
  behavioral and neural correlates, 238–240
  brain damage to left hemisphere, 239
  grounding in motor function neural systems, 234
automatic attention processing, 78, 89

Baddeley, A., 38, 109–110
Baldo, J.V., 237, 238
basal forebrain nuclei, and arousal system, 77

basal ganglia, 57
  damage, 56–57
Baum, S.H., 239
behavioral relevance principle, 206
behavioral therapy, and mood improvement, 160
Berthier, M.L., 206, 208
beta-adrenergic blocking agents, and language performance, 166
biomarkers, for impaired language performance, 164
Blumstein, Sheila, 256
Bogousslavsky, J., 157, 158
Bohlhalter, S., 192
Boston Diagnostic Aphasia Examination, 235
Boston Naming Test, 235, 237
bottleneck processing, 79
brain
  activation during passive observation of audiovisual stimuli, 232–233, 233*f*
  activation patterns, 115
  function mapping, 21*f*
  praxis, language and, 188–196
  structures of declarative memory system, 105–106
brain-language models, 13
  multifunctional, 18–20
  psycholinguistic models of interlinks, 15–18
brainstem, and arousal system, 77
Broca's aphasia, 4, 14*t*
Broca's area, 13, 17, 203, 232, 256
  and apraxia of speech, 197
  neural activation during lip reading, 193
  role in working memory-language interlinks, 115
Broca-Wernicke-Lichtheim-Geschwind lesion-deficit model of aphasia, 13
Brodmann's area, 192
  damage, 115
Brownsett, S.L.E., 57
Buchsbaum, B.R., 123
Buxbaum, L.J., 202

Cabeza, R., 261
  components approach, 113
Cahana-Amitay, D., 161, 162, 164, 261
Callan, D.E., 232
Caplan, D., 113
Caramazza, A., 195

Carpenter, P.A., 111
Caspari, I., 120
catastrophic reaction, 156
category clustering, 117
Category Test, 46*t*
Cato, A.M., 148
caudate, control function of, 20
central executive system, 109
cerebellum
 language networks in, 20
 paravermal, 57
 and procedural memory system, 106
cerebral artery, damage in aphasia, 47
cerebral plasticity, 263
channel function, of attention system, 81
Choe, Y., 242
cholinergic deficiency, and impaired verbal memory, 24
Christensen, S.C., 112–113, 118
citalopram, 160
Clark, N., 124
clock drawing test, 45
cocktail party effect, 75
Code, C., 159
Coelho, C., 53
cognitive control, neural effects, 57
cognitive domains, interaction with other, 238
cognitive factors, as treatment outcome predictors, 5
cognitive flexibility executive function, 44*t*
Cognitive Linguistic Quick Test (CLQT), 45, 54
cognitive rehabilitation, 55
Color Trails Tests, 52
communication, executive function and, 51–53
compensatory mechanisms, cognitive abilities as, 205
competition, neural bases in attention system, 83
complementary alternative medicine (CAM) therapies, 164
complex attention, 77–78
 mechanisms, 78–80
complex motor movement, 188
component process framework, 106–107, 261
concept fields, neuroanatomy of, 225
conduction aphasia, 4, 14*t*, 119
 and reduced working memory abilities, 121
confrontation naming, perseveration and, 49

conscious awareness, clearing information from, 111
constraint-based aphasia intervention (CILT), 208
constraint-based aphasia therapy, 206–208
constraint-induced movement therapy, 205
content of information, and retention, 105
continuous perseveration, 48
contralateral neglect, 80
control, 17
controlled attention, 78, 89
control system, prefrontal-based, 38
convergence zones, theory of, 255–256
corpus callosum, 224, 225
corticothalamic mechanism, and executive support for word-level processing, 41
cortisol levels
 for linguistic vs. nonlinguistic tasks, 163
 salivary, 164
Coslett, H.B., 92
Cowan, N., 110
Crocker, L.D., 148–149
Crosson, B., 57, 92, 116, 148

Dalla Volta, R., 189
Damasio, Antonio, 255
David, A.S., 208–209
declarative memory, 105–107
declarative/procedural model, 24
default mode network (DMN), connectivity of, 93
deletion inhibitory process, 111
depression, 146–147, 259
 acute and chronic stages, 158–159
 after stroke, 153–156
 and aphasia, 156–161
  neural and psychosocial factors, 157–159
  recovery and intervention effects, 159–161
 and cognitive function disruption, 149
 neural correlates on executive function, 152
 pharmacological agents for poststroke, 160
De Renzi, E., 197
dichotic listening, 74
Dick, A.S., 234
discourse processing
 and executive functions, 42
 neural correlates, 52–53
distributed neural networks, 17
divided attention, 76, 78

dopaminergic system, pharmacotherapy for, 93
dorsal anterior cingulate cortex, activation of, 58
dorsal vagal motor nucleus (DVN), 151*f*
dorsal/ventral account model, 15–16, 16*f*
dorsolateral prefrontal cortex (DLPFC)
    and discourse processing impairment, 53
    hypoactivation of, 152
dorsomedial (BA10) prefrontal regions, 42
dual tasks, 79
Duffau, H., 22–23, 256
Duncan, J., 83
duration of information, and retention, 105
dysexecutive syndrome, 39

Eickhoff, S.B., 83
Einstein, Albert, theory of relativity, 262
Eisner, F., 196
electroconvulsive therapy (ECT), 161
embedded processes model, for memory, 110
emblems, 190
embodiment theory, 195
emotion, 146–166
    altered, in aphasia, 155–156, 166
    definition, 147–149
    effects on cognition, 149–153
emotional behavioral index, for poststroke behavior, 157
emotional states, 259
emotion-cognition-brain interdependence, 150–153
energizing process, 83
episodic buffer, 110
episodic component, in declarative system, 105
errorless learning, 125, 126
    and neural network reshaping, 128
error patterns, in aphasia recovery, 123
escitalopram, 160
executive attention system, 81
executive dysfunction, 47–51
executive functions, 5, 36–37, 258
    and apraxia, 202
    assessing in aphasia, 43–47
    defining, 37–38
    and discourse processing, 42
    and functional communication, 51–53
    limitations on neural mappings, 42–43
    models of, 38–39
    neural correlates, 39–40, 52–53
    neural networks of, 44*t*
    prognostic values, 54–58
    reduced efficiency, 48
    semantic processing and, 40–41
    short-term memory and, 120
    testing in aphasic individuals, 45, 46*t*
executive shifting, impaired, 51–52
executive system, central, 109
explicit memory, 105–107, 125
eye-tracking study, 236
Eysenck, M.W., 162

Fadiga, L., 193
Fedorenko, E., 22, 84, 112
feedback, and treatment outcome, 125
Fillingham, J.K., 126
fixed module-specific neural organization, 17
focused attention, 77–78
focusing principle, 206
Francis, D.R., 124
Freedman, M.L., 124
Freud, Sigmund, neuroanatomy of concept fields, 225
Fridriksson, J., 52, 127, 193, 243
Friederici, A.D., 19, 115, 256
Friedmann, N., 121
frontal aging hypothesis, 39
frontal/basal-ganglia connections, and procedural memory system, 106
frontal cortex, neural organization of, 22
frontal gyrus, left inferior, 17–18
frontal lobes, and executive behaviors, 39
frontal networks
    associated with nonlinguistic functions, 18
    language, 17
frontoparietal structures, damage to, 203, 204
frontotemporal networks, and discourse processing, 42
functional integration, 93
functional localizer, 22
functional neuroanatomy models of language, 12, 13–27
fusiform gyrus, 227
Fuster, J.M., 39

Gainotti, G., 197
Gardner, H., 238
Gentilucci, M., 189
Geschwind, N., 199

gesture-language interlinks, cognitive
    mechanisms underlying, 189–191
gestures. *See also* tool use
    motor control of, 189
    recognition, and emotional meaning, 196
    role in aphasia treatment, 204–209
    symbolic, 200
gesture training, 205
Ghika-Schmid, F., 157
Gibson, K.R., 112
global aphasic syndrome, 14*t*
Goldenberg, G., 128
Goldstein, K., 146
Gonzalez-Rothi, L.J., 92
Graphic Pattern Generation, 46*t*, 48
gray matter volume, and age-based
    compensatory mechanisms, 26
Grodzinsky, Y., 22
Gutbrod, K., 117
Gvion, A., 121

Hagoort's framework, 17
Hamberger, M.J., 227, 228*f*
Hamilton Depression Rating Scale, 157
handedness, 198
Harnish, S.M., 240
Harris Wright, H., 118
Harvey, D.Y., 50
Hasher, L., 111
Hasson, U., 232
heart-rate variability, and neural network
    integrity, 150, 151*f*
Hebb, D.O., 108, 128
Hebbian plasticity, 205–206
Heilman, K.M., 199
Helm-Estabrooks, N., 90
hemispheric specialization, visual recognition
    vs. language, 224–225
Herrmann, M., 158, 159
Heschl's gyrus, reduction in neural
    activation, 232
Hessler, D., 231
Hickok, G., 192, 195, 204, 234, 235, 255
Hillis, A.E., 203
hippocampus
    and memory, 105
    and word learning, 127
Hitch, G., 109–110
Humphreys, G.W., 124

hypothalamic-pituitary-adrenal (HPA)
    axis, 77, 152
    stress reactivity mechanism, 163

Iaoboni, M., 193
ideational apraxia, 198
ideomotor apraxia, 198–199
images, high-context, 236
impaired switching/cognitive flexibility, 47
implicit learning, 125
implicit memory, 105–107
inferior frontal cortex, 149
inferior frontal gyrus, 166, 202, 259
    mirror neurons and, 193
inferior longitudinal fasciculus (IFG), and
    semantic control processes, 41
inferior parietal lobule, mirror neurons in, 192
information type, and memory
    classification, 104–105
inhibitory mechanisms, linking working
    memory and executive functions
    with, 111
initiation, motor component of, 57
input mechanisms, in apraxia models, 200
intelligence, and measure of executive
    function, 47
intention, 41
    treatment, 56
interactional synchrony, 196
interaction of cognitive phenomena, ix
interactive attentional system, 81
intraparietal sulcus, 202

James, W., 76
Jirak, D., 195
Just, M.A., 111

Kalinyak-Fliszar, M., 124
Kasselimis, D.S., 123
Kiran, S., 125, 237
Knoeferle, P., 229
Kobayashi, S., 201
Koenig-Bruhin, M., 124
Kurland, J., 209

Langner, R., 83
language
    in aging brain, 25–27
    attention relationship with, 79–80

language (cont.)
  creation, 263
  delocalized dynamic model of processing, 22–23
  and domain-general brain structure, 85f
  future directions for neural multifunctional models, 20–25
  long-term gains, 1
  neural comprehension networks, 15
  neural correlates of praxis and, 187
  neural multifunctionality of, 257–260
  neural organization of, 261–263
  neurobiology of, 5, 24
  praxis, and brain, 188–196
  production networks, 15
  social value assigned to, 159
  visual information use in performance, 226–235
language-based procedures, levels, 53
language connectome, 256–257
language-executive functions, neural correlates, 40–43
language function, and working memory, 111
language therapy
  neural changes in attention networks induced by, 93
  STM training effects on outcomes, 124
Laures-Gore, J.S., 162–163, 164
Laures, J.S., 164
learning
  in aphasia treatment, 125
  errorless, 125, 126
    and neural network reshaping, 128
  neural basis, 128
left anterior temporal cortex, and semantic errors, 122
left hemisphere
  brain damage
    and audiovisual processing, 239
    and motor movement voluntary control, 197
  role of preserved tissue, 264
left inferior frontal gyrus, 17–18
  and semantic control, 40–41
left inferior parietal cortex, 237
left inferior parietal lobe, 202
left parietal lobe, difficulties with tool-based gestures, 197
left precuneus, 241

left temporal lobe, 103–104
Lemmo, M., 197
"lexical gesture" model, 190
lexical network, 114
lexical perseveration, 49
Liepmann, H., 198
limbic system, 148
  interconnections with, 149
linguistic anxiety, 152, 161–162
linguistic function, anxiety and, 150–152
linguistic information, spreading activation of, 114, 114f
linguistic processes, memory functions and, 103–104
listening, dichotic, 74
long-term memory (LTM), 108, 259
  effects on language performance in aphasia, 117
  establishment of representation in, 125
long-term working memory, 113
Luchelli, F., 197
Luria, A., 146

MacDonald, M.C., 112–113
Mahon, B.Z., 195
Mahoney, K., 124
Makuuchi, M., 115
mammillary bodies, and memory, 105
Martin, N., 123
Martin, R., 124
Mayer, J.F., 118
McClung, J.S., 4
McGettigan, C., 196
McGurk effect, 230, 239
McKissok, S., 125
McNeill, D., 190
Meizner, M., 128
melodic intonation therapy, 265
memory, 5, 17, 259
  and aphasia recovery and treatment, 123–129
  deficits, and aphasia, 116–123
  multiple classifications, 104–107
  types, 107–116
  verbal short-term deficits, 108
memory functions, 103–129
  and linguistic processes, 103–104
memory-language interactions, behavioral and neural processes underlying, 104

memory-language model, development, 119
memory-related aphasia treatment, neural
    structures, 127–129
Menke, R., 128
mesencephalic reticular formation, and arousal
    system, 77
Mesulam, M.M., 231
Miceli, G., 125
mirror neurons, 192–195
    and aphasia, 203–204
mismatch negativity, 86
Miyake, A., 112
modality of information, and retention, 105
mood improvement, behavioral therapy
    and, 160
Moore, A.B., 116
Moscovitch, M., 113, 261
motivation
    anxiety and, 162
    emotion and, 149
    poststroke depression and anxiety
        impact, 154
motor circuits, in syntactic processing, 194
motor functions
    disruption, 186. *See also* apraxia
    and language function, 259
motor-linguistic integration, 260
motor programming, 209
motor speech perception, neural basis of, 193
motor systems
    role in predicting audiovisual effects, 234
    voluntary control. *See* praxis in aphasia
        recovery
multifunctional brain-language models,
    18–20
multifunctionality, 2–3, 262
    evidence for, 12–27
multifunctional modularity, 18
Murray, L.L., 88, 118, 165
Musacchia, G., 231
Myung, J., 203

Naeser, M., 263
naming deficit, 56
naming therapy, 91–92
    in aphasia, 209
n-back test, 118
negative emotions, processing words
    connoting, 148

negative words, cortical responses to, 148
neural correlates, evidence for, 114–116
neural mappings, limitations for executive
    functions, 42–43
neural multifunctionality, x, 2, 261, 265
    of language, 257–260
    future directions for models, 20–25
neural networks, 23
    distributed, 17
neural plasticity, conceptualization, 128
neural processes, in recovery, 2
neural reorganization, 56–58
neural substrates, of nonlinguistic functions, 2
Newman, S., 115
nondeclarative/procedural memory, 105–107
nonlinguistic functions, 4
    frontal networks associated with, 18
    neural substrates of, 2
nonverbal cues, exclusion from treatment, 207
nonverbal tasks, administration of, 45
noradrenergic system, pharmacotherapy
    for, 93
Norman, D.A., 38
nouns, older adults' impaired retrieval of, 25
nucleus ambiguus (NA), 151*f*

object naming, vs. action naming, 203
occipitoparietal regions, damage, 198
Ochipa, C., 199
Ofek, E., 148
Ojanen, V., 232
optic aphasia, 224
orienting attention system, 81
output mechanisms, in apraxia models, 200

pantomimes, 190
Papagno, C., 198
parallel processing, vs. serial processing, 79
parallel processing working memory (WM)
    system, 109–110, 110*f*
paravermal cerebellum, 57
parietal brain damage, 92
pars opercularis, 17, 19
pars triangularis, 17
Peoppel, D., 195
perseveration, 48–49
    subtypes linked to language
        performance, 49
persistent visual neglect, 80

278 | Index

personality, poststroke depression and anxiety impact, 154
pharmacological agents, 166
 and performance on standardized langauge tests, 207
 for poststroke depression, 160
pharmacotherapy
 for dopaminergic and noradrenergic systems, 93
 studies, 24
phonemic perseveration, 49
phonological cueing, 241
phonological input store, 109
phonological intervention, vs. semantic, 128
phonological loop, 109
 deficits, 115
phonological short-term memory, deficit patterns, 119–120
physiological brain activation, reduced, 86
pictures
 effect on language processing, 227–229
 naming, 237
 stimuli in assessment/treatment studies, 240–241
 visual processing, behavioral and neural correlates, 235–240
planning executive function, 44*t*
planum temporale, 123
Poeppel, David, 256
Porteus Mazes, 46*t*
Posner, M.I., 81
praxis in aphasia recovery, 186–209
 introduction, 186–188
 neural correlates of language and, 187
prefrontal cortex, 106
 damage, and language-related executive control deficits, 40
 and impaired semantic control, 50
 lesions in left, 238
prefrontal regions
 control system, 38
 and declarative information processing, 106
Price, C.J., 15, 19–20
process-specific alliances, 107, 261
program-of-action perseveration, 49
propranolol, 166, 259
psycholinguistic models of language, 2
psychological refractory period, 79

psychophysiological stress reactivity, in aphasia treatment, 164–166
Pulvelmüller, F., 193, 206, 208

Radanovic, M., 51
Raven's Colored Progressive Matrices, 44, 46*t*, 54, 238
Raymer, A.M., 205
Raz, N., 42
reaction times, declines in, 87
reading
 APT II to treat difficulties, 91
 complex syntax processing during, 19
reading span test, 120–121
reality, experience of, 255
recovery
 from aphasia, redefining, 263–266
 neural processes in, 2
 variability in patterns, 3
recurrent perseveration, 48
reflexive attention, 78
refractory effects, 50, 238
repetition tasks, overly rapid delay, and deficit language performance, 120
resource allocation function, 78
 deficit, 88–89
responsive naming, 228*f*
restraint inhibitory process, 111
retrieval, for linguistic information, 5
retrosplenial cortex, 148
Rey-Osterreith Complex Figure Test, 43
Rhodes, M.G., 112
right hemisphere
 attention mechanisms, 92
 damage, and language problems, 86
 and mediating attention processes, 80
 role in aphasia recovery, 264, 265*f*
 strokes, and attention deficits, 74
Rochon, E., 127
Rogalsky, C., 204
Rose, M., 191, 204, 206, 207
rostral frontal cortex, 148
Rothi, L.J., 199, 205
Roy, E.A., 200

salivary cortisol levels, 164
Sandberg, C., 237
Sarasson, S., 243
Saygin, A.P., 198, 204

scene-sentence matching, 229
Schmid, G., 239
Schoppe, K.J., 197
Schroeder, C.E., 231
Schwartz, M.F., 122
Scott, S.K., 196
secondary depression, 159
selective attention, 76, 77
　with dual-task paradigms, 87
self-agency, poststroke depression and anxiety impact, 154
semantic component, in declarative system, 105
semantic control, 49–51, 84
semantic intervention, vs. phonological, 128
semantic perseveration, 49
semantic process, 19
semantic processing, executive functions and, 40–41
sentence comprehension, 111
　working memory and, 111–112
sentence processing
　abilities in older adults, 25
　attention modulation role in, 84
　neural networks in service of, 116
　online, 115–116
　online and offline properties, 113
sentence-verification response times, 229
separate language resource theory, 121
Sequence Generating Test, 46t, 48
sequence learning, 106
sequential model of memory, 108
serial processing, vs. parallel processing, 79
Shallice, T., 38, 83
Shiffrin, R.M., 108
Shisler Marshall, R., 165
short-term memory (STM), 108, 116–117, 259
　assessment in aphasia, 117–118
　impaired, behavioral observations, 118–121
　verbal, 114
　vs. working memory, 109
　　neural correlates, 121–123
short-term/working memory-language interlinks, 114–116
sign language of deaf, 190
simple motor movement, 188
Skipper, J.I., 234
space-time phenomenon, 262
Spatt, J., 128
speech perception, motor theory of, 191–192

speech processing
　audiovisual information in, 230
　interaction among visual, attentional and, 231
　mediating, 19
Square, P., 200
staircase method, 125–126
Stanton, K., 242
state function, of attention system, 81
Stead, A., 236
stimulus novelty, 110
stress
　anxiety-induced dysregulation, 146–147
　psychophysiological reactivity in aphasia treatment, 164–166
　reactivity in aphasia, 161–166
stroke
　depression and anxiety after, 153–156
　pharmacological agents for depression after, 160
　right hemisphere, and attention deficits, 74
Stroop test, 44, 45, 78
stuck-in-set pattern of perseveration, 48
Studer-Eichenberger, F., 124
Stuss, D.T., 81
subcortical circuits, and executive functions, 39–40
superior frontal gyrus, activation of, 58
superior temporal gyri, 57
　structural integrity, 122–123
superior temporal sulcus, in multimodal processing, 232
supervisory attention system, 109
sustained attention, 76–77
switching/cognitive flexibility, impaired, 47
"switching cost," 47
symbolic gestures, 200
symbols, processing, 236
sympathetic nervous system (SNS), activation of, 77
synchronicity, motor processing of, 196
synonym judgment tasks, 237
syntactic processing
　motor circuits in, 194
　temporal cortex in, 19
Szalfarski, J.P., 241

Tanaka, Y., 166
temporal aspects of memory processing, 107

temporal cortex
  left anterior, and semantic errors, 122
  and procedural memory system, 106
  and STM deficits, 122
  in syntactic processing, 19
temporal gyri, 227, 237
temporal networks, support of mental lexicon, 24
temporal regions, 104
temporal tracking of speech envelope, 231
tertiary depression, 159
Test of Nonverbal Intelligence, 54–55
text coherence, processing of, 42
thalamic aphasia, 51
thalamocortical mechanism, and executive support for word-level processing, 41
thalamus, 57
  and arousal system, 77
  and memory, 105
Thayer, J.F., 150
Thompson-Schill, S.L., 50
time-locked, multiregional retroactivation, 255
timing, 262
tool use
  gestures and overlap of apraxia and aphasia, 200
  impaired pantomiming, 199
  study of, 189
Tower of Hanoi Test, 46t, 48
Tower of London, 46t
Townend, E., 157
Trail Making B test, 45
training, and attention deficits, 91
transcortical aphasia, 4, 14t
transcranial magnetic stimulation (TMS) protocol, 208
transitive gestures, deficient recognition, 202
tricyclic nortriptyline, 160

Ugawa, Y., 201
Ullman, M.T., 24–25
  declarative/procedural model, 107
uncinate fasciculus (UF), 19
  and semantic control processes, 41
unification, 17

Vallila-Rohter, S.M., 125
ventral-dorsal speech perception model, 195
ventral premotor area, mirror neurons in, 192
ventral stream, 15
ventral system, 202
ventral white matter tracts, 41
ventromedial (BA11) prefrontal regions, 42
verbal/nonverbal fluency executive function, 44t
verbal short-term memory, 114
  deficits in, 108
verbs, older adults' impaired retrieval of, 25
vigilance, 76
Virtual Planning Test, 46t
visemes, 229
visual aphasia treatment study, 243
visual components, aphasia assessment/treatment studies with, 240–243
visual information, use in language performance, 226–235
Visual Mood Analog Scale, 157
visual neglect, persistent, 80
visual processing, 260
  in aphasia recovery, 224–243
visual scenes
  effect on language processing, 227–229
  visual processing, behavioral and neural correlates, 235–240
Visual Search Test, 46t
visual-working memory-executive functions language interlinks, neural correlates, 23f
visuospatial sketchpad, 109
voluntary attention, 78
voxel-based lesion symptom mapping study, 122, 238

Wallace, S.E., 236
Wallesch, C.W., 158
Ward, J., 125
Waters, G.S., 113
Wechsler Memory Scale-Revised, 117
Weintraub, S., 81
Wernicke, C., neuroanatomy of concept fields, 225
Wernicke's aphasia, 4, 14t
Wernicke's area, 13
"what" pathway, 15
"where" pathway, 15
white matter
  and aphasic word comprehension deficits, 50
  integrity, and age-based compensatory mechanisms, 26

whole-brain phenomenon, language as, 262
Wilson, S.M., 193
Wisconsin Card Sorting Test (WCST), 43, 46t, 51, 52
Wisenburn, B., 124
word deafness, 239
word judgment, 237
word learning, hippocampus and, 127
word-level processing, executive support for, 41
word production, 57
   aphasia therapy study, 241
   gesturing support of, 191
   STM impairment and, 119
word recall, 110
word repetition, 201f
working memory, 259
   and language function, 111
   load effects, and judgment accuracy of rhymes and synonyms, 120
   multicomponent model of, 110f
   rehearsal mechanisms of, 115
   resource pools, 112
   vs. short-term memory (STM), 109
Wunderlich, A., 242

Yerkes-Dodson law, 162, 163
Yuan, P., 42

Zack, R.T., 111
Zelazo, P.D., 39
Ziegler, W., 239, 242
Zion Golumbic, E.M., 231